Learning Disabilities Sourcebook, 3rd Edition

Leukemia Sourcebook

Liver Disorders Sourcebook

Lung Disorders Sourcebook

Medical Tests Sourcebook, 3rd Edition

Men's Health Concerns Sourcebook, 2nd Edition

Mental Health Disorders Sourcebook, 4th Edition

Mental Retardation Sourcebook

Movement Disorders Sourcebook, 2nd Edition

Multiple Sclerosis Sourcebook

Muscular Dystrophy Sourcebook

Obesity Sourcebook

Osteoporosis Sourcebook

Pain Sourcebook, 3rd Edition

Pediatric Cancer Sourcebook

Physical & Mental Issues in Aging Sourcebook

Podiatry Sourcebook, 2nd Edition

Pregnancy & Birth Sourcebook, 2nd Edition

Prostate & Urological Disorders Sourcebook

Prostate Cancer Sourcebook

Reconstructive & Cosmetic Surgery Sourcebook

Rehabilitation Sourcebook

Respiratory Disorders Sourcebook, 2nd Edition

Sexually Transmitted Diseases Sourcebook, 3rd Edition

Sleep Disorders Sourcebook, 3rd Edition

Smoking Concerns Sourcebook

Sports Injuries Sourcebook, 3rd Edition

Stress-Related Disorders Sourcebook, 2nd Edition

Stroke Sourcebook, 2nd Edition

Surgery Sourcebook, 2nd Edition

Thyroid Disorders Sourcebook

Transplantation Sourcebook

Traveler's Health Sourcebook

Urinary Tract & Kidney Diseases & Disorders Sourcebook, 2nd Edition

Vegetarian Sourcebook

Women's Health Concerns Sourcebook, 3rd Edition

Workplace Health & Safety Sourcebook

Worldwide Health Sourcebook

Teens

Accident & Safety Information for Teens

Alcohol Information for Teens, 2nd Edition

Allergy Information for Teens

Asthma Information for Teens, 2nd Edition

Body Information for Teens

Cancer Information for Teens

Complementary & Alternative Medicine Information for Teens

Diabetes Information for Teens

Diet Information for Teens, 2nd Edition

Drug Information for Teens, 3rd Edition

Eating Disorders Information for Teens, 2nd Edition

Fitness Information for Teens, 2nd Edition

Learning Disabilities Information for Teens

Mental Health Information for Teens, 3rd Edition

Pregnancy Information for Teens

Sexual Health Information for Teens, 2nd Edition

Skin Health Information for Teens, 2nd Edition

Sleep Information for Teens

Sports Injuries Information for Teens, 2nd Edition

Stress Information for Teens

Suicide Information for Teens, 2nd Edition

Tobacco Information for Teens, 2nd Edition

Cancer
SOURCEBOOK
for Women

Fourth Edition

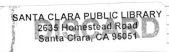

Health Reference Series

Fourth Edition

Cancer SOURCEBOOK for Women

Basic Consumer Health Information about Gynecologic Cancers and Other Cancers of Special Concern to Women, Including Cancers of the Breast, Cervix, Colon, Lung, Ovaries, Thyroid, and Uterus

Along with Facts about Benign Conditions of the Female Reproductive System, Cancer Risk Factors, Screening and Prevention Programs, Women's Issues in Cancer Treatment and Survivorship, Research Initiatives, a Glossary of Cancer Terms, and a Directory of Resources for Additional Help and Information

Edited by
Karen Bellenir

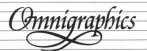

Omnigraphics

P.O. Box 31-1640, Detroit, MI 48231

Bibliographic Note
Because this page cannot legibly accommodate all the copyright notices, the Bibliographic Note portion of the Preface constitutes an extension of the copyright notice.

Edited by Karen Bellenir

Health Reference Series

Karen Bellenir, *Managing Editor*
David A. Cooke, MD, FACP, *Medical Consultant*
Elizabeth Collins, *Research and Permissions Coordinator*
Cherry Edwards, *Permissions Assistant*
EdIndex, Services for Publishers, *Indexers*

* * *

Omnigraphics, Inc.
Matthew P. Barbour, *Senior Vice President*
Kevin M. Hayes, *Operations Manager*

* * *

Peter E. Ruffner, *Publisher*

Copyright © 2010 Omnigraphics, Inc.

ISBN 978-0-7808-1139-3

Library of Congress Cataloging-in-Publication Data

Cancer sourcebook for women : basic consumer health information about gynecologic cancers and other cancers of special concern to women, including cancers of the breast, cervix, colon, lung, ovaries, thyroid, and uterus; along with facts about benign conditions of the female reproductive system, cancer risk factors, screening and prevention programs, women's issues in cancer treatment ... / edited by Karen Bellenir. -- 4th ed.
   p. cm.
   Summary: "Provides basic consumer health information about risk factors, prevention, diagnosis, and treatment of cancers of concern to women. Includes index, glossary of related terms, and other resources"--Provided by publisher.
   Includes bibliographical references and index.
   ISBN 978-0-7808-1139-3 (hardcover : alk. paper) 1. Generative organs, Female--Popular works. 2. Cancer in women--Popular works. I. Bellenir, Karen.
   RC280.G5C34 2010
   616.99'40082--dc22
                                                                    2010027636

Table of Contents

Visit www.healthreferenceseries.com to view *A Contents Guide to the Health Reference Series*, a listing of more than 15,000 topics and the volumes in which they are covered.

Part II: Breast Cancer

Part III: Gynecologic Cancers

Part IV: Other Cancers of Special Concern to Women

Part V: Diagnosing and Treating Cancer

Part VI: Coping with the Side Effects of Cancer and Cancer Treatments

Part VII: Women's Issues in Cancer Survivorship

Part VIII: Additional Help and Information

Preface

About This Book

According to the National Cancer Institute, cancer continues to take
a devastating toll. Among women in the United States, cancer is the
second-leading cause of death after heart disease. Medical researchers
fighting against cancer have made significant progress, however. In
recent years, cancer incidence rates have been stable, and—although
the annual rate of decline in cancer death rates among men have been
twice as large as the declines in women—mortality has decreased for
ten of the top 15 cancers in women. With improved cancer screening
programs and innovative treatments, women receiving a cancer diagnosis today have a better chance of overcoming their disease than
ever before.

Cancer Sourcebook for Women, Fourth Edition offers updated information about gynecologic cancers and other cancers of special
concern to women, including breast cancer, cancers of the female reproductive organs, and cancers responsible for the highest number of
deaths in women. It explains cancer risks—including lifestyle factors,
inherited genetic abnormalities, and hormonal medications—and
methods used to diagnose and treat cancer. Practical suggestions for
coping with the treatment side effects are provided, and a section on
cancer survivorship discusses methods for maintaining quality of life
during and after treatment. The book concludes with a glossary of
cancer-related terms, a directory of resources, and facts about locating support groups.

Women seeking additional information about other specific cancers, a wide variety of cancer-related topics, or disease management issues, may wish to consult the following additional volumes within Omnigraphics' *Health Reference Series*:

- *Breast Cancer Sourcebook, 3rd Edition* offers facts about breast health and breast cancer, including information about risk factors, prevention efforts, screening and diagnostic methods, treatment options, and post-treatment follow-up care.

- *Cancer Sourcebook, 5th Edition* discusses the prevention, diagnosis, and treatment of head and neck cancers, lung cancers, gastrointestinal cancers, genitourinary cancers, lymphomas, blood cell cancers, endocrine cancers, skin cancers, bone cancers, and metastatic cancers.

- *Cancer Survivorship Sourcebook* addresses such issues as the physical, educational, emotional, social, and financial needs of cancer patients beginning with diagnosis and continuing through treatment and beyond. It also includes facts about clinical trials and offers suggestions for dealing with the side effects of cancer treatments.

- *Disease Management Sourcebook* looks at how patients and their loved ones can cope with chronic and serious illnesses. It talks about navigating the health care system, communicating with health care providers, assessing health care quality, and making informed health care decisions.

- *Leukemia Sourcebook* details the symptoms, diagnosis, and treatments of adult and childhood forms of acute and chronic leukemia.

- *Women's Health Concerns Sourcebook, 3rd Edition* offers information about issues and trends in women's health and takes a focused look at health conditions of special concern to women, including endometriosis, uterine fibroids, menstrual irregularities, menopause, sexual dysfunction, and infertility.

How to Use This Book

This book is divided into parts and chapters. Parts focus on broad areas of interest. Chapters are devoted to single topics within a part.

Part I: Understanding Cancer Risks in Women describes the factors that place women in danger of developing some of the most common

types of cancers. Some of these risks, such as smoking and exposure to human papillomavirus, can be avoided or diminished by lifestyle choices. The presence of other risks, such as cancer-related genes or age, cannot be altered, but identifying and understanding them can help women make informed decisions about screening options and preventive measures.

Part II: Breast Cancer explains the processes by which cancer develops in the breast. It discusses risks specifically linked to breast cancer development and factors that have been found to be protective against breast cancer. Screening tools, including mammography and clinical breast exams, are discussed, and facts about the steps involved in diagnosing, staging, and treating breast cancer are included.

Part III: Gynecologic Cancers discusses cancers of a woman's reproductive organs. Individual chapters include information about symptoms, diagnosis, and treatment of cervical cancer, endometrial cancer, gestational trophoblastic tumors, ovarian cancer, uterine cancer, vaginal cancer, and vulvar cancer.

Part IV: Other Cancers of Special Concern to Women discusses cancers other than gynecologic cancers that have a higher prevalence among women than among men or that are responsible for the most cancer-related deaths among women. For example, although thyroid cancer occurs in both genders, women are nearly three times more likely to develop thyroid cancer than are men. Additionally, three of the top four cancer-related causes of death among women are from cancers that occur in men as well as in women: lung cancer, colorectal cancers, and pancreatic cancer.

Part V: Diagnosing and Treating Cancer explains the steps, tests, and procedures involved in making a cancer diagnosis and planning a course of treatment. Commonly used surgical procedures—such as hysterectomy, mastectomy, and cryosurgery—are described, and other treatment techniques, including chemotherapy and radiation therapy, are discussed. The part concludes with information for women who may be considering treatment through a clinical trial.

Part VI: Coping with the Side Effects of Cancer and Cancer Treatments offers practical suggestions for dealing with common adverse effects of various cancer treatments or symptomatic consequences related to the growth of the cancer itself. These include nausea, vomiting, other gastrointestinal symptoms, pain, lymphedema, anemia, and neuropathy. Tips are also included for dealing with issues related to the way

cancer treatments may affect physical appearance, thinking efficiencies, and energy levels.

Part VII: Women's Issues in Cancer Survivorship provides supportive information for women who have received a cancer diagnosis. It discusses maintaining the quality of daily life through proper nutrition, exercise, and attention to mental health issues. It also discusses questions about sexual intimacy, fertility, and pregnancy among women who have been treated for gynecologic cancers, and it includes facts about the need for ongoing medical care for long-term well-being.

Part VIII: Additional Help and Information offers a glossary of cancer-related terms, a directory of information resources, and suggestions for finding support groups.

Bibliographic Note

This volume contains documents and excerpts from publications issued by the following U.S. government agencies: Agency for Healthcare Research and Quality; Centers for Disease Control and Prevention (CDC); National Cancer Institute; National Women's Health Information Center; and the Office on Women's Health, U.S. Department of Health and Human Services.

In addition, this volume contains copyrighted documents from the following organizations: American College of Surgeons; American Society for Colposcopy and Cervical Pathology; American Society of Clinical Oncology; Canadian Cancer Society; Cancer Care, Inc.; Cancer Research UK; Cleveland Clinic Foundation; Cosmetic Executive Women Foundation's Cancer and Careers; Gynecologic Cancer Foundation; Imaginis Corporation; Macmillan Cancer Support; Moores Cancer Center, University of California–San Diego; National Cervical Cancer Public Education Campaign; National Comprehensive Cancer Network; Skin Cancer Foundation; Society of Laparoendoscopic Surgeons; Trustees of the University of Pennsylvania, OncoLink; and the Women's Cancer Network.

Full citation information is provided on the first page of each chapter or section. Every effort has been made to secure all necessary rights to reprint the copyrighted material. If any omissions have been made, please contact Omnigraphics to make corrections for future editions.

Acknowledgements

In addition to the organizations listed above, special thanks are due to Liz Collins, research and permissions coordinator; Cherry Edwards,

permissions assistant; Zachary Klimecki, editorial assistant; and Elizabeth Bellenir, prepress technician.

About the Health Reference Series

The *Health Reference Series* is designed to provide basic medical information for patients, families, caregivers, and the general public. Each volume takes a particular topic and provides comprehensive coverage. This is especially important for people who may be dealing with a newly diagnosed disease or a chronic disorder in themselves or in a family member. People looking for preventive guidance, information about disease warning signs, medical statistics, and risk factors for health problems will also find answers to their questions in the *Health Reference Series*. The *Series*, however, is not intended to serve as a tool for diagnosing illness, in prescribing treatments, or as a substitute for the physician/patient relationship. All people concerned about medical symptoms or the possibility of disease are encouraged to seek professional care from an appropriate health care provider.

A Note about Spelling and Style

Health Reference Series editors use *Stedman's Medical Dictionary* as an authority for questions related to the spelling of medical terms and the *Chicago Manual of Style* for questions related to grammatical structures, punctuation, and other editorial concerns. Consistent adherence is not always possible, however, because the individual volumes within the *Series* include many documents from a wide variety of different producers and copyright holders, and the editor's primary goal is to present material from each source as accurately as is possible following the terms specified by each document's producer. This sometimes means that information in different chapters or sections may follow other guidelines and alternate spelling authorities. For example, occasionally a copyright holder may require that eponymous terms be shown in possessive forms (Crohn's disease *vs.* Crohn disease) or that British spelling norms be retained (leukaemia *vs.* leukemia).

Locating Information within the Health Reference Series

The *Health Reference Series* contains a wealth of information about a wide variety of medical topics. Ensuring easy access to all the fact sheets, research reports, in-depth discussions, and other material contained within the individual books of the *Series* remains one of our

highest priorities. As the *Series* continues to grow in size and scope, however, locating the precise information needed by a reader may become more challenging.

A Contents Guide to the Health Reference Series was developed to direct readers to the specific volumes that address their concerns. It presents an extensive list of diseases, treatments, and other topics of general interest compiled from the Tables of Contents and major index headings. To access *A Contents Guide to the Health Reference Series*, visit www.healthreferenceseries.com.

Medical Consultant

Medical consultation services are provided to the *Health Reference Series* editors by David A. Cooke, MD, FACP. Dr. Cooke is a graduate of Brandeis University, and he received his M.D. degree from the University of Michigan. He completed residency training at the University of Wisconsin Hospital and Clinics. He is board-certified in Internal Medicine. Dr. Cooke currently works as part of the University of Michigan Health System and practices in Ann Arbor, MI. In his free time, he enjoys writing, science fiction, and spending time with his family.

Our Advisory Board

We would like to thank the following board members for providing guidance to the development of this *Series*:

- Dr. Lynda Baker, Associate Professor of Library and Information Science, Wayne State University, Detroit, MI
- Nancy Bulgarelli, William Beaumont Hospital Library, Royal Oak, MI
- Karen Imarisio, Bloomfield Township Public Library, Bloomfield Township, MI
- Karen Morgan, Mardigian Library, University of Michigan-Dearborn, Dearborn, MI
- Rosemary Orlando, St. Clair Shores Public Library, St. Clair Shores, MI

Health Reference Series Update Policy

The inaugural book in the *Health Reference Series* was the first edition of *Cancer Sourcebook* published in 1989. Since then, the *Series*

has been enthusiastically received by librarians and in the medical community. In order to maintain the standard of providing high-quality health information for the layperson the editorial staff at Omnigraphics felt it was necessary to implement a policy of updating volumes when warranted.

Medical researchers have been making tremendous strides, and it is the purpose of the *Health Reference Series* to stay current with the most recent advances. Each decision to update a volume is made on an individual basis. Some of the considerations include how much new information is available and the feedback we receive from people who use the books. If there is a topic you would like to see added to the update list, or an area of medical concern you feel has not been adequately addressed, please write to:

Editor
Health Reference Series
Omnigraphics, Inc.
P.O. Box 31-1640
Detroit, MI 48231
E-mail: editorial@omnigraphics.com

Part One

Understanding Cancer Risks in Women

Chapter 1

What Women Need to Know about Cancer

Cancer

Cancer is one of the most common causes of death in American women. But thanks to improved cancer screening and treatment, you have a better chance of beating cancer than ever before. About 66 percent of people diagnosed with cancer between 1996 and 2002 survived for at least five years. As the science of cancer detection and treatment continues to advance, even more people will survive cancer in the future.

What Is Cancer?

Cancer is a disease in which abnormal cells grow, divide, and spread, often forming a mass called a tumor. Although any abnormal growth is a tumor, some tumors are benign (not cancer) and some are malignant (cancer). Cancers may invade nearby tissues and metastasize, or spread to other parts of the body. Cancer can develop in almost any part of the body. In two types of cancer, leukemia and lymphoma, tumors do not form. Instead, cancer cells spread throughout the blood and the immune system, respectively.

Even if you haven't been diagnosed with cancer, it is important to know that there are steps you can take to reduce your chances of getting cancer, detect cancer early, and make sure you get the treatment you need.

Excerpted from "Cancer," *The Healthy Woman: A Complete Guide for All Ages*, Office on Women's Health, U.S. Health and Human Services, 2008, pp. 51–66.

3

What Causes Cancer?

A number of factors may affect your cancer risk—your chances of developing cancer in your lifetime. Your family history, personal history, and environment all play a part. Some risk factors are beyond your control, such as age and family history.

But you can change some aspects of your behavior or environment to reduce your risk. Keep in mind that most women with these risk factors will never have cancer.

Age is the most important risk factor for cancer. Most cancers—77 percent—occur in persons who are 55 years old or older. For this reason, you will need more tests and checkups to detect early signs of cancer as you get older.

Inherited Risk

Inherited genetic mutations, on their own, cause very few cancers. Several common types of cancer tend to run in families. These include breast cancer, ovarian cancer, colon cancer, melanoma, and lung cancer.

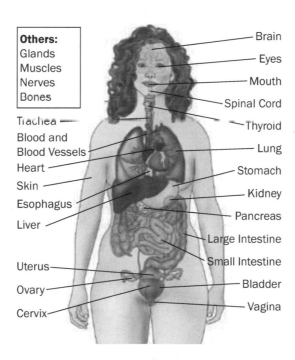

Others:
Glands
Muscles
Nerves
Bones

Trachea
Blood and
Blood Vessels
Heart
Skin
Esophagus
Liver
Uterus
Ovary
Cervix

Brain
Eyes
Mouth
Spinal Cord
Thyroid
Lung
Stomach
Kidney
Pancreas
Large Intestine
Small Intestine
Bladder
Vagina

Figure 1.1. Many areas of the body can be potentially affected by cancer.

4

However, environment and behavior also affect the development of these cancers.

If you have a family history of a certain type of cancer, it does not mean that you will develop that disease. Talk to your doctor about cancer in your family. You may need to take steps to reduce your risk or be screened more often or at an earlier age.

Tobacco Use

Tobacco use is one of the leading causes of cancer. It increases the risk of cancers of the lung, larynx, mouth, nose, pharynx, esophagus, pancreas, kidney, bladder, liver, cervix, and stomach. Tobacco use causes 30 percent of all cancer deaths and 87 percent of lung cancer deaths in the United States.

Smoking not only causes cancer in smokers, but it also may raise the risk of lung cancer for nonsmokers who breathe in secondhand smoke.

You can reduce your risk of lung cancer and other cancers by not smoking or using other tobacco products. You should also avoid secondhand smoke. If you currently smoke, quitting can lower your risk of cancer.

Genetic Mutations

Changes to a cell's DNA, called genetic mutations, may cause the cell to become cancerous. Most of the mutations that cause cancer are caused by the environment, behavior (such as smoking cigarettes), or chance. But some cancer-causing mutations are inherited.

Excessive Alcohol Intake

Drinking alcohol is a risk factor in cancers of the mouth, pharynx, esophagus, larynx, and liver. It may increase your risk of breast, colon, and rectal cancers.

When drinking alcohol is combined with tobacco use, the risks of mouth, pharyngeal, and esophageal cancers are further increased. However, low or moderate alcohol intake may lower your risk of heart disease.

You can reduce your risk by avoiding drinking alcohol to excess. If you drink alcohol, do it in moderation.

Ultraviolet (UV) Rays

The sun's UV rays cause most skin cancers. The amount of UV rays in sunlight depends on the time of day, season, and location. There

are more UV rays at midday, during the summer months, and at locations close to the equator. However, you may be exposed whenever you are outdoors during the day—even on cloudy days. Water and snow, which reflect sunlight back toward your skin, can also increase your UV exposure.

You can reduce your risk by protecting your skin from UV rays.

- Avoid sun exposure between 10 a.m. and 4 p.m., when the sun's rays are the most damaging.

- Wear protective clothing and a hat that shades your face.

- Avoid artificial UV rays from tanning beds or sunlamps.

- If you plan to spend time outside, apply sunscreen 30 to 60 minutes before you go out.

- Apply a broad-spectrum sunscreen with a sun protective factor (SPF) of at least 15. Reapply it after sweating or bathing.

Some Medications

The female hormones estrogen and progesterone affect the growth and development of certain cancers. Drugs that contain these female hormones affect cancer risk.

Menopausal hormone therapy (MHT) relieves the symptoms of menopause and may prevent osteoporosis. There are two types of MHT. Both types affect cancer risk:

- Estrogen-only MHT increases the risk of endometrial cancer and ovarian cancer. Progestin is added to MHT to reduce endometrial cancer risk.

- Combined MHT, which contains estrogen and progesterone or progestin, increases the risk of breast cancer. But it lowers the risk of colon cancer.

Birth control pills also contain female hormones. The pill lowers the risk of endometrial and ovarian cancers. But it may increase the risk of cervical, liver, and breast cancers. Today, birth control pills contain lower hormone levels than in the past. So the effects of the pill on cancer risk may be reduced.

Drugs used to suppress the immune system during an organ transplant may also lead to cancer, especially lymphoma. Chemotherapy drugs, used to treat many types of cancer, may cause leukemia. Cancer survivors are at higher risk of this disease. You can learn more

by talking to your doctor about the benefits and risks of these medications.

Substances in the Home, Workplace, and the Environment

- Some chemicals, particles, metals, radioactive materials, and other substances can increase your risk of developing cancer.
- Radon is a radioactive gas. It can build up in underground spaces, such as basements, if there is not enough airflow.
- Asbestos is a fibrous material that was widely used in building insulation until 1980.
- Secondhand smoke includes smoke from burning cigarettes and exhaled smoke.
- Air pollution is caused by substances and fine particles released into the air.
- Sources may include motor vehicles, power plants that burn fossil fuels, and factories.
- Chemicals and metals in pesticides, solvents (paint thinners, grease removers, and dry cleaning chemicals), and other substances may increase cancer risk.

Workers in agriculture, mining, manufacturing, and other industries may be exposed to carcinogens more often and at higher concentrations. Therefore, they may have an even greater cancer risk.

You can reduce your risk by avoiding or reducing your exposure to cancer causing substances at home and at work.

Infections

Some infections may increase your risk of developing cancer.

- Human papillomavirus (HPV) is the most common sexually transmitted infection in the United States. HPV is the primary cause of most cervical cancers. There is a new HPV vaccine available for girls and young women. This vaccine and regular screening can reduce infections and cancer risk.
- Hepatitis B and hepatitis C viruses may be transmitted by injected drug use, intimate sexual contact, or contact with infected blood. Infection may lead to liver cancer. These viruses are more common in Asia than in the United States. Because of this, Asian

7

American women who have recently immigrated have a higher risk of infection and liver cancer.

- *Helicobacter pylori* (*H. pylori*) bacteria cause a common stomach infection that increases the risk of developing stomach cancer. *H. pylori* is more common in developing countries than in the United States. Recent immigrants from Asia or Latin America have a greater chance of infection and risk for stomach cancer.

You can reduce your risk by taking steps to prevent infection when possible. Vaccines are available for HPV and the hepatitis B virus. If you think you may be at high risk for any of these infections, talk to your doctor about tests and treatments.

Breast and Ovarian Cancer: Inherited Risk Factors

Women with a family history of breast or ovarian cancer may inherit mutated genes that increase their risk of developing these diseases. Mutations of the BRCA1 or BRCA2 genes are most strongly linked to these cancers, but other genes also play a role. Inherited mutated genes cause only about five to 10 percent of breast and ovarian cancers. And even women who inherit these mutated genes may not develop cancer.

If you have a family history of breast or ovarian cancer, talk to your doctor. Genetic counseling can help you decide if testing for BRCA mutations might be helpful. If you do test positive, your doctor may suggest additional screening tests, taking tamoxifen or an aromatase inhibitor (a drug that reduces breast cancer risk), or surgery to remove the breasts or ovaries to prevent cancer.

Ten Most Common Cancers in American Women

- Breast cancer
- Lung cancer
- Colon and rectal cancers
- Endometrial cancer
- Non-Hodgkin lymphoma
- Melanoma (skin cancer)
- Ovarian cancer
- Thyroid cancer

- Pancreatic cancer
- Leukemia

Ten Cancers Responsible for the Most Deaths among American Women

- Lung cancer
- Breast cancer
- Colon and rectal cancers
- Pancreatic cancer
- Ovarian cancer
- Non-Hodgkin lymphoma
- Leukemia
- Endometrial cancer
- Brain tumors
- Myeloma

Finding Out If You Have Cancer

Cancer Symptoms

At first, cancer may not produce any symptoms. As a tumor grows, you may feel discomfort or pain at the tumor site, abnormal bleeding, fatigue, and weight loss. Other symptoms may depend on the location of the cancer.

Cancer Screening

Depending on your age and risk factors, you should be screened for some cancers. This is important even if you feel healthy. Screening can allow your doctor to find and remove abnormal cells before they turn into cancer. These tests can also detect cancer early, before you feel any symptoms.

Screening is not recommended for all women or for all types of cancer. Screening tests are not completely accurate, and they can have harms. Talk to your doctor about the benefits and harms of commonly used screening tests. Tests may produce false-positive results, meaning they may show you have cancer when you don't. This can cause

worry and unneeded medical procedures. Tests may also produce false-negative results that miss cancer. Your doctor will need to do more tests to confirm the results. Your primary care doctor may also refer you to an oncologist for more tests. An oncologist is a doctor who specializes in cancer.

The information below lists the screenings recommended for women with average risk for some common cancers. If you think you may have higher than average risk, talk to your doctor about your risk factors. You may need additional tests.

Breast Cancer

You should be screened for breast cancer on the following schedule:

- In your 20s and 30s, you should have a clinical breast exam every three years. After you turn 40, you should have a clinical breast exam every year.

- Starting at age 40, you should have mammograms (an x-ray examination of the breasts) every one to two years.

- At any age, you should be familiar with the normal feel and appearance of your breasts. Report any changes to your doctor right way.

Discuss breast cancer risk with your doctor. If you are at higher risk, you may need mammograms at an earlier age. You may also need more frequent exams or additional tests.

Cervical Cancer

Beginning three years after the start of sexual activity or at age 21, you should have a Pap test each year. A Pap test is a microscopic examination of cells taken from the cervix. After three normal tests, you only need to be tested every three years. If you are older than age 65 and have had three normal tests, you may choose to stop being testing. If you have had your cervix removed as part of a hysterectomy, you do not need to be screened (unless the hysterectomy was performed to treat cancer).

Colorectal Cancer

Beginning at age 50, you should be screened for colorectal cancer on one of the following schedules.

- You may have a fecal occult blood test (FOBT) (a test that checks for blood in the stool) once each year.

- Flexible sigmoidoscopy (examination of the lower colon) may be performed once every five years.

- FOBT each year may be combined with flexible sigmoidoscopy once every five years.

- You may have a colonoscopy (examination of the colon) every 10 years.

- Computed tomography (tuh-MOG-ruh-fee) (CT) scans of the colon ("virtual colonoscopy") are used at some medical centers for screening.

Talk to your doctor about which type of testing is best for you. If you are at high risk of colon cancer, your doctor may recommend additional testing.

Surviving Cancer

Thanks to improved screening and treatment, more and more women are surviving longer after a cancer diagnosis. Cancer may affect your health, emotions, work, and relationships long after your treatment ends. As a cancer survivor, you need to continue to take care of your physical and emotional health.

Talk to your doctor about any symptoms you have, such as pain, fatigue, or depression.

Set up a schedule for follow-up care with your doctor. At follow-up appointments, your doctor can address any side effects of treatment and check to see if the cancer has returned or spread.

Talk to your health care team about a wellness plan that can improve your health and may reduce the chances that your cancer will return.

Take care of your emotions and seek support when you need it.

Chapter 2

Common Gynecologic Conditions That Are Not Indicative of Cancer

Options for Treatment

If you have a problem that affects your uterus or another part of your reproductive system, this information is for you. It explains most of the problems that can affect a woman's reproductive system and ways the problems can be treated, including medication, surgery, and other kinds of treatments.

About the Uterus

The uterus is located in the lower abdomen between the bladder and the rectum. The uterus is also called the womb. It is pear-shaped, and the lower, narrow end of the uterus is the cervix. When a woman is pregnant, the baby grows in the uterus until he or she is born.

On each side of the uterus at the top are the fallopian tubes and ovaries. Together, the uterus, vagina, ovaries, and fallopian tubes make up the reproductive system.

In women who have not gone through menopause ("the change" or "change of life"), the ovaries produce the hormone estrogen at the beginning of the menstrual cycle. Estrogen helps to prepare the lining of the uterus (called the endometrium) for possible pregnancy. When

The information in this chapter is from "Common Uterine Conditions," Agency for Healthcare Research and Quality (www.ahrq.gov), 1997. Revised and updated by David A. Cooke, MD, FACP May 2010.

the uterus is ready, one of the ovaries releases an egg. The egg travels down the fallopian tube where it waits for possible fertilization.

If the woman becomes pregnant, the fertilized egg travels to the uterus where it attaches to the endometrium. If she does not, the endometrium and the unfertilized egg are discharged through the vagina during the woman's next period (menstruation).

Some of the problems that can affect your uterus are:

- Noncancerous growths in the uterus, called fibroids, which can cause pain and bleeding

- Endometriosis, a condition in which the tissue that forms the lining of the uterus grows outside the uterus

- Heavy bleeding each time you have your period or between periods

- Hormonal imbalances

- Unexplained pelvic pain

Treatment Options

Your doctor may have recommended that you have a hysterectomy or another kind of treatment. Before you decide what to do, it is important that you understand the problem and the different options you have for dealing with it.

The following information can help you think about your condition, learn about your treatment choices, and decide on some questions to ask your doctor.

Keep in mind that every woman is different and every situation is different. A good treatment choice for one woman may not be the best choice for another. That is why you should take these steps:

- Talk over your options carefully with your doctor.

- Ask questions until you understand what the doctor is telling you.

- Consider getting a second opinion.

- Work with your doctor to choose the treatment that is best for you.

You Are Not Alone

The first thing you need to know is that you are not alone. About one of every 10 women between the ages of 18 and 50 has this type of problem. Usually, the problem can be treated, and the symptoms can be relieved. Most women who have had treatment are satisfied

with the results and are glad to be free of pain or other unpleasant symptoms.

The first step in getting relief is to find out what the problem is.

Finding Out about the Problem

There are several ways your doctor can find out (diagnose) what is causing your symptoms. The most common include the following:

A Medical History

The first step in diagnosing your problem is a medical history. The doctor—or sometimes the nurse—will ask you questions about your medical history. This will include questions about your symptoms and any serious illnesses you have had, as well as whether you have ever had surgery, been pregnant, or had children. You also may be asked about the medical history of close family members.

If you have been using herbs, acupuncture, or other "natural remedies," be sure to tell your doctor about them.

The doctor may ask about your sex life. You may be uncomfortable talking about such personal matters, but it is important for your doctor to know if something that is happening in your sex life might be related to your condition.

A Vaginal Exam

The doctor will use instruments to look inside your cervix and uterus. The doctor will use a speculum to keep the walls of the vagina apart during the exam. Sometimes this exam is uncomfortable. You may feel a slight cramp, but it usually is not painful. If you are able to relax, you will be more comfortable. The doctor may look inside the vagina and cervix with a lighted tube.

A Pap Test (or Pap Smear)

During the vaginal exam, the doctor usually takes a sample of cells from the cervix with a wooden or plastic scraper, cotton swab, or small brush. The test is quick and usually painless. The cells are placed on a glass slide or in a small jar, which is sent to a lab. A Pap test is one way that doctors can find cancer of the cervix or dysplasia, which is a condition that sometimes can turn into cancer.

All women over 21 years of age should have a Pap test done every one to three years.

Testing for an infection called human papilloma virus (HPV) is frequently done on the same sample used for your Pap smear. Results of this test can help your doctor interpret your Pap smear results.

Laboratory Tests

The doctor will take a sample of your blood and a urine specimen and send them to a lab to be examined. The results of these tests will tell the doctor a lot about your general health.

Imaging Tests

There are many ways to look inside the body without surgery. X-rays are the most well known. Your doctor may also suggest an ultrasound test, CAT scan, or MRI. These tests help the doctor to learn more about your body and what is causing your problem.

Depending on your symptoms, the doctor may suggest an endometrial biopsy, dilation and curettage (D&C), or other tests to help diagnose your problem.

Noncancerous Uterine Conditions

After your medical history, examination, and tests are done, your doctor will explain your condition to you and talk about your options for treatment. Later in this chapter you will find a list of questions you may want to ask your doctor.

Surgery, medicine (including hormones), a combination of the two, or "watchful waiting" are the most common choices for dealing with most noncancerous uterine conditions. Watchful waiting means having no treatment but seeing the doctor regularly to keep track of your condition and discuss symptoms. After a period of watchful waiting, if you are still having problems, you may decide with your doctor to consider one or more treatment options.

There are always new treatments in development. Be sure to ask your doctor if there are any new treatments for your condition that are not described in this chapter.

Your doctor may recommend that you have a hysterectomy. Remember all treatments—including medicine, surgery, other types of treatments, and even a decision to wait or not be treated—have risks and benefits. Be sure to ask your doctor about the risks and benefits of each treatment option you are offered. Then you can work with your doctor to weigh your options and make an informed choice.

Fibroids

What are fibroids?

Fibroids are growths in the walls of the uterus. Sometimes, a fibroid is attached to the outside of the uterus by a stalk. Fibroids can be as small as a seed or a pea or as large as an orange or small melon. Although fibroids are called "tumors," they are not cancer. They are smooth muscle growths.

About two of every 10 women who have not gone through menopause have fibroids. The technical term for a fibroid tumor is leiomyoma.

Fibroids may cause no symptoms at all, or they may cause pain or bleeding. Fibroids may make it hard to pass urine if they grow large enough to press on the bladder.

Fibroids also can make it hard for you to get pregnant. Sometimes fibroids can cause problems with pregnancy, labor, or delivery, including miscarriage and premature birth.

How are fibroids treated?

You may have several treatments to choose from if you have fibroids. It depends on how big the fibroids are, where they are, and whether you are pregnant or want to become pregnant.

Watchful waiting may be all the treatment you need if your fibroid is small and you do not have any symptoms. You will need regular visits to your doctor for a pelvic exam to monitor the growth of the fibroid.

Nonsurgical treatments for fibroids include hormones and pain relief medicines.

Taking gonadotropin releasing hormone (GnRH) can cause fibroids to shrink. This may make surgery easier, or it may be used instead of an operation.

Your doctor may prescribe ibuprofen (for example, Advil), acetaminophen (for example, Tylenol), or another medicine to relieve pain.

Surgical treatments for fibroids include hysterectomy, myomectomy, and embolization.

Hysterectomy is usually recommended when the fibroids are causing symptoms, when they have grown rapidly, or when the fibroids are large (as large as a grapefruit).

Myomectomy is an operation to remove a fibroid tumor without taking out the uterus. This means that pregnancy is still possible, although a Cesarean section may be necessary.

Recovery time after a myomectomy is about three to four weeks. About 20 percent of women who undergo myomectomy need a blood

transfusion, about 30 percent have a fever after surgery, and many patients develop adhesions (scar tissue) in their pelvis in the months following surgery. These complications are more likely to occur when there is more than one fibroid and when the fibroids are large.

The growths may come back after a myomectomy, and repeat surgery may be necessary. If you are considering a myomectomy, be sure to ask the doctor how likely it is that new fibroids might grow after the surgery.

You also should ask your doctor how much experience he or she has in doing this procedure. Not all gynecologists have been trained to perform myomectomies.

Another option is laser surgery, which usually is an outpatient procedure. With laser surgery, the doctor uses a high-intensity light to remove small fibroids.

Depending on the location of the fibroid, it may be possible to remove it during a laparoscopy. Or, the doctor may put a thin tube (called a hysteroscope) with a laser through the vagina and into the uterus. The tube may have a small scraper to scrape away the fibroid from the wall of the uterus.

Embolization is a newer procedure that can often treat problematic fibroids without performing major surgery. A thin tube known as a catheter is inserted into an artery in the leg, and is threaded under x-ray guidance to the blood vessels that supply the fibroid. Bits of material are placed in the fibroid's blood vessel with the catheter, which cause the vessel to clot off and close. Without a blood supply, the fibroid will wither and disappear.

Embolization can be a good alternative to surgery, but it is not an option for all patients. The size and location of the fibroids are factors, as are other medical problems that the patient might have. Embolization is usually performed by interventional radiologists, rather than gynecologists.

Endometriosis

What is endometriosis?

Endometrial tissue lines the uterus. Each month, in tune with the menstrual cycle, the endometrial tissue thickens and is shed during menstruation.

If you have endometriosis, it means that the same kind of tissue that lines your uterus is also growing in other parts of your body, usually in the abdomen. This can cause scar tissue to build up around your organs.

Endometriosis may cause severe pain and abnormal bleeding, usually around the time of your period. Pain during intercourse is another common symptom. However, it is possible to have endometriosis and not have any symptoms. Endometriosis is a leading cause of infertility (inability to get pregnant). Often it is not diagnosed until a woman has trouble getting pregnant.

Endometriosis will lessen after menopause and during pregnancy, since the growth of endometrial tissue depends on estrogen. If you have endometriosis and take estrogen-replacement therapy after menopause, the tissue may grow back.

The only way to be sure that you have endometriosis is through a surgical procedure, laparoscopy. Endometriosis can be a chronic condition and may return even after treatment with medicine or surgery.

How can endometriosis be treated?

There are several options for treating endometriosis. The best treatment for you may depend on whether you want to relieve pain, increase your chances of getting pregnant, or both. It is important to work with your doctor to weigh the benefits and risks of each treatment.

Nonsurgical treatments include medicine, including hormones. There are two types of hormone therapy: those that will make your body think it is pregnant and those that will make your body think it is in menopause. Both are meant to stop the body from producing the messages that cause the endometrial tissue to grow. Birth control pills may be used for a few months to try to shrink the adhesions in women who want to become pregnant. Other hormones—GnRH and danazol—also may help relieve the pain of endometriosis.

Doctors sometimes prescribe pain relievers, such as ibuprofen (for example, Advil and Motrin) or, for severe pain, codeine.

Other nonsurgical options include watchful waiting and changes in diet and exercise.

Several types of surgery are used to treat endometriosis, including the following:

- Laser laparoscopy, in which a cut is made in the abdomen and adhesions are removed, either by laser beams or electric cauterization.

- Hysterectomy, which may not cure endometriosis. Unless the ovaries are removed also, they will continue to produce estrogen. This may encourage endometrial tissue to grow in other areas of the body.

- Bowel resection, which means taking out a section of the bowel, if endometriosis is affecting the bowel.

- Cutting certain nerves, called the sacral nerves, in the lower back to relieve pain.

Endometrial Hyperplasia

What is hyperplasia?

Hyperplasia is a condition in which the lining of the uterus becomes too thick, which results in abnormal bleeding. Hyperplasia is thought to be caused by too much estrogen.

Depending on your age and how long you have had hyperplasia, your doctor may want to do a biopsy before beginning treatment to rule out cancer.

Hyperplasia may be seen with or without atypia. Atypia is an abnormal appearance of the uterine cells on endometrial biopsy.

Hyperplasia without atypia usually does not lead to uterine cancer. Hyperplasia with atypia indicates an increased risk of developing uterine cancer.

How is hyperplasia treated?

Hormone treatment with birth control pills or progesterone helps the majority of women with endometrial hyperplasia.

Placement of a hormone-releasing intrauterine device (IUD) can also be effective for treatment of endometrial hyperplasia.

Hysterectomy is sometimes recommended to treat hyperplasia. Generally, this is preferred if atypia is seen on biopsy, in older women, or in women who cannot or do not wish to take hormone therapy.

Because some types of hyperplasia can lead to cancer, your doctor will watch your condition carefully if you choose not to have a hysterectomy.

Uterine Prolapse

What is uterine prolapse?

If you have uterine prolapse, it means that your uterus has tilted or slipped. Sometimes it slips so far down that it reaches into the vagina. This happens when the ligaments that hold the uterus to the wall of the pelvis become too weak to hold the uterus in its place.

Uterine prolapse can cause feelings of pressure and discomfort. Urine may leak.

How is uterine prolapse treated?

Treatment choices depend on how weak the ligaments have become, your age, health, and whether you want to become pregnant.

Options that do not involve an operation include the following:

- Exercises (called Kegel exercises) can help to strengthen the muscles of the pelvis. How to do Kegel exercises: Tighten your pelvic muscles as if you are trying to hold back urine. Hold the muscles tight for a few seconds and then release them. Repeat this exercise up to 10 times. Repeat the Kegel exercises up to four time each day.

- Taking estrogen to limit further weakening of the muscles and tissues that support the uterus.

- Inserting a pessary—which is a rubber, diaphragm-like device— around the cervix to help prop up the uterus. The pessary does have drawbacks. It may dislodge or cause irritation, it may interfere with intercourse, and it must be removed regularly for cleaning.

- Watchful waiting.

Surgical treatments include tightening the weakened muscles without taking out the uterus. This is usually done through the vagina, but it also can be done through the abdomen. Although this is a type of surgery, it is not as extensive as a hysterectomy.

Doctors usually recommend a hysterectomy if symptoms are bothersome or if the uterus has dropped so far that it is coming through the vagina.

Ovarian Cysts

What are ovarian cysts?

Ovarian cysts are small, fluid-filled sacs that usually are not malignant. They may not cause any symptoms, or they may be quite painful. Sometimes, ovarian cysts appear in connection with the menstrual cycle, and they may go away on their own in a few months. When these cysts grow large, they may cause feelings of pressure or fullness.

Although most ovarian cysts are benign (not cancer), they must be taken very seriously. A sonogram will show whether a cyst is fluid-filled or has solid matter in it. If it is solid, it may be related to endometriosis, or it may be cancerous.

What are the treatments for ovarian cysts?

If you have not yet gone through menopause, you may not need any treatment, unless the cyst is very big or causing pain. Sometimes, taking birth control pills will make the cyst smaller. Surgery may be needed if the cyst is causing symptoms or is more than two inches across.

If surgery is needed, often the cyst can be removed without removing the ovary. Even if one ovary has to be removed, it is still possible to become pregnant as long as one ovary remains.

After menopause, the risk of ovarian cancer increases. Surgery to remove an ovarian cyst is usually recommended in this case. Your doctor will probably want to do a biopsy to see if cancer is present.

If you have gone through menopause and you have an ovarian cyst, talk with your doctor about what will be done during surgery. Make sure you understand whether he or she plans to remove just the cyst, the cyst and the ovary, or to do a hysterectomy. Talk over the options with your doctor and make your own wishes known.

Treatment options include the following:

- Watchful waiting
- Hormone therapy to reduce the size of the cyst
- Cystectomy to remove the cyst
- Oophorectomy to remove the affected ovary
- Hysterectomy (This usually is not necessary unless the cyst is cancerous)

Pelvic Inflammatory Disease

Pelvic inflammatory disease (PID) is caused by an infection that starts in the vagina. Most often, it is caused by a sexually transmitted disease (STD). The infection spreads upward into the uterus, fallopian tubes, and pelvis.

Women who use intrauterine devices (IUDs) are at increased risk for PID. Rarely, the bacteria that cause PID enter the body during childbirth or abortion.

PID can cause pelvic pain and fevers. It also may cause infertility (inability to get pregnant) because of damage to the fallopian tubes. Sacs of pus, called abscesses, may form in the pelvis. Sometimes the vagina will discharge a pus-like substance.

If PID is not treated, pain may be so intense that it is hard to walk. The infection may spread into the bloodstream and throughout the body, causing fever, chills, joint infections, and sometimes death.

How is PID treated?

- If you have PID and it is the result of an STD, you and your sexual partner will be given drugs called antibiotics to treat the infection.
- If an abscess has formed, it may need to be drained.
- Treatment may include hospitalization.
- An operation may be done to help heal scar tissue.
- If the disease cannot be stopped in any other way, you may need surgery to remove the infected organs.

Severe Menstrual Pain

What is severe menstrual pain?

Some women have extreme cramping just before and during their period. The technical term for this is dysmenorrhea. If you have this kind of pain, you should seek treatment. Severe menstrual pain may be a symptom of endometriosis.

What can be done about severe menstrual pain?

Several types of medicine are used to treat painful cramps:

- Over-the-counter pain relievers, such as aspirin, ibuprofen, naproxen (for example, Aleve), or acetaminophen may be helpful.
- If over-the-counter medicines don't work, your doctor can give you a prescription for a stronger pain reliever, such as codeine.
- Birth control pills or other medicines may be used to reduce cramping.
- Surgery usually is not necessary if severe menstrual pain is the only problem.

Very Heavy Menstrual Bleeding

What is very heavy menstrual bleeding?

As you get closer to menopause, it may be hard to tell when your period is going to start. The time between your periods may be longer or shorter than usual. When it does start, bleeding may be very heavy and last for several weeks.

You may have dysfunctional uterine bleeding or DUB. DUB most often affects women over 45. Usually it is caused by an imbalance in the chemicals in the body (hormones) that control the menstrual cycle.

Younger women also may have heavy bleeding. Usually it is because of an irregular menstrual cycle. A woman may go for several months without a period, but the lining of her uterus continues to build up. When finally her body sheds the uterine lining, she may have very heavy bleeding.

The symptoms can be very upsetting and may make you feel limited in the things you can do. Sometimes, the symptoms are a sign of a more serious problem.

Your doctor will probably do a blood test. Depending on the results, your medical history, and your age, the doctor may recommend that you have a biopsy to rule out endometrial hyperplasia.

What treatments are used for very heavy menstrual bleeding?

- Birth control pills or other medicines may be helpful.

- Another choice is watchful waiting.

- A surgical procedure called endometrial ablation may help to relieve very heavy menstrual bleeding. Endometrial ablation causes sterility (inability to become pregnant), but it does not trigger menopause. The long-term effects of endometrial ablation are unknown.

Do you have a bleeding disorder?

If you have very heavy periods (lasting more than seven days or soaking more than one pad or tampon every two to three hours), frequent or long-lasting nosebleeds, easy bruising, or prolonged oozing of blood after dental work, you may have a bleeding disorder such as von Willebrand Disease. This is not the same as very heavy menstrual bleeding, but it can be an underlying cause.

Chronic Pelvic Pain

What is chronic pelvic pain?

If you feel intense pain in your pelvis, but the doctor can find no cause, you may have chronic pelvic pain.

How is chronic pelvic pain treated?

Options that do not involve surgery include combination thera-py—including anti-inflammatory medicines that contain ibuprofen, birth control pills, physical therapy, and nutritional and psychological counseling—may be helpful. Depending on the severity of the pain, watchful waiting may be another option.

Surgical options include surgery to take out scar tissue that may be causing pain. This is called adhesiolysis.

Hysterectomy may be an option for women whose pelvic veins are persistently swollen or when all other measures have been tried without success. However, it does not always relieve the pain.

Cutting certain nerves in the lower back to help relieve pain.

Chapter 3

Does Cancer Run in Your Family?

Family Genetics

While all cancers are caused by the disruption of genes, we know that approximately 5–10% of cancers are related to specific inherited genetic abnormalities.

There are scientific methods to identify some of these inherited defects and show whether some people have an increased chance of developing certain types of cancer. These cancers happen more often in some families than in others.

There are tests available that can identify if you are at increased risk. Let your healthcare provider know if any of your close relatives (parents, brothers, sisters, and children) have ever been diagnosed with cancer. Genetic testing should always be carried out at a clinic that also provides supportive counselling and education. Some people may decide not to take genetic testing when they understand the implications to their personal situation.

The fact that one or two family members have been diagnosed with cancer does not mean that you will also develop cancer. This is especially true if the family member is not a first-degree relative or if the

This chapter includes text from "Family Genetics," "Genetic Changes and Family Genetics," "Genetic Risk Assessment," "Understanding Your Risk," and "Cancers That Are Known to Be Hereditary," © 2009 Canadian Cancer Society. All rights reserved. Reprinted with permission. Accessed August 7, 2009. To view these documents along with additional information, visit http://www.cancer.ca/Canada-wide .aspx?sc_lang=en.

cancers are of different types. It is important to discuss screening with your doctor if you have a family history of cancer.

Genetic Changes and Family Genetics

It is not entirely clear whether a family's pattern of cancer is due to chance, similarities in the lifestyle choices of family members, or hereditary factors passed from parents to children through genes.

Understanding Genes and Inheritance

People from the same family share many characteristics. For example, parents pass on physical traits to their children like eye color, hair color, and body shape. Also, brothers and sisters may have similar personalities, and they may be good at the same kinds of activities. Our parents pass characteristics on to us through units of information called genes.

Our bodies are made up of cells. Genes are present in every cell and guide how each cell develops and functions. Over the past few years, scientists have learned a great deal about how changes in our genes (gene mutations) can influence our health.

Gene mutations can occur in two ways. They can be inherited from a parent or they can be the result of changes that occur during a person's lifetime. Every cell has the ability to spot these changes and fix them before they are passed on to new cells through the normal process of cell development. Sometimes a cell's ability to make these repairs fails and the altered gene may be passed on. Certain gene mutations that are passed on may increase the risk of developing cancer.

Genetic Risk Assessment

Genetic risk assessment is the evaluation of your personal risk for cancer, based on your family medical history. Genetic risk assessment is done by a genetic counsellor and includes discussions about your family history of cancer and recommendations for future action. Genetic testing that can identify if there is a gene mutation may follow genetic risk assessment.

If you are thinking about genetic risk assessment, consider the following issues:

Personal Preference

Research has shown that people have strong and differing opinions about genetic risk assessment. Some people want to know about their

risk while others prefer not to know. It is important to respect individual wishes. For people who want to know details about their risk, it can be upsetting if they are not provided with all the facts. Others who do not want to know their risks may be upset if they are given too much information. It is important that you know where you stand and that you let others know your wishes.

Psychological Impact

Genetic risk assessment is not completely understood. Having a genetic risk assessment may make you experience a wide range of emotions. You may worry about the impact the information may have on your job, your relationships and on your family. Or, genetic risk assessment might lessen anxiety as you learn more. Genetic counsellors and other healthcare professionals can help you deal with your emotions.

Confidentiality

You may be concerned about who will know about the results of your genetic risk assessment. It is important to know that there are some rules and procedures in place to help avoid the misuse of this information. Your genetic risk assessment will be kept confidential. Information about you or your genetic risk assessment is not released without your written consent. A genetic counsellor can answer your questions and concerns.

Sharing Information with Your Family

You will want to think carefully about telling other members of your family about the results of your genetic risk assessment. Some people have found that the best thing to do is to let their family members know they have had genetic risk assessment and to share the results if their relatives want to know.

Insurance and Employment

Should insurance companies ask people who are at greater risk for developing cancer to pay higher health or life insurance premiums? Should insurance companies seek any information about the history of inherited cancer and genetic testing at all? As genetic testing for cancer moves to regular clinical services in Canada, results from the test might be used to predict a person's future health risks and deny them life insurance or employment opportunities. It is still too early

to know how these questions will be answered. You may wish to talk to a genetic counsellor about your rights and responsibilities.

Concerns about Children

Research has shown that many people are especially concerned about their children's inherited risk for developing cancer. It is very upsetting to think that you may have passed on a gene mutation to your child. It is important to remember that through genetics research we are continually improving methods of cancer prevention, detection, and treatment, and this will benefit our children in the future. Knowing about an inherited increased risk for developing cancer can help our children become more aware of the importance of preventive and/or early detection measures.

Learning about Your Family's Health History

One way to learn if cancer runs in your family is to look at your family tree of cancer history. You will need to go back through as many generations as possible and find out which of your relatives had cancer. You will then need to collect as much information as you can about the type of cancer your relatives had and their ages when they were diagnosed with cancer. This may be difficult because medical records were not kept as well in the past as they are today. You may also need to contact health facilities (hospitals and cancer clinics). Genetic counsellors may be able to help you collect this information by providing you with the necessary consent forms so that medical records may be released to you.

Genetic Counselling

Once you have obtained a family tree of cancer history, it will be studied to see if your family qualifies for genetic counselling or a special research study. At the genetic counselling session you will meet with a genetic counsellor and other healthcare professionals. The genetic counsellor will provide information about genes and how they function and about the specific cancer causing genes that may have been identified. A genetic risk assessment is provided along with recommendations for cancer screening and/or monitoring. The genetic counsellor will also discuss how genetic testing for cancer may affect you and your family.

Genetic Testing

Genetic testing is a scientific process that involves special laboratory procedures. Scientists have recently developed methods of genetic

testing to tell if there are changes to a gene. Genetic testing may be able to identify if we carry a gene mutation that puts us at an increased risk for developing cancer long before the cancer actually develops.

Not everyone is eligible for genetic testing. There are several reasons why individuals may not be offered genetic testing. These will be discussed with you at a genetic counselling session.

Understanding Your Risk

It is important for you to know the level of your risk for developing cancer because it may help you to decide what type of healthcare action to take. We talk about risk of developing cancer as:

- risk factors which may contribute to the random development of cancer over our lifetime;

- the chance of having an inherited gene mutation.

Lifetime Risk

Lifetime risk is often discussed in relation to the risk of individuals in the general population. Many of us have heard that one in nine Canadian women will develop breast cancer in her lifetime. This statement means that if we kept track of a group of 1000 Canadian girl babies all through their lives, we would find that 111 of them (one in nine) would have been diagnosed with breast cancer at some point during that time. It does not mean that if nine Canadian women were together in a room then one of them would have breast cancer at that moment.

Lifetime risk may be stated in percentages. For example, you may be told that you have a 15% risk of developing cancer. This statement means that you have a 15% chance of being diagnosed with cancer sometime during your lifetime.

Risk Factors

Risk factors are anything that might increase our chance of developing a disease like cancer. Cancer is not a single disease, but a large group of diseases. Most cancers develop as a result of gene mutations that develop in the cells during a person's lifetime.

Cancer develops gradually as a result of a complex mix of risk factors related to:

- lifestyle (tobacco use, diet, exposure to sunlight);

- the environment;

- heredity;

- chance;

- age;

- gender.

Some risk factors can be avoided—we can choose not to smoke. Some cannot—we cannot choose the genes that we inherit through birth.

Many people who develop cancer have no known risk factors. Even if a person has one or more risk factors, it is impossible to know exactly how much they may contribute to developing cancer later in life.

Inherited Gene Mutations

While all cancers could be considered to be genetic—as they are triggered by altered genes—only a small portion of cancers (up to 10%) are passed on from one family generation to another. The risk of having an inherited gene mutation is generally talked about in relation to one of three groups: low, medium or high.

A cancer might be considered hereditary for a family if:

- the cancer is present in a number of generations;

- family members have developed cancer when they were younger than 50 years of age or at a younger age than usual for that type of cancer;

- family members have had more than one type of cancer.

Depending on your risk of developing cancer, cancer specialists may advise certain preventive and/or early detection measures. These recommendations may be made with or without genetic testing.

Taking Action to Reduce Your Risk

Preventive Measures

Preventive measures help reduce the chance to develop cancer. Research into cancer risk prevention provides us with information about how to lower our risk for developing cancer. You may:

- choose to have surgery;

- be given medication that may reduce your risk;

- wish to make some lifestyle changes.

Early Detection Measures

Early detection measures help to discover signs of cancer as early as possible. These methods could include a combination of:

- examinations done by a doctor;
- self-examinations you do on your own;
- clinical tests (like mammography, ultrasound).

Cancers That Are Known to Be Hereditary

There are some cancers that occur more often in some families than in others.

Studies have shown that breast and ovarian cancer often show up over many generations in one family. An inherited gene mutation that increases a woman's risk of developing breast cancer usually increases her risk of ovarian cancer as well. As a result, the two risks are often estimated together.

Colon cancer is another type of cancer that is often seen in members of the same family. Gene mutations associated with colon cancer may also increase the risk for developing other cancers like:

- cancer of the uterus;
- cancer of the rectum (lower end of the large bowel that links it to the anus);
- stomach cancer;
- cancer of the urinary tract;
- ovarian cancer.

Other cancers that may occur within the same family include:

- prostate cancer;
- familial medullary thyroid carcinoma;
- retinoblastoma;
- Wilm's tumour;
- some forms of leukemia;
- pancreatic cancer.

Research is continuing to find genes that may put people at higher risk of developing other types of cancer.

When you want to know more about inherited risk of cancer, e-mail the Canadian Cancer Society (info@cis.cancer.ca) or call an information specialist at their Cancer Information Service 888-939-3333.

Chapter 4

What Women Need to Know about Smoking and Cancer Risk

Chapter Contents

Section 4.1

Smoking and Cancer

Excerpted from "Highlights: Smoking Among Adults in the United
States: Cancer," Centers for Disease Control and Prevention (CDC), 2004;
and "Women and Tobacco," CDC, May 2009.

Smoking among Adults in the United States

- Cancer is the second leading cause of death and was among the
  first diseases causally linked to smoking.

- Lung cancer is the leading cause of cancer death, and cigarette
  smoking causes most cases.

- Compared to nonsmokers, men who smoke are about 23 times
  more likely to develop lung cancer and women who smoke are
  about 13 times more likely. Smoking causes about 90% of lung
  cancer deaths in men and almost 80% in women.

- In 2003, an estimated 171,900 new cases of lung cancer occurred
  and approximately 157,200 people died from lung cancer.

- The 2004 Surgeon General's report adds more evidence to previous conclusions that smoking causes cancers of the oral cavity,
  pharynx, larynx, esophagus, lung, and bladder.

- Cancer-causing agents (carcinogens) in tobacco smoke damage
  important genes that control the growth of cells, causing them to
  grow abnormally or to reproduce too rapidly.

- Cigarette smoking is a major cause of esophageal cancer in the
  United States. Reductions in smoking and smokeless tobacco use
  could prevent many of the approximately 12,300 new cases and
  12,100 deaths from esophageal cancer that occur annually.

- The combination of smoking and alcohol consumption causes
  most laryngeal cancer cases. In 2003, an estimated 3800 deaths
  occurred from laryngeal cancer.

- In 2003, an estimated 57,400 new cases of bladder cancer were
  diagnosed and an estimated 12,500 died from the disease.

- For smoking-attributable cancers, the risk generally increases with the number of cigarettes smoked and the number of years of smoking, and generally decreases after quitting completely.

- Smoking cigarettes that have a lower yield of tar does not substantially reduce the risk for lung cancer.

- Cigarette smoking increases the risk of developing mouth cancers. This risk also increases among people who smoke pipes and cigars.

- Reductions in the number of people who smoke cigarettes, pipes, cigars, and other tobacco products or use smokeless tobacco could prevent most of the estimated 30,200 new cases and 7,800 deaths from oral cavity and pharynx cancers annually in the United States.

New Cancers Confirmed by This Report

- The 2004 Surgeon General's report newly identifies other cancers caused by smoking, including cancers of the stomach, cervix, kidney, and pancreas and acute myeloid leukemia.

- In 2003, an estimated 22,400 new cases of stomach cancer were diagnosed, and an estimated 12,100 deaths were expected to occur.

- Former smokers have lower rates of stomach cancer than those who continue to smoke.

- For women, the risk of cervical cancer increases with the duration of smoking.

- In 2003, an estimated 31,900 new cases of kidney cancer were diagnosed, and an estimated 11,900 people died from the disease.

- In 2003, an estimated 30,700 new cases of pancreatic cancer were diagnosed, attributing to 30,000 deaths. The median time from diagnosis to death from pancreatic cancer is about three months.

- In 2003, approximately 10,500 cases of acute myeloid leukemia were diagnosed in adults.

- Benzene is a known cause of acute myeloid leukemia, and cigarette smoke is a major source of benzene exposure. Among U.S. smokers, 90% of benzene exposures come from cigarettes.

Women and Tobacco

Health Effects and Mortality

- Cigarette smoking kills an estimated 178,000 women in the United States annually. The three leading smoking-related causes of death in women are lung cancer (45,000), heart disease (40,000), and chronic lung disease (42,000).

- Ninety percent of all lung cancer deaths in women smokers are attributable to smoking. Since 1950, lung cancer deaths among women have increased by more than 600 percent. By 1987, lung cancer had surpassed breast cancer as the leading cause of cancer-related deaths in women.

- Women who smoke have an increased risk for other cancers, including cancers of the oral cavity, pharynx, larynx (voice box), esophagus, pancreas, kidney, bladder, and uterine cervix. Women who smoke double their risk for developing coronary heart disease and increase by more than tenfold their likelihood of dying from chronic obstructive pulmonary disease.

- Cigarette smoking increases the risk for infertility, preterm delivery, stillbirth, low birth weight, and sudden infant death syndrome (SIDS).

- Postmenopausal women who smoke have lower bone density than women who never smoked. Women who smoke have an increased risk for hip fracture than never smokers.

National Estimates of Tobacco Use

- An estimated 18.1% of adult U.S. women aged 18 years or older (slightly less than one of five) are current cigarette smokers. Cigarette smoking estimates for women by age are as follows: 18–24 years (20.7%), 25–44 years (21.4%), 45–64 years (18.8%), and 65 years or older (8.3%).

- Prevalence of cigarette smoking is highest among women who are American Indians or Alaska Natives (26.8%), followed by whites (20%), African Americans (17.3%), Hispanics (11.1%), and Asians [excluding Native Hawaiians and other Pacific Islanders] (6.1%).

- Cigarette smoking estimates are highest for women with a general educational development (GED) diploma (38.8%) or 9–11

years of education (29.0%), and lowest for women with an undergraduate college degree (9.6%) or a graduate college degree (7.4%).

- Smoking prevalence is higher among women living below the poverty level (26.9%) compared with women living at or above the poverty level (17.6%).

- An estimated 18% of pregnant women aged 15–44 years smoke cigarettes, compared with 30% of nonpregnant women of the same age.

- The use of cigars and smokeless tobacco among females is generally low—1.9% of females 12 or older are current cigar smokers, and 0.3% are current smokeless tobacco users.

Section 4.2

Questions and Answers About Women and Smoking

Excerpted from "Women and Smoking: Questions and Answers," National Cancer Institute (www.cancer.gov), February 27, 2008.

Are women who smoke at increased risk of health problems?

Yes. Women and men who smoke are at increased risk of developing cancer, heart disease, and lung disease and of dying prematurely.

A pregnant smoker is at higher risk of having her baby born too early and with an abnormally low weight. A woman who smokes during or after pregnancy increases her infant's risk of death from sudden infant death syndrome (SIDS).

In addition, some studies suggest that women who smoke are more likely to experience irregular or painful periods. Smokers are more likely than nonsmokers to go through menopause at a younger age. Women who smoke after menopause have lower bone density and a higher risk of hip fracture than do women who don't smoke.

Does smoking increase cancer risk in women?

Yes. Smoking causes cancers of the lung, esophagus, larynx (voice box), mouth, throat, kidney, bladder, pancreas, stomach, and cervix, as well as acute myeloid leukemia. In 1987, lung cancer surpassed breast cancer to become the leading cause of cancer death in U.S. women. Unlike early breast cancer and many other types of cancer, lung cancer is rarely curable. Most deaths from lung cancer among U.S. women are caused by smoking.

What are the immediate benefits of quitting smoking for women?

The immediate health benefits of quitting smoking are substantial. Within a few hours, the level of carbon monoxide in the blood begins to decline. (Carbon monoxide, a colorless, odorless gas found in cigarette smoke, reduces the blood's ability to carry oxygen.) Heart rate and blood pressure, which were abnormally high while smoking, begin to return to normal. Within a few weeks, women who quit smoking have improved circulation, don't produce as much phlegm, and don't cough or wheeze as often. Women can also expect significant improvements in lung function within several months of quitting.

Also, women who quit smoking reduce the risk of infertility, and pregnant women who quit early in their pregnancy reduce the risk of the baby being born too early and with an abnormally low weight.

What are the long-term benefits of quitting smoking for women?

Quitting smoking dramatically reduces the risk of developing an illness caused by smoking:

- The risk of death from heart disease is substantially reduced within one or two years after quitting, and eventually becomes the same as that of nonsmokers.

- The risk of death from lung cancer and other lung diseases declines steadily, beginning about five years after quitting.

- Quitting smoking as early in life as possible is likely to reduce the risk of fractures that would be caused by smoking in old age.

- Regardless of age, women can substantially reduce the risk of disease, including cancer, by quitting smoking. For women who have already developed cancer, quitting smoking helps the body

to heal and to respond to cancer treatment, and quitting reduces the risk of developing a second cancer.

Is the National Institutes of Health (NIH) supporting research on women, tobacco, and cancer?

Yes. The NIH is funding research that aims to prevent and reduce tobacco use among women, and to increase the survival rates of women suffering from cancers caused by smoking. The National Cancer Institute (NCI), a component of the NIH and the nation's lead agency for cancer research, formed the Women, Tobacco, and Cancer Working Group to stimulate scientific research and suggest approaches to prevent tobacco-related cancers among women in the United States and around the world. The Working Group, a public/private partnership that met in 2003, discussed the issues and made recommendations for progress in this area.

The health effects of smoking in women are an area of concern for many other NIH agencies, including the National Institute on Drug Abuse, the National Institute of Dental and Craniofacial Research, the National Institute of Child Health and Human Development, the John E. Fogarty International Center, and the National Center for Complementary and Alternative Medicine. Some current and recent NIH-funded research projects in this area include the following:

- A survey of tobacco use among pregnant women in several developing countries.

- A study of the use of nicotine replacement products among pregnant smokers.

- A program to help women remain smoke free after giving birth.

- An examination of the effectiveness of the nicotine patch in male and female smokers.

In addition, the NCI is funding studies to investigate the effects of smoking and quitting on various cancers, including those of the lung, breast, uterus, and cervix. Studies are also investigating genetic/molecular differences between women and men and their effect on cancer risk.

Section 4.3

Smoking Cessation

Excerpted from "Cessation," and "How To Quit Smoking,"
Centers for Disease Control and Prevention,
May 29, 2009.

Nicotine is the psychoactive drug in tobacco products that produces dependence. Most smokers are dependent on nicotine, and smokeless tobacco use can also lead to nicotine dependence. Nicotine dependence is the most common form of chemical dependence in the United States. Research suggests that nicotine is as addictive as heroin, cocaine, or alcohol. Examples of nicotine withdrawal symptoms include irritability, anxiety, difficulty concentrating, and increased appetite. Quitting tobacco use is difficult and may require multiple attempts, as users often relapse because of withdrawal symptoms. Tobacco dependence is a chronic condition that often requires repeated intervention.

Health Benefits of Cessation

People who stop smoking greatly reduce their risk of dying prematurely. Benefits are greater for people who stop at earlier ages, but cessation is beneficial at all ages.

Smoking cessation lowers the risk for lung and other types of cancer. The risk for developing cancer declines with the number of years of smoking cessation.

Risk for coronary heart disease, stroke, and peripheral vascular disease is reduced after smoking cessation. Coronary heart disease risk is substantially reduced within one to two years of cessation.

Cessation reduces respiratory symptoms, such as coughing, wheezing, and shortness of breath. The rate of decline in lung function is slower among persons who quit smoking.

Women who stop smoking before or during pregnancy reduce their risk for adverse reproductive outcomes such as infertility or having a low-birth-weight baby.

Quitting Interest and Behavior Among Tobacco Users

Among current U.S. adult smokers, 70% report that they want to quit completely. In 2006, an estimated 19.2 million (44.2%) adult smokers had stopped smoking for at least one day during the preceding 12 months because they were trying to quit.

An estimated 45.7 million adults were former smokers in 2006.

More than 54% of current high school cigarette smokers in the United States tried to quit smoking within the preceding year.

Tobacco Use Cessation Methods

Brief clinical interventions by health care providers can increase the chances of successful cessation, as can counseling and behavioral cessation therapies. Treatments with more person-to-person contact and intensity (for example, more time with counselors) are more effective. Individual, group, or telephone counseling are all effective.

Pharmacological therapies found to be effective for treating tobacco dependence include nicotine replacement products (e.g., gum, inhaler, patch) and non-nicotine medications, such as bupropion SR (Zyban®) and varenicline tartrate (Chantix™).

Resources

The Tobacco Control Research Branch of the NCI established the Smokefree.gov website in collaboration with the Centers for Disease Control and Prevention and the American Cancer Society to help people quit smoking. The website (www.smokefree.gov) provides an online guide, "Clearing the Air: Quit Smoking Today," for smokers interested in quitting. The guide covers thinking about quitting, preparing to quit, quitting, and staying quit.

"Clearing the Air: Quit Smoking Today" is also available as a print publication. Other publications available from the website include the following:

- Clear Horizons for smokers over age 50.

- Forever Free™ for smokers who have recently quit.

- Guía para Dejar de Fumar for Spanish-speaking smokers.

- Pathways to Freedom for African American smokers.

The National Cancer Institute's (NCI) Smoking Quitline offers a wide range of services, including individualized counseling, printed

information, referrals to other sources, and recorded messages. Smoking cessation counselors are available to answer smoking-related questions in English or Spanish, Monday through Friday, 9:00 a.m. to 4:30 p.m., local time. Smoking cessation counselors are also available through LiveHelp (an online instant messaging service) at http://www.cancer.gov/help on the internet. LiveHelp is available Monday through Friday, 9:00 a.m. to 11:00 p.m., Eastern time.

- Telephone: 877-448-7848 (877-44U-QUIT)

- Internet website: http://www.cancer.gov

Online Government Resources

Smokefree.gov
A website dedicated to helping you quit smoking.
http://www.ahrq.gov/consumer/tobacco/helpsmokers.htm

1-800-QUIT-NOW
A free, phone-based service with educational materials and coaches that can help you quit smoking or chewing tobacco.
http://1800quitnow.cancer.gov

Help for Smokers and Other Tobacco Users
Booklet that tells you about ways you can quit.
http://www.ahrq.gov/consumer/tobacco/helpsmokers.htm

I QUIT! What to Do When You're Sick of Smoking, Chewing, or Dipping
A booklet that will help you quit all tobacco products.
http://www.cdc.gov/tobacco/quit_smoking/how_to_quit/iquit/index.htm

Pathways to Freedom: Winning the Fight Against Tobacco
Guide that addresses tobacco issues specific to African Americans.
http://www.cdc.gov/tobacco/quit_smoking/how_to_quit/pathways/index.htm

Questions and Answers About Smoking Cessation
A fact sheet from the National Cancer Institute.
http://www.cancer.gov/cancertopics/factsheet/tobacco/cessation

Quit Smoking
Tools and guides to help you quit smoking.
http://www.ahrq.gov/consumer/index.html#smoking

Quit Tips
Five tips to help you quit.
http://www.cdc.gov/tobacco/quit_smoking/how_to_quit/quit_tips/index
.htm

Tobacco Cessation—You Can Quit Smoking Now!
The latest information to help you quit from the Surgeon General's
website.
http://www.surgeongeneral.gov/tobacco/

You Can Quit Smoking
A consumer guide to help you become tobacco free.
http://www.cdc.gov/tobacco/quit_smoking/how_to_quit/you_can_quit/
index.htm

Other Online and Telephone Resources

American Cancer Society
Guide to quitting smoking.
http://www.cancer.org/docroot/home/index.asp/docroot/PED/content/
PED_10_13X_Guide_for_Quitting_Smoking.asp

American Heart Association
800-AHA-USA1
 http://www.amhrt.org/presenter.jhtml?identifier=1200000

American Legacy Foundation—Quit Plan
A five-day plan to get ready to quit.
URL: http://women.americanlegacy.org/quit/index.cfm

American Lung Association
800-LUNG-USA
http://www.lungusa.org

Chapter 5

Facts about Human Papillomavirus (HPV) and Cancer Risk

Chapter Contents

Section 5.1

HPV Facts

What is HPV?

HPV is the short form for human papillomavirus. HPV is a family of very common viruses that cause almost all cervical cancers, plus a variety of other problems like common warts, genital warts, and plantar warts. HPV also causes cancers of the vulva, vagina, anus, and cancers of the head and neck. Both women and men become infected with HPV types that cause cervical cancer through sexual intercourse and sexual contact.

Are there different kinds of HPV?

There are over 100 strains of the HPV virus, with over 35 known different HPV types that infect the genital tract. At least 15 of these can lead to cervical cancer. The most common cancer-causing types of the virus are 16 and 18. This is important to know because these two types alone cause about 70% of all cervical cancer. The cervical cancer vaccine protects against these two types 100% of the time.

How does HPV work?

An HPV infection rarely leads to cervical cancer. In most women infected with HPV, the cells in the cervix return to normal after the body's immune system destroys the HPV infection without the woman ever having any signs or symptoms of the HPV. However, some HPV infections do not go away and may remain present in the cervical cells for years. Long-standing infection can lead to changes in the cells that can progress to cancer. It is these cell changes that a Pap test can detect. When the HPV virus is not treated, the cells will continue to

change until they become cervical cancer. Because it can last so long in your body before any cell changes occur, it is difficult to know who transmitted the HPV to you. Don't make assumptions and blame your current partner.

How common is HPV?

HPV is the most common sexually transmitted infection. It is common in all sexually active people. At least 70% of sexually active people will get HPV at some time in their lives. HPV is most common in young women and men who are in their late teens and early 20s. The CDC estimates that there are 6.2 million new infections each year in the United States. Since it is so common, there is nothing to be ashamed about. If you are diagnosed with HPV, talk to your health care provider about it. Get answers to your questions.

What are the signs and symptoms of HPV?

Most women and men do not know when they are infected with HPV. There are usually no symptoms. Anyone who has ever had genital contact with another person, not just sexual intercourse, can get HPV. Both men and women can get it—and pass it on to their sex partners without even realizing it. An abnormal Pap test result is usually a woman's first clue of an infection, but most HPV-infected women do not ever have an abnormal Pap test result. HPV is not HIV or herpes. They are different viruses with different symptoms.

How can I protect against HPV infection?

The only sure way to prevent HPV infection is to abstain from all sexual activity. Sexually active adults can reduce their risk by being in a mutually faithful relationship with someone who has had no other or few sex partners, or by limiting their number of sex partners. But even persons with only one lifetime sex partner can get HPV if their partner has had previous partners.

Do condoms protect against HPV?

Recent studies suggest that condoms provide some protection against the HPV infection. However, since condoms do not cover all areas of the body involved in sexual contact that can be the source of the spread of HPV, they do not offer complete protection. However, in addition to HPV protection, they do reduce the risk of HIV and other

sexually transmitted disease when used all the time and in the right way.

What are the factors that increase your risk for HPV?

You are more likely to get HPV if you smoke, if you start having sex at a young age, or if you have many sex partners or your sex partner has many sex partners.

How do I know if I have HPV?

The only way to know if you have an HPV infection is if your health care provider tests you for the virus. This may be done directly from the Pap test container or by using an additional swab at the time of the Pap test. Your health care provider may or may not perform the HPV test, depending on many factors including your age and risk factors. The only way to tell if a cancer-causing type of HPV infection has caused the cells in your cervix to change is to have a Pap test. Signs of an HPV infection may appear weeks, months, or years after the first infection, which is why it is important to have regular Pap tests and HPV tests as recommended by your health care provider.

Why isn't there an HPV test for men?

The diseases that HPV causes in women do not happen in men. So the test results will not be helpful for a man.

I've been told I have HPV. How do I know if or when it has cleared up?

Most HPV infections will clear on their own. Those women that have long-standing HPV infections are more at risk for developing cervical precancerous lesions or cervical cancer. There is no shot or pill that is available to clear your HPV infection. Hopefully, as in most women, your body's immune system will clear your HPV infection on its own. If your health care provider is performing an HPV test on you, and your test is negative, it is likely that your infection cleared.

Should I get an HPV Test?

The HPV test detects high-risk or cancer-causing types of HPV that can cause changes in your cervical cells. However, this test cannot tell you the exact type of high-risk HPV. Women 30 years of age and older

can have both the Pap test and the HPV test for cervical cancer screening. The HPV test can also be used to help understand the meaning of a borderline abnormal Pap test. In that situation, your health care provider may do an HPV test to find out more about the abnormal cells. However, if your Pap test shows a definite pre-cancerous abnormality, an HPV test is not needed. Virtually all of these changes are caused by HPV. You can assume the HPV test will be positive.

Is there a cure for HPV?

Currently, there is no cure for the virus. There are treatments for the cervical changes that HPV can cause. If your Pap and HPV tests show that cells in your cervix have changed, you should discuss treatment options with your health care provider.

Can you prevent HPV?

Good news! There is now a vaccine to prevent HPV infection. Girls and women ages nine to 26 can protect themselves from HPV and cervical changes related to HPV by getting the cervical cancer vaccine.

How does the vaccine work?

The cervical cancer vaccine takes prevention a giant leap forward by blocking the first step along the pathway to cervical cancer, HPV infection. The vaccine is given in the arm or thigh three times—at the first visit, two months later and four months after that. The best protection is achieved after all three shots are given. It is not known at this time whether booster shots will be needed later. Studies show that the vaccine is extremely safe. There are no live viruses in the vaccine. The most common side effects are redness and soreness where the shot was given. Headaches (like when you have a cold or fever) are also common. Fever can also occur. Over the counter pain and fever medications will help if you have symptoms. As with any new medication, safety issues will continue to be monitored.

Remember, you can prevent cervical cancer:

- Vaccinate early
- Pap test regularly
- HPV test when recommended

Section 5.2

HPV Prevalence in U.S. Women

Excerpted from "Study Estimates Overall HPV Prevalence in
U.S. Women," National Cancer Institute (www.cancer.gov), 2007.

Data from the National Health and Nutrition Examination Survey (NHANES) published in the February 28, 2007, *Journal of the American Medical Association* (*JAMA*) have provided the first national estimate of the prevalence of human papillomavirus (HPV) infection among women in the United States aged 14 to 59. Investigators found that a total of 26.8 percent of women overall tested positive for one or more strains of HPV.

Overall prevalence included both low-risk and high-risk HPV types. Low-risk types of HPV can cause genital warts or other nonmalignant conditions. High-risk types of HPV can cause cervical cancer, and up to 70 percent of cervical cancers worldwide are caused by two high-risk strains alone—HPV types 16 and 18.

"We think it's important to let women know how common [HPV] is," says Dr. Eileen Dunne from the Centers for Disease Control and Prevention, lead author of the study.

All women aged 14 to 59 selected to participate in the 2003–2004 NHANES, designed to collect health and nutrition measurements from a representative sample of the U.S. population, were eligible to participate in the HPV study. Most eligible women submitted self-collected cervicovaginal swab samples, 1,921 of which could be used for DNA extraction and HPV detection and typing.

Overall, 26.8 percent of women tested positive for one or more strains of HPV. Prevalence of HPV was highest in women ages 20–24. Among all participating women, the prevalence of high-risk types of HPV was 15.2 percent. The prevalence of HPV types 6, 11, 16, and 18 (the types targeted by the HPV vaccine Gardasil) was 3.4 percent overall, translating to an estimated 3.1 million exposed women in the studied age groups.

An important limitation of this study, explains Dr. Philip Castle, an investigator in the National Cancer Institute's Division of Cancer Epidemiology and Genetics, is that "this prevalence study is only a

snapshot of HPV in the country, but doesn't tell us anything about total lifetime exposure to HPV or the risk of precancer and cancer. Risk is not testing positive at one time point—it's the persistence of carcinogenic types of HPV."

Persistence of HPV infection —how long the virus remains active in a woman's body—is key to whether exposure to a high-risk type of HPV leads to cervical cancer. "If an infection from specific oncogenic HPV types does not clear within a period of time (about six months), it puts that woman at greater risk for cervical precursor lesions," explains Dr. Dunne.

"There's a lot of misunderstanding about HPV's complex natural history," Dr. Dunne continues. "It's not that if you get the infection, you get the disease. It's a common infection, and a lot of them clear [on their own]. The important thing is that women have routine cervical cancer screening with Pap tests, and appropriate groups of women receive the preventative vaccine that's now available."

The baseline data provided by this study may help researchers determine the public-health impact of HPV vaccination, explain the authors. However, "This is one piece of the big puzzle," says Dr. Dunne. "Looking at diseases such as genital warts, cervical cancer precursors, and cervical cancer will also be necessary to monitor vaccine impact."

"What we need...is a surveillance program that's linked to HPV vaccination uptake over a long period of time, so we can see the impact, and also any potential adverse effects, of an HPV vaccine," agrees Dr. Castle. "By monitoring benefits and risks of HPV vaccination, we can optimize the use of HPV vaccines to achieve the greatest good for women."

Section 5.3

Questions and Answers about the HPV Vaccine

Excerpted from, "Human Papillomavirus (HPV) Vaccines: Questions and Answers," National Cancer Institute (www.cancer.gov), October 22, 2009.

What are human papillomaviruses?

Human papillomaviruses (HPVs) are a group of more than 100 related viruses. They are called papillomaviruses because certain types may cause warts, or papillomas, which are benign (noncancerous) tumors. The HPVs that cause the common warts that grow on hands and feet are different from those that cause growths in the throat or genital area. Some types of HPV are associated with certain types of cancer. These are called "high-risk," oncogenic, or carcinogenic HPVs.

Of the more than 100 types of HPV, more than 30 types can be passed from one person to another through sexual contact. Transmission can occur in the genitals, anal, or mouth regions. Although HPVs are usually transmitted sexually, doctors cannot say for certain when infection occurred. About six million new genital HPV infections occur each year in the United States. Most HPV infections occur without any symptoms and go away without any treatment over the course of a few years. However, HPV infections sometimes persist for many years, with or without causing detectable cell abnormalities.

Do HPV infections cause cancer?

Infection with certain types of HPV is the major cause of cervical cancer. Almost all women will have an HPV infection at some point, but very few will develop cervical cancer. The immune system of most women will usually suppress or eliminate HPVs. Only HPV infections that are persistent (do not go away over many years) can lead to cervical cancer. In 2009, more than 11,000 women in the United States will be diagnosed with this type of cancer and about 4,000 will die from it. Cervical cancer strikes nearly half a million women each year worldwide, claiming more than a quarter of a million lives. Studies have

found that HPV infection is also a strong risk factor for oropharyngeal cancer (cancer that forms in tissues of the oropharynx, which is the middle part of the throat and includes the soft palate, the base of the tongue, and the tonsils). Studies also suggest that HPVs may play a role in cancers of the anus, vulva, vagina, and penis.

Can HPV infection be prevented?

The surest way to eliminate risk for genital HPV infection is to refrain from any genital contact with another individual.

For those who choose to be sexually active, a long-term, mutually monogamous relationship with an uninfected partner is the strategy most likely to prevent genital HPV infection. However, it is difficult to determine whether a partner who has been sexually active in the past is currently infected.

It is not known how much protection condoms provide against HPV infection, because areas not covered by a condom can be infected by the virus. Although the effect of condoms in preventing HPV infection is unknown, condom use has been associated with a lower rate of cervical cancer, an HPV-associated disease.

The U.S. Food and Drug Administration (FDA) has approved two vaccines to prevent HPV infections: Gardasil® and Cervarix®. Both vaccines are highly effective in preventing persistent infections with HPV types 16 and 18, two high-risk HPVs that cause most (70 percent) cervical cancers. Gardasil also prevents infection with HPV types 6 and 11, which cause virtually all (90 percent) genital warts. In addition, there is some initial evidence that Cervarix provides partial protection against a few other HPV types that can cause cancer, but further evaluation is required before the magnitude and impact of this effect is understood.

What are Gardasil and Cervarix?

The Gardasil vaccine, which is produced by Merck & Co., Inc. (Merck), is called a quadrivalent vaccine because it protects against four HPV types: 6, 11, 16, and 18. Gardasil is given through a series of three injections into muscle tissue over a six-month period. The FDA has approved Gardasil for use in females for the prevention of cervical cancer, and some vulvar and vaginal cancers, caused by HPV types 16 and 18 and for use in males and females for the prevention of genital warts caused by HPV types 6 and 11. The vaccine is approved for these uses in females and males ages nine to 26.

Cervarix is produced by GlaxoSmithKline (GSK). It is called a bivalent vaccine because it targets two HPV types: 16 and 18. This vaccine

is also given in three doses over a six-month period. The FDA has approved Cervarix for use in females ages 10 to 25 for the prevention of cervical cancer caused by HPV types 16 and 18.

Both Gardasil and Cervarix are based on technology developed in part by National Cancer Institute (NCI) scientists. NCI, a component of the National Institutes of Health, licensed the technology to two pharmaceutical companies—Merck and GSK—to develop HPV vaccines for widespread distribution.

Neither of these HPV vaccines has been proven to provide complete protection against persistent infection with other HPV types, although some initial results suggest that both vaccines might provide partial protection against a few additional HPV types that can cause cervical cancer. Overall, therefore, about 30 percent of cervical cancers will not be prevented by these vaccines. Also, in the case of Gardasil, 10 percent of genital warts will not be prevented by the vaccine. Neither vaccine prevents other sexually transmitted diseases, and they do not treat HPV infection or cervical cancer.

Because the vaccines do not protect against all HPV infections that cause cervical cancer, it is important for vaccinated women to continue to undergo cervical cancer screening as recommended for women who have not been vaccinated.

How do HPV vaccines work?

The HPV vaccines work like other immunizations that guard against viral infection. The investigators hypothesized that the unique surface components of HPV might create an antibody-response that is capable of protecting the body against infection and that these components could be used to form the basis of a vaccine. These surface components can interact with one another to form virus-like particles (VLP) that are noninfectious and stimulate the immune system to produce antibodies that can prevent the complete papillomavirus from infecting cells. They are thought to protect primarily by causing the production of antibodies that prevent infection and, consequently, the development of cervical cell changes (as seen on Pap tests) that may lead to cancer. Although these vaccines can help prevent HPV infection, they do not help eliminate existing HPV infections.

How effective are the HPV vaccines?

Gardasil and Cervarix are highly effective in preventing infection with the types of HPV they target. Studies have shown that both

Gardasil and Cervarix prevent nearly 100 percent of the precancerous cervical cell changes caused by the types of HPV targeted by the vaccine for up to four years after vaccination among women who were not infected at the time of vaccination.

Why are these vaccines important?

Widespread vaccination has the potential to reduce cervical cancer deaths around the world by as much as two-thirds, if all women were to get the vaccine and if protection turns out to be long-term. In addition, the vaccines can reduce the need for medical care, biopsies, and invasive procedures associated with follow-up from abnormal Pap tests, thus helping to reduce health care costs and anxieties related to abnormal Pap tests and follow-up procedures.

How safe are the HPV vaccines?

Before any vaccine is licensed, the FDA must determine that it is both safe and effective. Both Gardasil and Cervarix have been tested in tens of thousands of people in the United States and many other countries. Thus far, no serious side effects have been shown to be caused by the vaccines. The most common problems have been brief soreness and other local symptoms at the injection site. These problems are similar to ones commonly experienced with other vaccines. The vaccines have not been sufficiently tested during pregnancy and, therefore, should not be used by pregnant women.

A recent safety review by the FDA and the Centers for Disease Control and Prevention (CDC) considered adverse side effects related to Gardasil immunization that have been reported to the Vaccine Adverse Events Reporting System since the vaccine was licensed. The rates of adverse side effects in the safety review were consistent with what was seen in safety studies carried out before the vaccine was approved and were similar to those seen with other vaccines. However, a higher proportion of syncope (fainting) and venous thrombolic events (blood clots) were seen with Gardasil than are usually seen with other vaccines. Falls after syncope may sometimes cause serious injuries, such as head injuries. These can largely be prevented by keeping the vaccinated person seated for up to 15 minutes after vaccination. The FDA and CDC have reminded health care providers that, to prevent falls and injuries, all vaccine recipients should remain seated or lying down and be closely observed for 15 minutes after vaccination.

How long do the vaccines protect against infection?

The duration of immunity is not yet known. Research is being conducted to find out how long protection will last. Phase III clinical trials have shown that Gardasil and Cervarix can provide protection against HPV16 for four years. Smaller studies have suggested that protection is likely to last for longer than four years, but it is not known if protection conferred through vaccination will be lifelong.

Will booster vaccinations be needed?

Studies are under way to determine whether booster vaccinations (supplementary doses of a vaccine, usually smaller than the initial dose or doses, that are given to maintain immunity) are necessary.

Who should get these vaccines?

Both Gardasil and Cervarix are proven to be effective only if given before infection with HPV, so it is recommended that they be given before an individual is sexually active. The FDA's licensing decision includes information about the age and sex for recipients of the vaccine. The FDA approved Gardasil for use in females ages nine to 26 and approved Cervarix for use in females ages 10 to 25.

Data from Merck show high efficacy of Gardasil in males for preventing genital warts associated with HPV6 and HPV11, the two HPV types that cause most genital warts. The FDA approved Gardasil for use in males ages nine to 26 to prevent genital warts caused by HPV6 and HPV11

In addition to the benefits that exist for cervical cancer prevention in females and the prevention of warts in both males and females, there may be additional benefits to vaccination. These include a possible reduction in risk of anal and oropharyngeal cancers in males and females, as well as penile cancer in males, although clinical trials have not directly evaluated these possibilities.

After a vaccine is licensed by the FDA, the Advisory Committee on Immunization Practices (ACIP) makes additional recommendations to the Secretary of the U.S. Department of Health and Human Services and the Director of the CDC on who should receive the vaccine, at what age, how often, the appropriate dose, and situations in which it should not be administered. ACIP is made up of 15 experts in fields associated with immunization. ACIP provides advice on the most effective ways to use vaccines to prevent diseases. ACIP recommends that Gardasil be given routinely to girls ages 11 to 12. The

recommendations also allow for the vaccination of girls beginning at nine years of age and the vaccination of girls and women ages 13 to 26. An ACIP policy for Cervarix is expected within the next few months. It is also expected that ACIP will make recommendations about use of the vaccine in males. The cost-benefit ratio of vaccinating males is under debate because HPV-associated cancers are rarer in men than women.

Should the vaccines be given to people who are already infected with HPV?

Although the preventive vaccines currently under study have been found to be generally safe when given to women who are already infected with HPV, it is important for women to know that the vaccines protect against infection, and provide maximum benefit, for a woman who is vaccinated before she is sexually active. This is because these vaccines do not treat infections. For example, one recent study found that Cervarix was not effective in helping women who are already infected to clear the infection. However, because very few young women have been infected with all HPV types that are included in the vaccines, it is possible that women may still get residual benefit from vaccination even if they have been infected with one or more of the types included in the vaccines. This possibility has not yet been formally studied.

It is not feasible to prescreen all women to see who has been exposed to the HPV types in the vaccines. At present, there is no generally available test to tell whether an individual has been exposed to HPV. The currently approved HPV DNA test shows only whether a woman has a current HPV infection and identifies the HPV type. It does not provide information on past infections. The decision to vaccinate or not, based on likelihood of prior exposure to these HPV types, is being discussed by ACIP and other advisory groups.

Should women who already have cervical cell changes get the vaccines?

Gardasil and Cervarix appear to be safe in women who have cervical abnormalities, but it is not expected that the vaccine would help clear the abnormalities because it has been shown that the vaccine does not treat established infections. Women should talk with their health care providers about treatment for abnormal cervical cell changes.

Do women who have been vaccinated still need to have Pap tests?

Yes. Because these vaccines do not protect against all HPV types that can cause cancer, Pap tests continue to be essential to detect cervical cancers and precancerous changes. In addition, Pap tests are critically important for women who have not been vaccinated or who are already infected with HPV.

How much do these vaccines cost, and will insurance pay for it?

The retail price of Gardasil is approximately $120 per dose and $360 for the full series. Individual or group insurance plans are subject to state laws, which generally establish coverage based on recommendations from the ACIP. Medicaid coverage is in accordance with the ACIP standard, and immunizations are a mandatory service under Medicaid for eligible individuals under age 21. Medicaid also includes the Vaccines for Children Program, which provides immunization services for children 18 and under who are Medicaid eligible, uninsured, under-insured, and receiving immunizations through a Federally Qualified Health Center or Rural Health Clinic, or who are Native American or Alaska Native.

What research is being done on HPV?

Researchers at the National Cancer Institute (NCI) and elsewhere are studying how high risk HPV types cause precancerous changes in normal cells and how these changes can be prevented or managed most efficiently. NCI is conducting a community-based clinical trial of the Cervarix HPV vaccine in Costa Rica, where cervical cancer rates are high. This study is designed to obtain information about the vaccine's longer-term safety, the extent and duration of protection, the immune mechanisms of protection, and the natural history of infection with HPV types other than the types included in the vaccine. NCI is also collaborating with other researchers on second-generation preventive vaccines and on therapeutic HPV vaccines, which would prevent the development of cancer among women previously infected with HPV. The ideal vaccine strategy would combine a preventive and therapeutic vaccine.

Laboratory research has indicated that HPVs produce proteins known as E5, E6, and E7. These proteins interfere with the cell functions that normally prevent excessive growth. For example, HPV E6

interferes with the human protein p53, which acts to keep tumors from growing. A better understanding of how these proteins interact may help researchers develop ways to interrupt the process by which HPV infection can lead to the growth of abnormal cells.

Researchers at the NCI and elsewhere are also studying what people know and understand about HPVs and cervical cancer, the best way to communicate to the public about the latest research results, and how doctors are talking with their patients about HPVs. This research will help to ensure that the public receives accurate information about HPVs that is easily understood and will facilitate access to appropriate tests for those who need them.

Chapter 6

Cancer Risks Associated with Hormonal Medications

Chapter Contents

Section 6.1

Oral Contraceptives and Cancer Risk

Excerpted from "Oral Contraceptives and Cancer Risk:
Questions and Answers," National Cancer Institute (www.cancer.gov),
May 4, 2006.

Oral contraceptives (OCs) first became available to American women in the early 1960s. The convenience, effectiveness, and reversibility of action of birth control pills (popularly known as "the pill") have made them the most popular form of birth control in the United States. However, concerns have been raised about the role that the hormones in OCs might play in a number of cancers and how hormone-based OCs contribute to their development. Sufficient time has elapsed since the introduction of OCs to allow investigators to study large numbers of women who took birth control pills for many years.

This chapter addresses only what is known about OC use and the risk of developing cancer. It does not deal with other serious side effects of OC use, such as the increased risk of cardiovascular disease for certain groups of women. Recently, alternative methods of delivering hormones for contraception have been developed, including a topical patch, vaginal ring, and intrauterine delivery system, but these products are too new to have been tested in clinical trials (research studies) for long-term safety and other effects. They also are not covered in this fact sheet.

What types of oral contraceptives are available in the United States? Why do researchers believe that oral contraceptives may influence cancer risk?

Currently, two types of OCs are available in the United States. The most commonly prescribed OC contains two man-made versions of natural female hormones (estrogen and progesterone) that are similar to the hormones the ovaries normally produce. This type of pill is often called a "combined oral contraceptive." The second type of OC available in the United States is called the minipill. It contains only a type of progesterone.

Estrogen stimulates the growth and development of the uterus at puberty, causes the endometrium (the inner lining of the uterus) to thicken during the first half of the menstrual cycle, and influences breast tissue throughout life, but particularly from puberty to menopause.

Progesterone, which is produced during the last half of the menstrual cycle, prepares the endometrium to receive the egg. If the egg is fertilized, progesterone secretion continues, preventing release of additional eggs from the ovaries. For this reason, progesterone is called the "pregnancy-supporting" hormone, and scientists believe that it has valuable contraceptive effects. The man-made progesterone used in OCs is called progestogen or progestin.

Because medical research suggests that some cancers depend on naturally occurring sex hormones for their development and growth, scientists have been investigating a possible link between OC use and cancer risk. Researchers have focused a great deal of attention on OC users over the past 40 years. This scrutiny has produced a wealth of data on OC use and the development of certain cancers, although results of these studies have not always been consistent. The risk of endometrial and ovarian cancers is reduced with the use of OCs, while the risk of breast and cervical cancers is increased.

How do oral contraceptives affect breast cancer risk?

A woman's risk of developing breast cancer depends on several factors, some of which are related to her natural hormones. Hormonal factors that increase the risk of breast cancer include conditions that may allow high levels of hormones to persist for long periods of time, such as beginning menstruation at an early age (before age 12), experiencing menopause at a late age (after age 55), having a first child after age 30, and not having children at all.

A 1996 analysis of worldwide epidemiologic data conducted by the Collaborative Group on Hormonal Factors in Breast Cancer found that women who were current or recent users of birth control pills had a slightly elevated risk of developing breast cancer. The risk was highest for women who started using OCs as teenagers. However, ten or more years after women stopped using OCs, their risk of developing breast cancer returned to the same level as if they had never used birth control pills, regardless of family history of breast cancer, reproductive history, geographic area of residence, ethnic background, differences in study design, dose and type of hormone, or duration of use. In addition, breast cancers diagnosed in women after

ten or more years of not using OCs were less advanced than breast cancers diagnosed in women who had never used OCs. To conduct this analysis, the researchers examined the results of 54 studies. The analysis involved 53,297 women with breast cancer and 100,239 women without breast cancer. More than 200 researchers participated in this combined analysis of their original studies, which represented about 90 percent of the epidemiological studies throughout the world that had investigated the possible relationship between OCs and breast cancer.

The findings of the Women's Contraceptive and Reproductive Experiences (Women's CARE) study were in contrast to those described above. The Women's CARE study examined the use of OCs as a risk factor for breast cancer in women ages 35 to 64. Researchers interviewed 4,575 women who were diagnosed with breast cancer between 1994 and 1998, and 4,682 women who did not have breast cancer. Investigators collected detailed information about the participants' use of OCs, reproductive history, health, and family history. The results, which were published in 2002, indicated that current or former use of OCs did not significantly increase the risk of breast cancer. The findings were similar for white and black women. Factors such as longer periods of use, higher doses of estrogen, initiation of OC use before age 20, and OC use by women with a family history of breast cancer were not associated with an increased risk of the disease.

In a National Cancer Institute (NCI)-sponsored study published in 2003, researchers examined risk factors for breast cancer among women ages 20 to 34 compared with women ages 35 to 54. Women diagnosed with breast cancer were asked whether they had used OCs for more than six months before diagnosis and, if so, whether the most recent use had been within five years, five to ten years, or more than ten years. The results indicated that the risk was highest for women who used OCs within five years prior to diagnosis, particularly in the younger group.

How do oral contraceptives affect ovarian and endometrial cancer risk?

Studies have consistently shown that using OCs reduces the risk of ovarian cancer. In a 1992 analysis of 20 studies of OC use and ovarian cancer, researchers from Harvard Medical School found that the risk of ovarian cancer decreased with increasing duration of OC use. Results showed a 10–12% percent decrease in risk after one year of use, and approximately a 50% decrease after five years of use.

Researchers have studied how the amount or type of hormones in OCs affects ovarian cancer risk reduction. One of the studies used in the Harvard analysis, the Cancer and Steroid Hormone Study (CASH), found that the reduction in ovarian cancer risk was the same regardless of the type or amount of estrogen or progestin in the pill. A more recent analysis of data from the CASH study, however, indicated that OC formulations with high levels of progestin reduced ovarian cancer risk more than preparations with low progestin levels. In another recent study, the Steroid Hormones and Reproductions (SHARE) study, researchers investigated new, lower-dose progestins that have varying androgenic properties (testosterone-like effects). They found no difference in ovarian cancer risk between androgenic and nonandrogenic pills.

OC use in women at increased risk of ovarian cancer due to BRCA1 and BRCA2 genetic mutations has been studied. One study showed a reduction in risk, but a more recent study showed no effect.

The use of OCs has been shown to significantly reduce the risk of endometrial cancer. This protective effect increases with the length of time OCs are used, and continues for many years after a woman stops using OCs.

How do oral contraceptives affect cervical cancer risk?

Evidence shows that long-term use of OCs (five or more years) may be associated with an increased risk of cancer of the cervix (the narrow, lower portion of the uterus). Although OC use may increase the risk of cervical cancer, human papillomavirus (HPV) is recognized as the major cause of this disease. Approximately 14 types of HPV have been identified as having the potential to cause cancer, and HPVs have been found in 99 percent of cervical cancer biopsy specimens worldwide.

A 2003 analysis by the International Agency for Research on Cancer (IARC) found an increased risk of cervical cancer with longer use of OCs. Researchers analyzed data from 28 studies that included 12,531 women with cervical cancer. The data suggested that the risk of cervical cancer may decrease after OC use stops. In another IARC report, data from eight studies were combined to assess the effect of OC use on cervical cancer risk in HPV-positive women. Researchers found a fourfold increase in risk among women who had used OCs for longer than five years. Risk was also increased among women who began using OCs before age 20 and women who had used OCs within the past five years. The IARC is planning a study to reanalyze all data related to OC use and cervical cancer risk.

How do oral contraceptives affect liver cancer risk?

Several studies have found that OCs increase the risk of liver cancer in populations usually considered low risk, such as white women in the United States and Europe who do not have liver disease. In these studies, women who used OCs for longer periods of time were found to be at increased risk for liver cancer. However, OCs did not increase the risk of liver cancer in Asian and African women, who are considered high risk for this disease. Researchers believe this is because other risk factors, such as hepatitis infection, outweigh the effect of OCs.

Section 6.2

Menopausal Hormone Replacement Therapy Use and Cancer

Excerpted from "Menopausal Hormone Replacement Therapy Use and Cancer," National Cancer Institute, January 5, 2007. The complete text of this document, including references and resources for additional information, can be found online at http://www.cancer.gov/cancertopics/factsheet/Risk/menopausal-hormones.

What is menopause?

Menopause is the time in a woman's life when menstruation (having a period) ends. It is part of a biological process that begins, for most women, in their mid-thirties. During this time, the ovaries gradually produce lower levels of natural sex hormones—estrogen and progesterone. Estrogen promotes the normal development of a woman's breasts and uterus, controls the cycle of ovulation (when an ovary releases an egg into a fallopian tube), and affects many aspects of a woman's physical and emotional health.

Progesterone controls menstruation and prepares the lining of the uterus to receive the fertilized egg.

"Natural menopause" occurs when a woman has her last menstrual period, or stops menstruating, and is considered complete when menstruation has stopped for one year. This usually occurs between

ages 45 and 55, with variations in timing from woman to woman. Women who undergo surgery to remove both ovaries (an operation called bilateral oophorectomy) experience "surgical menopause"—an immediate end to menstruation caused by lack of hormones produced by the ovaries.

By the time a woman has reached natural menopause, estrogen output has decreased significantly. Even though low levels of this hormone are produced by other organs after menopause, these levels are only about one-tenth of the level found in premenopausal women. Progesterone is nearly absent in menopausal women.

What are menopausal hormones and why are they used?

Doctors may recommend menopausal hormones to counter some of the problems often associated with the onset of menopause (hot flashes, night sweats, sleeplessness, and vaginal dryness) or to prevent some long-term conditions that are more common in postmenopausal women, such as osteoporosis (a condition characterized by a decrease in bone mass and density, causing bones to become fragile). Menopausal hormone use (sometimes referred to as hormone replacement therapy or postmenopausal hormone use) usually involves treatment with either estrogen alone or estrogen in combination with progesterone or progestin, a synthetic hormone with effects similar to those of progesterone. Among women who are prescribed menopausal hormones, women who have undergone a hysterectomy (surgery to remove the uterus and, sometimes, the cervix) are generally given estrogen alone. Women who have not undergone this surgery are given estrogen plus progestin, which is known to have a lower risk of causing endometrial cancer (cancer of the lining of the uterus).

How does medical research determine the benefits and risks of taking menopausal hormones?

Researchers commonly conduct two very different, yet important types of studies with people to examine the benefits and risks of hormone use: clinical trials and observational studies. In clinical trials, the participants are given either hormones or placebos (look-alike pills that do not contain any drug) to determine the effect of the hormones on various conditions and diseases. In observational studies, the investigators do not try to affect the outcome; they compare the health status of women taking hormones to that of women not taking hormones.

69

What has medical research found out about the risks and benefits of hormone use after menopause?

The most comprehensive evidence about the risks and benefits of taking hormones after menopause to prevent disease comes from the Women's Health Initiative (WHI) Hormone Program, which was sponsored by the National Heart, Lung, and Blood Institute (NHLBI) and the National Cancer Institute (NCI), parts of the National Institutes of Health (NIH). This research program examined the effects of menopausal hormones on women's health. The WHI Hormone Program involved two studies—the use of estrogen plus progestin for women with a uterus (the Estrogen-plus-Progestin Study), and the use of estrogen alone for women without a uterus (the Estrogen-Alone Study). In both hormone therapy studies, women were randomly assigned to receive either the hormone medication being studied or the placebo.

The WHI Estrogen-plus-Progestin Study was stopped in July 2002, when investigators reported that the overall risks of estrogen plus progestin, specifically Prempro™, outweighed the benefits. The researchers found that use of this estrogen-plus-progestin pill increased the risk of breast cancer, heart disease, stroke, blood clots, and urinary incontinence. However, the risk of colorectal cancer and hip fractures was lower among women using estrogen plus progestin than among those taking the placebo. In addition, the WHI Memory Study showed that estrogen plus progestin doubled the risk for developing dementia (a decline in mental ability in which the patient can no longer function independently on a day-to-day basis) in postmenopausal women age 65 and older. The risk increased for all types of dementia, including Alzheimer disease.

The WHI Estrogen-Alone Study, which involved Premarin™, was stopped in February 2004, when the researchers concluded that estrogen alone increased the risk of stroke and blood clots. In contrast with the WHI Estrogen-plus-Progestin Study, the risk of breast cancer was decreased in women using estrogen alone compared with those taking the placebo. Use of estrogen alone did not increase or decrease the risk of colorectal cancer. Similar to the results seen in the Estrogen-plus-Progestin Study, women using estrogen alone had an increased risk of urinary incontinence and a decreased risk of hip fractures.

Another large epidemiologic study, the Million Women Study, enrolled 1.3 million women in the United Kingdom. This study evaluated health outcomes in women using and not using menopausal hormones. Several analyses have been published to date, and many more are expected in the future.

How does menopausal hormone use affect breast cancer risk and survival?

The WHI Estrogen-plus-Progestin Study concluded that estrogen plus progestin increases the risk of invasive breast cancer. After five years of follow-up, women taking these hormones had a 24 percent increase in breast cancer risk compared with women taking the placebo. The increase amounted to an additional eight cases of breast cancer for every 10,000 women taking estrogen plus progestin for one year compared with 10,000 women taking the placebo.

A detailed analysis of data from the WHI Estrogen-plus-Progestin Study showed that, among women taking estrogen plus progestin, the breast cancers were slightly larger and diagnosed at more advanced stages compared with breast cancers in women taking the placebo. Among women taking estrogen plus progestin, 25.4% of the cancers had spread outside the breast to nearby organs or lymph nodes compared with 16.0% among nonusers. Women taking estrogen plus progestin also had more abnormal mammograms (breast x-rays that require additional evaluation) than the women taking the placebo.

The WHI Estrogen-Alone Study concluded that taking estrogen did not increase the risk of breast cancer in women with a prior hysterectomy, at least for the seven years of follow-up in the study. Further analysis of data from the study indicated a 20% decrease in risk of breast cancer in women taking estrogen alone, although this decrease was seen mainly in the occurrence of early-stage breast cancer and ductal breast cancer (a specific type that begins in the lining of the milk ducts in the breast). The observed reduction amounted to six fewer cases of breast cancer for every 10,000 women taking estrogen for one year compared with 10,000 nonusers, but this lower incidence was not statistically significant; that is, the lower incidence could have arisen by chance rather than being related to estrogen-alone use. The Estrogen-Alone Study also showed a substantial increase in the frequency of abnormal mammograms.

A comprehensive review of data from 51 epidemiological (population) studies published in the 1980s and 1990s found a statistically significant increase in breast cancer risk among current or recent users of any hormone replacement therapy compared with the risk among nonusers. Most women in the analysis (88%) had used estrogen alone, and data for estrogen-plus-progestin users was not analyzed separately. Analysis of the pooled data also showed that the risk of breast cancer increased with increasing duration of hormone use, and

71

this effect was more prominent in women with low body weight or a low body mass index. However, breast cancers in hormone users were less likely to have spread to other parts of the body compared with the breast cancers in nonusers. The increase in breast cancer risk largely, if not completely, disappeared about five years after cessation of hormone use.

As part of the Million Women Study, researchers examined six types of breast cancer among users and nonusers of menopausal hormones. The results showed that the effects of hormone use varied among breast cancer types. Overall, breast cancer risk was significantly increased among current users, although the risk was lower among women with higher body mass index.

What are the effects of hormone use on the risk of endometrial cancer?

Studies have shown that long-term exposure of the uterus to estrogen alone increases a woman's risk of endometrial cancer. The risk associated with estrogen plus progestin appears to be much less, but some data suggest that the risk is still increased compared with the risk for nonusers. The long-term effects of estrogen plus progestin on endometrial cancer risk remain uncertain.

The WHI Estrogen-plus-Progestin Study showed that endometrial cancer rates for women taking estrogen plus progestin daily were the same as or possibly less than those for women taking the placebo pill. Uterine bleeding, however, was a common side effect, leading to more frequent biopsies and ultrasounds for women taking estrogen plus progestin compared with those taking a placebo.

The Million Women Study confirmed a lower risk of endometrial cancer in women taking estrogen plus progestin in comparison with those taking estrogen only or tibolone, a synthetic steroid that is not available in the United States.

How does menopausal hormone use affect the risk of ovarian cancer?

Several observational studies have found that the use of estrogen alone is associated with a slightly increased risk of ovarian cancer for women who used this hormone for ten or more years. One observational study that followed 44,241 menopausal women for approximately 20 years concluded that women who used estrogen alone for ten or more years were twice as likely to develop ovarian cancer compared with

women who did not use menopausal hormones. Another large observational study also found an association between estrogen use and death due to ovarian cancer. In this study, the increased risk appeared to be limited to women who used estrogen for ten or more years.

The results from the Million Women Study showed that women currently using menopausal hormones had an increased risk of developing ovarian cancer and a 20 percent likelihood of dying from the disease compared with nonusers. However, the increased risk disappeared after hormone use stopped.

Data from the WHI Estrogen-plus-Progestin Study indicate that there may be an increased risk of ovarian cancer with use of estrogen plus progestin. After 5.6 years of follow-up, a 58% increased risk of ovarian cancer was reported in women using estrogen plus progestin compared with nonusers, but the increased risk was not statistically significant. One observational study suggested that regimens of estrogen plus progestin do not increase the risk of ovarian cancer if progestin is used for more than 15 days per month, but this study was too small to draw firm conclusions. More research is needed to clarify the relationship between menopausal hormone use, particularly for estrogen plus progestin, and the risk of ovarian cancer.

How does menopausal hormone use affect the risk of colorectal cancer?

After five years of follow-up of women taking estrogen plus progestin, the WHI Estrogen-plus-Progestin Study reported a 37% reduction in colorectal cancer cases compared with women taking the placebo. On average, the researchers found that if a group of 10,000 women takes estrogen plus progestin for a year, six fewer cases of colon cancer will occur than in a group of nonusers. These findings are consistent with observational studies, which have suggested that the use of postmenopausal hormones may reduce the risk of colorectal cancer. The WHI Estrogen-Alone Study concluded that estrogen alone had no significant effect on colorectal cancer risk.

Should women with a history of cancer take menopausal hormones?

One of the roles of naturally occurring estrogen is to promote the normal growth of cells in the breast and uterus. For this reason, it is generally believed that menopausal estrogen use by women who have already been diagnosed with breast cancer may promote further tumor

growth. Studies of hormone use to treat menopausal symptoms in breast cancer survivors have produced conflicting results.

In one trial, 434 breast cancer survivors receiving either estrogen alone or estrogen plus progestin were followed for two years before the study was stopped because researchers concluded that even short-term use of hormone replacement therapy posed an unacceptable risk of breast cancer recurrence. Among these study participants, 26 women in the group receiving hormone replacement therapy had another occurrence of breast cancer compared with seven women in the group receiving no hormone replacement therapy. In another study, which included 378 women who were followed for four years, 11 women receiving hormone replacement therapy had another occurrence of breast cancer compared with 13 women receiving no hormone replacement therapy, so the risk of breast cancer recurrence was not increased. A review of 15 studies comprising a total of 1,416 breast cancer survivors and 1,998 women without a history of breast cancer found no increase in risk of cancer recurrence with hormone replacement therapy use.

There is limited research on the risks associated with menopausal hormone use by women who have had other cancers, particularly gynecological cancers. One review of the published research found that no firm conclusion could be drawn about the safety of hormone use in women with a history of cancer. However, survivors of gastric and bladder cancer and meningioma may be at higher risk of a recurrence. Survivors of gynecological cancers may be at higher risk because these cancers tend to be more hormone-dependent, but more studies are needed.

Does the way in which hormones are administered make a difference?

Most of the data on the long-term health effects of hormones come from studies in which hormones (estrogen alone or estrogen plus progestin) are administered orally in the form of pills. Hormones in the form of transdermal patches or gels are also used to treat menopause-related symptoms. Estrogen-containing vaginal creams and rings can be used specifically for vaginal dryness. Progesterone is also available as a pill or gel. The amount of estrogen that enters the bloodstream from estrogen-containing vaginal creams and rings depends on the types of hormones and the dose. Generally, vaginal administration of hormones results in lower levels of circulating hormones compared with an equivalent oral dose. Because the vaginal epithelium (thin

layer of tissue that covers the vagina) responds to very small doses of estrogen, low-dose estrogen-containing creams or gels can be used.

What should women do if they are concerned about taking menopausal hormones?

Although menopausal hormones have short-term benefits such as relief from hot flashes and vaginal dryness, several health concerns are associated with their use. Women should discuss with their health care provider whether to take menopausal hormones and what alternatives may be appropriate for them. The U.S. Food and Drug Administration (FDA) currently advises women to use menopausal hormones for the shortest time and at the lowest dose possible to control symptoms. The FDA publication Menopause and hormones provides additional information about the risks and benefits of hormone use for menopausal symptoms.

What are the alternatives for women who choose not to take menopausal hormones?

To decrease the risk of chronic disease, women can adopt a healthy lifestyle by exercising regularly, eating a healthy diet, limiting the consumption of alcohol, and not starting to smoke or, for smokers, trying to quit. Eating foods rich in calcium and vitamin D or taking dietary supplements containing these nutrients can help prevent osteoporosis. Results from the WHI showed that taking calcium and vitamin D supplements provided some benefit in preserving bone mass and preventing hip fractures, particularly in women age 60 and older. Although generally well tolerated, these supplements were associated with an increased risk of kidney stones. Other drugs, such as alendronate (Fosamax®), raloxifene (Evista®), and risedronate (Actonel®), have been shown to prevent bone loss. In addition, parathyroid hormone (Forteo®) is approved by the FDA for osteoporosis treatment.

Short-term menopause-related problems may go away on their own and frequently require no therapy at all. Local therapy for specific symptoms, such as vaginal dryness and urinary bladder conditions, is available. Some women seek relief from menopausal symptoms with nonprescription complementary and alternative therapies containing estrogen-like compounds. Some sources of these estrogen-like compounds include soy-based products, whole grain cereal, oilseeds (primarily flaxseed), legumes, and the botanical black cohosh. The benefits and risks of most of these agents have not been proven, however.

Women should talk with their doctor about the option best for them.

What research still needs to be done?

Unresolved questions include whether different forms of the hormones, lower doses, different hormones, or different methods of administration are safer or more effective; whether risks and/or benefits persist after women stop taking hormones; whether women might be able to take hormones safely for a short period of time; and whether certain subgroups of women, including women with a history of cancer, might be at higher or lower risk than the general population.

Section 6.3

Diethylstilbestrol Exposure and Cancer Risk

Excerpted from "DES: Questions and Answers," National Cancer Institute (www.cancer.gov), November 29, 2006.

What is DES?

DES (diethylstilbestrol) is a synthetic form of estrogen, a female hormone. It was prescribed between 1938 and 1971 to help women with certain complications of pregnancy. Use of DES declined following studies in the 1950s that showed it was not effective in preventing pregnancy complications. When given during the first five months of a pregnancy, DES can interfere with the development of the reproductive system in a fetus. For this reason, although DES and other estrogens may be prescribed for some medical problems, they are no longer used during pregnancy.

What health problems might DES-exposed daughters have?

In 1971, DES was linked to clear cell adenocarcinoma in a small number of daughters of women who had used DES during pregnancy.

This uncommon cancer of the vagina or cervix is usually diagnosed between age 15 and 25 in DES-exposed daughters. Some cases have been reported in women in their thirties and forties. The risk to women older than age 40 is still unknown because the women first exposed to DES in utero are just reaching their fifties and information about their risk has not been gathered. The overall risk of an exposed daughter to develop this type of cancer is estimated to be approximately one in 1,000 (0.1 percent). Although clear cell adenocarcinoma is extremely rare, it is important that DES-exposed daughters be aware of the risk and have regular physical examinations.

Scientists found a link between DES exposure before birth and an increased risk of developing abnormal cells in the tissue of the cervix and vagina. Physicians use a number of terms to describe these abnormal cells, including dysplasia, cervical intraepithelial neoplasia, and squamous intraepithelial lesions. These abnormal cells resemble cancer cells in appearance; however, they do not invade nearby healthy tissue as cancer cells do. Although these conditions are not cancer, they may develop into cancer if left untreated. DES-exposed daughters should have a yearly Pap test and pelvic exam to check for abnormal cells. DES-exposed daughters may also have structural changes in the vagina, uterus, or cervix, as well as irregular menstruation and an increased risk of miscarriage, ectopic (tubal) pregnancy, infertility, and premature births.

Evidence from a recent study suggests that daughters of women who took DES during pregnancy may have a slightly increased risk of breast cancer after age 40. The risk of breast cancer for DES-exposed women over age 40 was 1.9 times the risk of breast cancer for unexposed women of the same ages. The increased risk association was present for all breast cancer risk factors examined, and did not differ by tumor receptor status, tumor size, or lymph node involvement.

Although this evidence suggests that prenatal DES exposure increases the risk of breast cancer, breast cancer is still a relatively rare event among DES-exposed women. For every 1,000 DES-exposed women aged 45 to 49, four new cases of breast cancer per year would be expected, compared with two new cases per year in every 1,000 unexposed women.

While the greater risk above age 40 is statistically significant, that is, is more than would be expected to happen by chance alone, it is still based on relatively small numbers. The actual risk could be quite a bit lower or higher. Therefore, additional research is needed to be sure that the increased risk was caused by DES.

What health problems might DES-exposed sons have?

There is some evidence that DES-exposed sons may have testicular abnormalities, such as undescended testicles or abnormally small testicles. The risk for testicular or prostate cancer is unclear; studies of the association between DES exposure in utero and testicular cancer have produced mixed results. In addition, investigations of abnormalities of the urogenital system among DES-exposed sons have not produced clear answers.

What health problems might DES-exposed mothers have?

Women who used DES may have a slightly increased risk of breast cancer. Current research indicates that the risk of breast cancer in DES-exposed mothers is approximately 30% higher than the risk for women who have not been exposed to this drug. This risk has been stable over time, and does not seem to increase as the mothers become older. Additional research is needed to clarify this issue and whether DES-exposed mothers are at higher risk for any other types of cancer.

How can people find out if they took DES during pregnancy or were exposed to DES in utero?

It has been estimated that five to 10 million people were exposed to DES during pregnancy. Many of these people are not aware that they were exposed. A woman who was pregnant between 1938 and 1971 and had problems or a history of problems during pregnancy may have been given DES or a similar drug. Women who think they used a hormone such as DES during pregnancy, or people who think that their mother used DES during pregnancy, can contact the attending physician or the hospital where the delivery took place to request a review of the medical records. If any pills were taken during pregnancy, obstetrical records should be checked to determine the name of the drug. Mothers and children have a right to this information.

However, finding medical records after a long period of time can be difficult. If the doctor has retired or died, another doctor may have taken over the practice as well as the records. The county medical society or health department may know where the records have been stored. Some pharmacies keep records for a long time and can be contacted regarding prescription dispensing information. Military

medical records are kept for 25 years. In many cases, however, it may be impossible to determine whether DES was used.

What should DES-exposed daughters do?

It is important for women who believe they may have been exposed to DES before birth to be aware of the possible health effects of DES and inform their doctor of their exposure. It is important that the physician be familiar with possible problems associated with DES exposure, because some problems, such as clear cell adenocarcinoma, are likely to be found only when the doctor is looking for them. A thorough examination may include the following:

- **Pelvic examination:** A doctor performs a physical examination of the reproductive organs. An examination of the rectum also should be done.

- **Palpation:** As part of a pelvic examination, the doctor feels the vagina, uterus, cervix, and ovaries for any lumps. Often palpation provides the only evidence that an abnormal growth is present.

- **Pap test:** A routine cervical Pap test is not adequate for DES-exposed daughters. The cervical Pap test must be supplemented with a special Pap test of the vagina called a "four-quadrant" Pap test, in which cell samples are taken from all sides of the upper vagina.

- **Iodine staining of the cervix and vagina:** An iodine solution is used to temporarily stain the linings of the cervix and vagina to detect adenosis (a noncancerous but abnormal growth of glandular tissue) or other abnormal tissue.

- **Colposcopy:** In colposcopy, a magnifying instrument is used to view the vagina and cervix. Some doctors do not perform colposcopy routinely. However, if the Pap test result is not normal, it is very important to check for abnormal tissue.

- **Biopsy:** Small samples of any tissue that appears abnormal on colposcopy are removed and examined under a microscope to see whether cancer cells are present.

- **Breast examinations:** Researchers are continuing to study whether DES-exposed daughters have a higher risk of breast cancer than unexposed daughters; therefore, DES-exposed daughters should continue to rigorously follow the routine breast cancer screening recommendations for their age group.

What should DES-exposed mothers do?

A woman who took DES while pregnant (or suspects she may have taken it) should inform her doctor. She should try to learn the dosage, when the medication was started, and how it was used. She also should inform her children who were exposed before birth so that this information can be included in their medical records. DES-exposed mothers should have regular breast cancer screenings and yearly medical checkups that include a pelvic examination and a Pap test.

What should DES-exposed sons do?

DES-exposed sons should inform their physician of their exposure and be examined periodically. While the level of risk of developing testicular cancer is unclear among DES-exposed sons, males with undescended testicles or unusually small testicles have an increased risk of developing testicular cancer, whether or not they were exposed to DES.

Is it safe for DES-exposed daughters to use oral contraceptives or hormone replacement therapy?

Each woman should discuss this important question with her doctor. Although studies have not shown that the use of birth control pills or hormone replacement therapy are unsafe for DES-exposed daughters, some doctors believe these women should avoid these medications because they contain estrogen. Structural changes in the vagina or cervix should cause no problems with the use of other forms of contraception, such as diaphragms or spermicides.

What is the focus of current research on DES exposure?

Researchers continue to study DES-exposed daughters as they move into the menopausal years. The cancer risks for exposed daughters and sons are also being studied to determine if they differ from the unexposed population. In addition, researchers are studying possible health effects on the grandchildren of mothers who were exposed to DES during pregnancy (also called third-generation daughters or DES granddaughters).

Two published studies have examined DES granddaughters for possible abnormalities. A 1995 study found that the age menstruation began was not affected by the mother's exposure to DES. In a 2002 study, researchers compared DES granddaughters' pelvic exams to

the results of their mothers' first pelvic exams. None of the grand-daughters' pelvic exams showed changes usually associated with DES exposure. The researchers concluded that third-generation effects of in utero DES exposure are unlikely.

A recent and larger study using questionnaires to daughters of mothers who were exposed in utero to DES (granddaughters), how-ever, shows a slight effect on menstrual periods—later attainment of menstrual regularization and more irregular periods—in the exposed granddaughters compared with the unexposed granddaughters. Also, there was a suggestion that infertility was greater among the exposed, and the exposed tended to have fewer births. Because a number of these associations are based on small numbers of events, researchers will continue to study these women to further clarify these findings.

Researchers are also following up on the observation that exposure to DES may lead to an increased risk of breast cancer. A 2006 analy-sis found that DES exposure in utero was associated with a slightly increased risk of breast cancer. The experience of the women thus far suggests that increased risk might be restricted to women age 40 or older. Further follow-up is needed to confirm this and to characterize risk as the women age.

A study published in 2003 found little support for the hypothesis that in utero exposure to DES influences the psychosexual characteris-tics (the likelihood of ever having been married, age at first intercourse, number of sexual partners, and having had a same-sex sexual partner in adulthood) of adult men and women.

Part Two

Breast Cancer

Chapter 7

What You Need to Know about Breast Cancer

Breast cancer is the most common type of cancer among women in the United States (other than skin cancer). Each year in the United States, more than 192,000 women are diagnosed with breast cancer. Breast cancer also develops in men. Each year, about 2,000 men in this country learn they have breast cancer.

The Breasts and Cancer

Inside a woman's breast are 15 to 20 sections called lobes. Each lobe is made of many smaller sections called lobules. Lobules have groups of tiny glands that can make milk. After a baby is born, a woman's breast milk flows from the lobules through thin tubes called ducts to the nipple. Fat and fibrous tissue fill the spaces between the lobules and ducts.

The breasts also contain lymph vessels. These vessels are connected to small, round masses of tissue called lymph nodes. Groups of lymph nodes are near the breast in the underarm (axilla), above the collarbone, and in the chest behind the breastbone.

Cancer begins in cells, the building blocks that make up tissues. Tissues make up the breasts and other parts of the body. Normal cells grow and divide to form new cells as the body needs them. When normal cells grow old or get damaged, they die, and new cells take their place. Sometimes, this process goes wrong. New cells form when the

Excerpted from "What You Need to Know about Breast Cancer," National Cancer Institute (www.cancer.gov), October 15, 2009.

body doesn't need them, and old or damaged cells don't die as they should. The buildup of extra cells often forms a mass of tissue called a lump, growth, or tumor.

Tumors in the breast can be benign (not cancer) or malignant (cancer). Benign tumors are not as harmful as malignant tumors. Benign tumors are rarely a threat to life. they can be removed and usually don't grow back. They don't invade the tissues around them, and they don't spread to other parts of the body.

Malignant tumors, on the other hand, may be a threat to life. They often can be removed, but sometimes they grow back again. Malignant tumors can invade and damage nearby organs and tissues (such as the chest wall), and they can spread to other parts of the body.

Breast cancer cells can spread by breaking away from the original tumor. They enter blood vessels or lymph vessels, which branch into all the tissues of the body. The cancer cells may be found in lymph nodes near the breast. The cancer cells may attach to other tissues and grow to form new tumors that may damage those tissues. The spread of cancer is called metastasis.

Breast Cancer Risk Factors

When you're told that you have breast cancer, it's natural to wonder what may have caused the disease. But no one knows the exact causes of breast cancer. Doctors seldom know why one woman develops breast cancer and another doesn't.

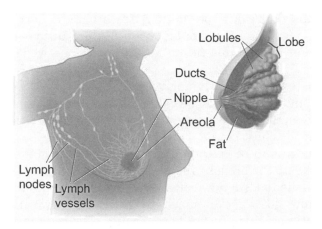

Figure 7.1. This picture shows the lobes and ducts inside the breast. It also shows the lymph nodes near the breast. (Source: National Caner Institute)

Doctors do know that bumping, bruising, or touching the breast does not cause cancer. And breast cancer is not contagious. You can't catch it from another person.

Doctors also know that women with certain risk factors are more likely than others to develop breast cancer. A risk factor is something that may increase the chance of getting a disease. Some risk factors (such as drinking alcohol) can be avoided. But most risk factors (such as having a family history of breast cancer) can't be avoided. Studies have found the following risk factors for breast cancer:

- **Age:** The chance of getting breast cancer increases as you get older. Most women are over 60 years old when they are diagnosed.

- **Personal health history:** Having breast cancer in one breast increases your risk of getting cancer in your other breast. Also, having certain types of abnormal breast cells (atypical hyperplasia, lobular carcinoma in situ [LCIS], or ductal carcinoma in situ [DCIS]) increases the risk of invasive breast cancer. These conditions are found with a breast biopsy.

- **Family health history:** Your risk of breast cancer is higher if your mother, father, sister, or daughter had breast cancer. The risk is even higher if your family member had breast cancer before age 50. Having other relatives (in either your mother's or father's family) with breast cancer or ovarian cancer may also increase your risk.

- **Certain genome changes:** Changes in certain genes, such as BRCA1 or BRCA2, substantially increase the risk of breast cancer. Tests can sometimes show the presence of these rare, specific gene changes in families with many women who have had breast cancer, and health care providers may suggest ways to try to reduce the risk of breast cancer or to improve the detection of this disease in women who have these genetic changes. Also, researchers have found specific regions on certain chromosomes that are linked to the risk of breast cancer. If a woman has a genetic change in one or more of these regions, the risk of breast cancer may be slightly increased. The risk increases with the number of genetic changes that are found. Although these genetic changes are more common among women than BRCA1 or BRCA2, the risk of breast cancer is far lower.

- **Radiation therapy to the chest:** Women who had radiation therapy to the chest (including the breasts) before age 30 are at an increased risk of breast cancer. This includes women treated

with radiation for Hodgkin lymphoma. Studies show that the younger a woman was when she received radiation treatment, the higher her risk of breast cancer later in life.

- **Reproductive and menstrual history:** The older a woman is when she has her first child, the greater her chance of breast cancer, and women who never had children are at an increased risk of breast cancer. Women who had their first menstrual period before age 12 are at an increased risk of breast cancer. Women who went through menopause after age 55 are at an increased risk of breast cancer. Women who take menopausal hormone therapy for many years have an increased risk of breast cancer.

- **Race:** In the United States, breast cancer is diagnosed more often in white women than in African American/black, Hispanic/Latina, Asian/Pacific Islander, or American Indian/Alaska Native women.

- **Breast density:** Breasts appear on a mammogram (breast x-ray) as having areas of dense and fatty (not dense) tissue. Women whose mammograms show a larger area of dense tissue than the mammograms of women of the same age are at increased risk of breast cancer.

- **History of taking DES:** DES (diethylstilbestrol) was given to some pregnant women in the United States between about 1940 and 1971. (It is no longer given to pregnant women.) Women who took DES during pregnancy may have a slightly increased risk of breast cancer. The possible effects on their daughters are under study.

- **Being overweight or obese after menopause:** The chance of getting breast cancer after menopause is higher in women who are overweight or obese.

- **Lack of physical activity:** Women who are physically inactive throughout life may have an increased risk of breast cancer.

- **Drinking alcohol:** Studies suggest that the more alcohol a woman drinks, the greater her risk of breast cancer.

Having a risk factor does not mean that a woman will get breast cancer. Most women who have risk factors never develop breast cancer.

Many other possible risk factors have been studied. For example, researchers are studying whether women who have a diet high in fat

or who are exposed to certain substances in the environment have an increased risk of breast cancer. Researchers continue to study these and other possible risk factors.

Symptoms

Early breast cancer usually doesn't cause symptoms. But as the tumor grows, it can change how the breast looks or feels. The common changes include the following:

- A lump or thickening in or near the breast or in the underarm area

- A change in the size or shape of the breast

- Dimpling or puckering in the skin of the breast

- A nipple turned inward into the breast

- Discharge (fluid) from the nipple, especially if it's bloody

- Scaly, red, or swollen skin on the breast, nipple, or areola (the dark area of skin at the center of the breast; the skin may have ridges or pitting so that it looks like the skin of an orange)

You should see your health care provider about any symptom that does not go away. Most often, these symptoms are not due to cancer. Another health problem could cause them. If you have any of these symptoms, you should tell your health care provider so that the problems can be diagnosed and treated.

Detection and Diagnosis

Your doctor can check for breast cancer before you have any symptoms. During an office visit, your doctor will ask about your personal and family medical history. You'll have a physical exam. Your doctor may order one or more imaging tests, such as a mammogram.

Doctors recommend that women have regular clinical breast exams and mammograms to find breast cancer early. Treatment is more likely to work well when breast cancer is detected early.

Clinical Breast Exam

During a clinical breast exam, your health care provider checks your breasts. You may be asked to raise your arms over your head, let them hang by your sides, or press your hands against your hips.

Your health care provider looks for differences in size or shape between your breasts. The skin of your breasts is checked for a rash, dimpling, or other abnormal signs. Your nipples may be squeezed to check for fluid.

Using the pads of the fingers to feel for lumps, your health care provider checks your entire breast, underarm, and collarbone area. A lump is generally the size of a pea before anyone can feel it. The exam is done on one side and then the other. Your health care provider checks the lymph nodes near the breast to see if they are enlarged.

If you have a lump, your health care provider will feel its size, shape, and texture. Your health care provider will also check to see if the lump moves easily. Benign lumps often feel different from cancerous ones. Lumps that are soft, smooth, round, and movable are likely to be benign. A hard, oddly shaped lump that feels firmly attached within the breast is more likely to be cancer, but further tests are needed to diagnose the problem.

Mammogram

A mammogram is an x-ray picture of tissues inside the breast. Mammograms can often show a breast lump before it can be felt. They also can show a cluster of tiny specks of calcium. These specks are called microcalcifications. Lumps or specks can be from cancer, precancerous cells, or other conditions. Further tests are needed to find out if abnormal cells are present.

If the mammogram shows an abnormal area of the breast, your doctor may order clearer, more detailed images of that area. Doctors use diagnostic mammograms to learn more about unusual breast changes, such as a lump, pain, thickening, nipple discharge, or change in breast size or shape. Diagnostic mammograms may focus on a specific area of the breast. They may involve special techniques and more views than screening mammograms.

Other Imaging Tests

If an abnormal area is found during a clinical breast exam or with a mammogram, the doctor may order other imaging tests:

- **Ultrasound:** A woman with a lump or other breast change may have an ultrasound test. An ultrasound device sends out sound waves that people can't hear. The sound waves bounce off breast tissues. A computer uses the echoes to create a picture. The picture may show whether a lump is solid, filled with fluid (a cyst),

or a mixture of both. Cysts usually are not cancer. But a solid lump may be cancer.

- **MRI:** MRI (magnetic resonance imaging) uses a powerful magnet linked to a computer. It makes detailed pictures of breast tissue. These pictures can show the difference between normal and diseased tissue.

Biopsy

A biopsy is the removal of tissue to look for cancer cells. A biopsy is the only way to tell for sure if cancer is present.

You may need to have a biopsy if an abnormal area is found. An abnormal area may be felt during a clinical breast exam but not seen on a mammogram. Or an abnormal area could be seen on a mammogram but not be felt during a clinical breast exam. In this case, doctors can use imaging procedures (such as a mammogram, an ultrasound, or MRI) to help see the area and remove tissue.

Your doctor may refer you to a surgeon or breast disease specialist for a biopsy. The surgeon or doctor will remove fluid or tissue from your breast in one of several ways:

- **Fine-needle aspiration biopsy:** Your doctor uses a thin needle to remove cells or fluid from a breast lump.

- **Core biopsy:** Your doctor uses a wide needle to remove a sample of breast tissue.

- **Skin biopsy:** If there are skin changes on your breast, your doctor may take a small sample of skin.

- **Surgical biopsy:** Your surgeon removes a sample of tissue. An incisional biopsy takes a part of the lump or abnormal area. An excisional biopsy takes the entire lump or abnormal area.

A pathologist will check the tissue or fluid removed from your breast for cancer cells. If cancer cells are found, the pathologist can tell what kind of cancer it is. The most common type of breast cancer is ductal carcinoma. It begins in the cells that line the breast ducts. Lobular carcinoma is another type. It begins in the lobules of the breast.

Lab Tests with Breast Tissue

If you are diagnosed with breast cancer, your doctor may order special lab tests on the breast tissue that was removed:

- **Hormone receptor tests:** Some breast tumors need hormones to grow. These tumors have receptors for the hormones estrogen, progesterone, or both. If the hormone receptor tests show that the breast tumor has these receptors, then hormone therapy is most often recommended as a treatment option.

- **HER2/neu test:** HER2/neu protein is found on some types of cancer cells. This test shows whether the tissue either has too much HER2/neu protein or too many copies of its gene. If the breast tumor has too much HER2/neu, then targeted therapy may be a treatment option.

It may take several weeks to get the results of these tests. The test results help your doctor decide which cancer treatments may be options for you.

Staging

If the biopsy shows that you have breast cancer, your doctor needs to learn the extent (stage) of the disease to help you choose the best treatment. The stage is based on the size of the cancer, whether the cancer has invaded nearby tissues, and whether the cancer has spread to other parts of the body. Staging may involve blood tests and other tests:

- **Bone scan:** The doctor injects a small amount of a radioactive substance into a blood vessel. It travels through the bloodstream and collects in the bones. A machine called a scanner detects and measures the radiation. The scanner makes pictures of the bones. The pictures may show cancer that has spread to the bones.

- **CT scan:** Doctors sometimes use CT (computed tomography) scans to look for breast cancer that has spread to the liver or lungs. An x-ray machine linked to a computer takes a series of detailed pictures of your chest or abdomen. You may receive contrast material by injection into a blood vessel in your arm or hand. The contrast material makes abnormal areas easier to see.

- **Lymph node biopsy:** The stage often is not known until after surgery to remove the tumor in your breast and one or more lymph nodes under your arm. Surgeons use a method called sentinel lymph node biopsy to remove the lymph node most likely to have breast cancer cells. The surgeon injects a blue dye, a radioactive substance, or both near the breast tumor. Or the surgeon

may inject a radioactive substance under the nipple. The surgeon then uses a scanner to find the sentinel lymph node containing the radioactive substance or looks for the lymph node stained with dye. The sentincl node is removed and checked for cancer cells. Cancer cells may appear first in the sentinel node before spreading to other lymph nodes and other places in the body.

These tests can show whether the cancer has spread and, if so, to what parts of your body. When breast cancer spreads, cancer cells are often found in lymph nodes under the arm (axillary lymph nodes). Also, breast cancer can spread to almost any other part of the body, such as the bones, liver, lungs, and brain.

When breast cancer spreads from its original place to another part of the body, the new tumor has the same kind of abnormal cells and the same name as the primary (original) tumor. For example, if breast cancer spreads to the bones, the cancer cells in the bones are actually breast cancer cells. The disease is metastatic breast cancer, not bone cancer. For that reason, it is treated as breast cancer, not bone cancer. Doctors call the new tumor "distant" or metastatic disease.

Treatment

Women with breast cancer have many treatment options. The treatment that's best for one woman may not be best for another. The options are surgery, radiation therapy, hormone therapy, chemotherapy, and targeted therapy. You may receive more than one type of treatment.

- Surgery and radiation therapy are types of local therapy. They remove or destroy cancer in the breast.

- Hormone therapy, chemotherapy, and targeted therapy are types of systemic therapy. The drug enters the bloodstream and destroys or controls cancer throughout the body.

The treatment that's right for you depends mainly on the stage of the cancer, the results of the hormone receptor tests, the result of the HER2/neu test, and your general health.

You may want to talk with your doctor about taking part in a clinical trial, a research study of new treatment methods. Clinical trials are an important option for women at any stage of breast cancer.

Your doctor can describe your treatment choices, the expected results, and the possible side effects. Because cancer therapy often damages healthy cells and tissues, side effects are common. Before

treatment starts, ask your health care team about possible side effects, how to prevent or reduce these effects, and how treatment may change your normal activities.

You may want to know how you will look during and after treatment. You and your health care team can work together to develop a treatment plan that meets your medical and personal needs.

Your doctor may refer you to a specialist, or you may ask for a referral. Specialists who treat breast cancer include surgeons, medical oncologists, and radiation oncologists. You also may be referred to a plastic surgeon or reconstructive surgeon. Your health care team may also include an oncology nurse and a registered dietitian.

Breast Reconstruction

Some women who plan to have a mastectomy decide to have breast reconstruction. Other women prefer to wear a breast form (prosthesis) inside their bra. Others decide to do nothing after surgery. All of these options have pros and cons. What is right for one woman may not be right for another. What is important is that nearly every woman treated for breast cancer has choices.

Breast reconstruction may be done at the same time as the mastectomy, or later on. If radiation therapy is part of the treatment plan, some doctors suggest waiting until after radiation therapy is complete.

If you are thinking about breast reconstruction, you should talk to a plastic surgeon before the mastectomy, even if you plan to have your reconstruction later on.

There are many ways for a surgeon to reconstruct the breast. Some women choose to have breast implants, which are filled with saline or silicone gel. You also may have breast reconstruction with tissue that the plastic surgeon removes from another part of your body. Skin, muscle, and fat can come from your lower abdomen, back, or buttocks. The surgeon uses this tissue to create a breast shape.

The type of reconstruction that is best for you depends on your age, body type, and the type of cancer surgery that you had. The plastic surgeon can explain the risks and benefits of each type of reconstruction.

Nutrition and Physical Activity

It's important for you to take very good care of yourself before, during, and after cancer treatment. Taking care of yourself includes eating well and staying as active as you can.

94

You need the right amount of calories to maintain a good weight. You also need enough protein to keep up your strength. Eating well may help you feel better and have more energy.

Sometimes, especially during or soon after treatment, you may not feel like eating. You may be uncomfortable or tired. You may find that foods don't taste as good as they used to. In addition, the side effects of treatment (such as poor appetite, nausea, vomiting, or mouth blisters) can make it hard to eat well. On the other hand, some women treated for breast cancer may have a problem with weight gain.

Your doctor, a registered dietitian, or another health care provider can suggest ways to help you meet your nutrition needs.

Many women find that they feel better when they stay active. Walking, yoga, swimming, and other activities can keep you strong and increase your energy. Exercise may reduce nausea and pain and make treatment easier to handle. It also can help relieve stress. Whatever physical activity you choose, be sure to talk to your doctor before you start. Also, if your activity causes you pain or other problems, be sure to let your doctor or nurse know.

Follow-Up Care

You'll need regular checkups after treatment for breast cancer. Checkups help ensure that any changes in your health are noted and treated if needed. If you have any health problems between checkups, you should contact your doctor.

Your doctor will check for return of the cancer. Also, checkups help detect health problems that can result from cancer treatment.

You should report any changes in the treated area or in your other breast to the doctor right away. Tell your doctor about any health problems, such as pain, loss of appetite or weight, changes in menstrual cycles, unusual vaginal bleeding, or blurred vision. Also talk to your doctor about headaches, dizziness, shortness of breath, coughing or hoarseness, backaches, or digestive problems that seem unusual or that don't go away. Such problems may arise months or years after treatment. They may suggest that the cancer has returned, but they can also be symptoms of other health problems. It's important to share your concerns with your doctor so that problems can be diagnosed and treated as soon as possible.

Checkups usually include an exam of the neck, underarm, chest, and breast areas. Since a new breast cancer may develop, you should have regular mammograms. You probably won't need a mammogram of a reconstructed breast or if you had a mastectomy without reconstruction. Your doctor may order other imaging procedures or lab tests.

Sources of Support

Learning that you have breast cancer can change your life and the lives of those close to you. These changes can be hard to handle. It's normal for you, your family, and your friends to need help coping with the feelings that such a diagnosis can bring.

Concerns about treatments and managing side effects, hospital stays, and medical bills are common. You may also worry about caring for your family, keeping your job, or continuing daily activities.

Several organizations offer special programs for women with breast cancer. Women who have had the disease serve as trained volunteers. They may talk with or visit women who have breast cancer, provide information, and lend emotional support. They often share their experiences with breast cancer treatment, breast reconstruction, and recovery.

You may be afraid that changes to your body will affect not only how you look but also how other people feel about you. You may worry that breast cancer and its treatment will affect your sexual relationships. Many couples find it helps to talk about their concerns. Some find that counseling or a couples' support group can be helpful.

Here's where you can go for support:

- Doctors, nurses, and other members of your health care team can answer questions about treatment, working, or other activities.

- Social workers, counselors, or members of the clergy can be helpful if you want to talk about your feelings or concerns. Often, social workers can suggest resources for financial aid, transportation, home care, or emotional support.

- Support groups also can help. In these groups, women with breast cancer or their family members meet with other patients or their families to share what they have learned about coping with the disease and the effects of treatment. Groups may offer support in person, over the telephone, or on the internet. You may want to talk with a member of your health care team about finding a support group. Keep in mind that each woman is different. Ways that one woman deals with cancer may not be right for another. You may want to ask your health care provider about advice you receive from other women with breast cancer.

- Information specialists at 800-4-CANCER (800-422-6237) and at LiveHelp (http://www.cancer.gov/help) can help you locate programs, services, and publications. They can send you a list of organizations that offer services to women with cancer.

Chapter 8

Understanding the Risk of Breast Cancer

Chapter Contents

Section 8.1

Probability of Breast Cancer in American Women

Excerpted from "Probability of Breast Cancer in American Women,"
National Cancer Institute (www.cancer.gov), October 5, 2006.

The National Cancer Institute's (NCI) Surveillance, Epidemiology, and End Results (SEER) Program has published its SEER Cancer Statistics Review 1975–2003. This report estimates that, based on current rates, 12.7 percent of women born in the United States today will develop breast cancer at some time in their lives. This estimate is based on breast cancer statistics for the years 2001 through 2003.

This estimate means that, if the current rate stays the same, women born now have an average risk of 12.7 percent (often expressed as "1 in 8") of being diagnosed with breast cancer at some time in their lives. On the other hand, the chance that they will never have breast cancer is 87.3 percent (expressed as "7 in 8").

In the 1970s, the lifetime risk of being diagnosed with breast cancer in the United States was just under 10 percent (often expressed as "1 in 10"). The estimated lifetime risk has generally been rising gradually since then; this year, the estimated risk decreased slightly.

The last five annual SEER reports show these estimates of lifetime risk:

- 13.4 percent for 1997 through 1999 ("1 in 7.45," often expressed as "1 in 7")

- 13.5 percent for 1998 through 2000 ("1 in 7.40," often expressed as "1 in 7")

- 13.4 percent for 1999 through 2001 ("1 in 7.47," often expressed as "1 in 7")

- 13.2 percent for 2000 through 2002 ("1 in 7.56," often expressed as "1 in 8")

- 12.7 percent for 2001 through 2003 ("1 in 7.87," often expressed as "1 in 8")

SEER statisticians expect some variability from year to year. Slight changes, such as the one reported this year, may be explained by a variety of factors, including minor changes in risk factor levels in the population, slight changes in screening rates, or just random variability inherent in the data.

The estimated probability of being diagnosed with breast cancer for specific age groups and for specific time periods is generally more informative than lifetime probabilities. Estimates by decade of life are less influenced by changes in life expectancy and incidence rates. The SEER report estimates the risk of developing breast cancer in 10-year age intervals. These calculations factor in the proportion of women who live to each age. In other words, they take into account that not all women live to older ages, when breast cancer risk becomes the greatest.

A woman's chance of being diagnosed with breast cancer is described as follows:

- From age 30 through age 39 . . . . . . 0.43 percent (often expressed as "1 in 233")

- From age 40 through age 49 . . . . . . 1.44 percent (often expressed as "1 in 69")

- From age 50 through age 59 . . . . . . 2.63 percent (often expressed as "1 in 38")

- From age 60 through age 69 . . . . . . 3.65 percent (often expressed as "1 in 27")

These probabilities are averages for the whole population. An individual woman's breast cancer risk may be higher or lower, depending on a number of factors, including her family history, reproductive history, race/ethnicity, and other factors that are not yet fully understood. To calculate an individual's estimated risk, see the Breast Cancer Risk Assessment Tool at http://www.cancer.gov/bcrisktool/ on the internet.

Section 8.2

Breast Cancer Risk and Protective Factors

Excerpted from PDQ® Cancer Information Summary. National Cancer Institute; Bethesda, MD. "Breast Cancer Prevention (PDQ®): Patient Version." Updated 10/2009. Available at: http://cancer.gov. Accessed July 23, 2009.

Avoiding cancer risk factors such as smoking, being overweight, and lack of exercise may help prevent certain cancers. Increasing protective factors such as quitting smoking, eating a healthy diet, and exercising may also help prevent some cancers. Talk to your doctor or other health care professional about how you might lower your risk of cancer.

Risk Factors

The following risk factors may increase the risk of breast cancer:

Estrogen (Endogenous)

Endogenous estrogen is a hormone made by the body. It helps the body develop and maintain female sex characteristics. Being exposed to estrogen over a long time may increase the risk of breast cancer. Estrogen levels are highest during the years a woman is menstruating. A woman's exposure to estrogen is increased in the following ways:

- **Early menstruation:** Beginning to have menstrual periods at age 11 or younger increases the number of years the breast tissue is exposed to estrogen.

- **Late menopause:** The more years a woman menstruates, the longer her breast tissue is exposed to estrogen.

- **Late pregnancy or never being pregnant:** Because estrogen levels are lower during pregnancy, breast tissue is exposed to more estrogen in women who become pregnant for the first time after age 35 or who never become pregnant.

Hormone Replacement Therapy/Hormone Therapy

Hormones that are made outside the body, in a laboratory, are called exogenous hormones. Estrogen, progestin, or both may be given to replace the estrogen no longer produced by the ovaries in postmenopausal women or women who have had their ovaries removed. This is called hormone replacement therapy (HRT) or hormone therapy (HT) and may be given in one of the following ways:

- Combination HRT/HT is estrogen combined with progesterone or progestin. This type of HRT/HT increases the risk of developing breast cancer.

- Estrogen-only therapy may be given to women who have had a hysterectomy. It is not known if this type of HRT/HT increases the risk of breast cancer.

Exposure to Radiation

Radiation therapy to the chest for the treatment of cancers increases the risk of breast cancer, starting ten years after treatment and lasting for a lifetime. The risk of developing breast cancer depends on the dose of radiation and the age at which it is given. The risk is highest if radiation treatment was used during puberty. For example, radiation therapy used to treat Hodgkin disease by age 16, especially radiation to the chest and neck, increases the risk of breast cancer.

Radiation therapy to treat cancer in one breast does not appear to increase the risk of developing cancer in the other breast.

For women who are at risk of breast cancer due to inherited changes in the BRCA1 and BRCA2 genes, exposure to radiation, such as that from chest x-rays, may further increase the risk of breast cancer, especially in women who were x-rayed before 20 years of age.

Obesity

Obesity increases the risk of breast cancer in postmenopausal women who have not used hormone replacement therapy.

Alcohol

Drinking alcohol increases the risk of breast cancer. The level of risk rises as the amount of alcohol consumed rises.

Inherited Risk

Women who have inherited certain changes in the BRCA1 and BRCA2 genes have a higher risk of breast cancer, and the breast cancer may develop at a younger age.

Protective Factors

The following protective factors may decrease the risk of breast cancer:

Exercise

Exercising four or more hours a week may decrease hormone levels and help lower breast cancer risk. The effect of exercise on breast cancer risk may be greatest in premenopausal women of normal or low weight. Care should be taken to exercise safely, because exercise carries the risk of injury to bones and muscles.

Estrogen (Decreased Exposure)

Decreasing the length of time a woman's breast tissue is exposed to estrogen may help prevent breast cancer. Exposure to estrogen is reduced in the following ways:

- **Pregnancy:** Estrogen levels are lower during pregnancy. The risk of breast cancer appears to be lower if a woman has her first full-term pregnancy before she is 20 years old.

- **Breastfeeding:** Estrogen levels may remain lower while a woman is breastfeeding.

- Ovarian ablation: The amount of estrogen made by the body can be greatly reduced by removing one or both ovaries, which make estrogen. Also, drugs may be taken to lower the amount of estrogen made by the ovaries.

- **Late menstruation:** Beginning to have menstrual periods at age 14 or older decreases the number of years the breast tissue is exposed to estrogen.

- **Early menopause**: The fewer years a woman menstruates, the shorter the time her breast tissue is exposed to estrogen.

Selective Estrogen Receptor Modulators

Selective estrogen receptor modulators (SERMs) are drugs that act like estrogen on some tissues in the body, but block the effect of

estrogen on other tissues. Tamoxifen is a SERM that belongs to the family of drugs called antiestrogens. Antiestrogens block the effects of the hormone estrogen in the body. Tamoxifen lowers the risk of breast cancer in women who are at high risk for the disease. This effect lasts for several years after drug treatment is stopped.

Taking tamoxifen increases the risk of developing other serious conditions, including endometrial cancer, stroke, cataracts, and blood clots, especially in the lungs and legs. The risk of developing these conditions increases with age. Women younger than 50 years who have a high risk of breast cancer may benefit the most from taking tamoxifen. Talk with your doctor about the risks and benefits of taking this drug.

Raloxifene is another SERM that helps prevent breast cancer. In postmenopausal women with osteoporosis (decreased bone density), raloxifene lowers the risk of breast cancer for women at both high risk and low risk of developing the disease. It is not known if raloxifene would have the same effect in women who do not have osteoporosis. Like tamoxifen, raloxifene may increase the risk of blood clots, especially in the lungs and legs, but does not appear to increase the risk of endometrial cancer.

Other SERMs are being studied in clinical trials.

Aromatase Inhibitors

Aromatase inhibitors lower the risk of new breast cancers in postmenopausal women with a history of breast cancer. In postmenopausal women, taking aromatase inhibitors decreases the amount of estrogen made by the body. Before menopause, estrogen is made by the ovaries and other tissues in a woman's body, including the brain, fat tissue, and skin. After menopause, the ovaries stop making estrogen, but the other tissues do not. Aromatase inhibitors block the action of an enzyme called aromatase, which is used to make all of the body's estrogen. Possible harms from taking aromatase inhibitors include osteoporosis and effects on brain function (such as talking, learning, and memory).

Prophylactic Mastectomy

Some women who have a high risk of breast cancer may choose to have a prophylactic mastectomy (the removal of both breasts when there are no signs of cancer). The risk of breast cancer is lowered in these women. However, it is very important to have a cancer risk assessment and counseling about all options for possible prevention

before making this decision. In some women, prophylactic mastectomy may cause anxiety, depression, and concerns about body image.

Prophylactic Oophorectomy

Some women who have a high risk of breast cancer may choose to have a prophylactic oophorectomy (the removal of both ovaries when there are no signs of cancer). This decreases the amount of estrogen made by the body and lowers the risk of breast cancer. However, it is very important to have a cancer risk assessment and counseling before making this decision. The sudden drop in estrogen levels may cause the onset of symptoms of menopause, including hot flashes, trouble sleeping, anxiety, and depression. Long-term effects include decreased sex drive, vaginal dryness, and decreased bone density. These symptoms vary greatly among women.

Fenretinide

Fenretinide is a type of vitamin A called a retinoid. When given to premenopausal women who have a history of breast cancer, fenretinide may lower the risk of forming a new breast cancer. Taken over time, fenretinide may cause night blindness and skin disorders. Women must avoid pregnancy while taking this drug because it could harm a developing fetus.

Section 8.3

Alcohol and Breast Cancer Risk

Excerpted from "Alcohol and Breast Cancer Risk: New Findings,"
National Cancer Institute (www.cancer.gov), April 30, 2008. Adapted
from the *NCI Cancer Bulletin*, vol. 5/no. 9, April 29, 2008.

While the potential health benefits of moderate alcohol consumption have garnered a lot of public attention, alcohol's impact on cancer risk has received much less. Epidemiological studies have consistently found that heavy drinking can increase the risk of liver, head and neck, and esophageal cancers, and even moderate drinking has been shown to increase the risk of breast cancer.

At the 2008 American Association for Cancer Research (AACR) annual meeting in San Diego, two new studies were presented that shed additional light on the alcohol-breast cancer connection, including one study that linked alcohol consumption with a significantly increased risk of the most common type of breast cancer.

Even though these studies grabbed headlines, researchers stress that important questions remain unanswered, such as which women who drink are at greatest risk, and what biological mechanism(s) alcohol might trigger to cause breast cancer. In short, researchers are still accumulating evidence that can form the basis for personalized clinical recommendations.

Nevertheless, some recommendations have already been made. As part of a far larger report on cancer prevention released last year, a consensus panel formed by the American Institute for Cancer Research (AICR) concluded: "The evidence on cancer justifies a recommendation not to drink alcoholic drinks."

The AICR report also acknowledged, however, the consistent findings that moderate alcohol consumption can protect against heart disease, and offered that, if individuals choose to drink, women should limit their consumption to one alcoholic beverage per day and men to two.

But even a highly consistent association between alcohol intake and breast cancer risk "is not the same as saying causality has been proven," says Dr. Arthur Schatzkin, chief of the Nutritional Epidemiology Branch

in the National Cancer Institute's (NCI) Division of Cancer Epidemiology and Genetics. The same, he adds, holds true for the protection against heart disease.

"The breast cancer risks involved with alcohol are indeed modest; nothing like the magnitude of the risks between smoking and lung cancer or HPV [human papilloma virus] and cervical cancer," Dr. Schatzkin continues. "So it's difficult to be absolutely certain from the available studies that it's not some other biologic or behavioral factors associated with moderate drinking that are the real etiologic agents in breast cancer."

The important point, he stresses, is that "Drinking alcohol is an entirely avoidable risk factor," especially for women with established risks like a family history of breast cancer.

Studies dating back to the 1920s show that alcohol consumption and mortality risk are represented by a J-shaped curve: Risk of death is somewhat elevated in teetotalers, dips for moderate drinkers, and then climbs steadily as consumption increases.

According to long-term studies performed by Dr. Arthur Klatsky and colleagues at Kaiser Permanente in Oakland, California, the vast bulk of the benefit of light-to-moderate alcohol consumption is due to an apparent protective effect against cardiovascular disease, primarily in middle-aged people.

Incidence data presented by NCI researchers at the AACR meeting were somewhat consistent with a J-curve, at least in terms of excessive alcohol consumption. Based on an analysis of more than 180,000 women in the NIH-AARP Diet and Health Study, they found that women who consumed three or more alcoholic drinks a day had more than a 50% increased risk of ER+/PR+ breast cancer, while women who drank smaller amounts also had an elevated risk, regardless of alcohol type.

The results, Dr. Klatsky notes, are mostly consistent with data from his studies and support the hypothesis that alcohol may increase breast cancer risk via an effect on estrogen. However, the results are not entirely consistent and highlight the difficulty in establishing a risk "threshold," Dr. Klatsky explains.

"Our data show that women who report having just several drinks a week don't have an increased [breast cancer] risk, and the risk begins somewhere between that and two drinks per day," he says.

In addition to the interplay between alcohol and estrogen, research has focused on several genes that code for the enzyme alcohol dehydrogenase (ADH), which is involved in alcohol metabolism. ADH initiates the breakdown of alcohol into acetaldehyde, ethanol's first metabolite, which is carcinogenic in animal models.

At the AACR meeting, researchers from Georgetown University's Lombardi Comprehensive Cancer Center and the State University of New York at Buffalo, using data from the Western New York Exposure and Breast Cancer Study, reported finding an increased breast cancer risk among postmenopausal women who drank and had variations in a gene that codes for ADH. The more the women reported drinking, the greater their risk.

"This is what we're really trying to get at now," says Lombardi's Deputy Director, Dr. Peter Shields, who co-led the study. "We're assuming that there are certain genetic susceptibilities. There's some evidence for it, but not enough studies to say that, for women who drink, certain genes put you at increased risk of breast cancer."

But other molecular players may be at work. Dr. Shields' lab has received funding from the Department of Defense to take a more systematic look at four potential causal mechanisms suggested by previous studies. These include the alcohol-estrogen link and the role of acetaldehyde, as well as alcohol-induced oxidative damage and disruption of folic acid pathways.

"We want to take this type of beverage that many women are going to drink," Dr. Shields says, "and figure out when they are really putting themselves at risk."

Chapter 9

Genes Associated with Breast Cancer

BRCA1 and BRCA2: Cancer Risk and Genetic Testing

What are BRCA1 and BRCA2?

BRCA1 and BRCA2 are human genes that belong to a class of genes known as tumor suppressors. In normal cells, BRCA1 and BRCA2 help ensure the stability of the cell's genetic material (DNA) and help prevent uncontrolled cell growth. Mutation of these genes has been linked to the development of hereditary breast and ovarian cancer.

The names BRCA1 and BRCA2 stand for breast cancer susceptibility gene 1 and breast cancer susceptibility gene 2, respectively.

How do BRCA1 and BRCA2 gene mutations affect a person's risk of cancer?

Not all gene changes, or mutations, are deleterious (harmful). Some mutations may be beneficial, whereas others may have no obvious effect (neutral). Harmful mutations can increase a person's risk of developing a disease, such as cancer.

A woman's lifetime risk of developing breast and/or ovarian cancer is greatly increased if she inherits a harmful mutation in BRCA1 or BRCA2. Such a woman has an increased risk of developing breast and/

Excerpted from "BRCA1 and BRCA2: Cancer Risk and Genetic Testing," National Cancer Institute (NCI, www.cancer.gov), May 29, 2009; and "CHEK2 Gene Carries Risk of Breast Cancer," NCI, September 25, 2006.

or ovarian cancer at an early age (before menopause) and often has multiple, close family members who have been diagnosed with these diseases. Harmful BRCA1 mutations may also increase a woman's risk of developing cervical, uterine, pancreatic, and colon cancer. Harmful BRCA2 mutations may additionally increase the risk of pancreatic cancer, stomach cancer, gallbladder and bile duct cancer, and melanoma.

Men with harmful BRCA1 mutations also have an increased risk of breast cancer and, possibly, of pancreatic cancer, testicular cancer, and early-onset prostate cancer. However, male breast cancer, pancreatic cancer, and prostate cancer appear to be more strongly associated with BRCA2 gene mutations.

The likelihood that a breast and/or ovarian cancer is associated with a harmful mutation in BRCA1 or BRCA2 is highest in families with a history of multiple cases of breast cancer, cases of both breast and ovarian cancer, one or more family members with two primary cancers (original tumors that develop at different sites in the body), or an Ashkenazi (Eastern European) Jewish background. However, not every woman in such families carries a harmful BRCA1 or BRCA2 mutation, and not every cancer in such families is linked to a harmful mutation in one of these genes. Furthermore, not every woman who has a harmful BRCA1 or BRCA2 mutation will develop breast and/or ovarian cancer.

According to estimates of lifetime risk, about 12.0 percent of women (120 out of 1,000) in the general population will develop breast cancer sometime during their lives compared with about 60 percent of women (600 out of 1,000) who have inherited a harmful mutation in BRCA1 or BRCA2 (4, 5). In other words, a woman who has inherited a harmful mutation in BRCA1 or BRCA2 is about five times more likely to develop breast cancer than a woman who does not have such a mutation.

Lifetime risk estimates for ovarian cancer among women in the general population indicate that 1.4 percent (14 out of 1,000) will be diagnosed with ovarian cancer compared with 15 to 40 percent of women (150–400 out of 1,000) who have a harmful BRCA1 or BRCA2 mutation.

Do inherited mutations in other genes increase the risk of breast and/or ovarian tumors?

Yes. Mutations in several other genes, including TP53, PTEN, STK11/LKB1, CDH1, CHEK2, ATM, MLH1, and MSH2, have been associated

with hereditary breast and/or ovarian tumors. However, the majority of hereditary breast cancers can be accounted for by inherited mutations in BRCA1 and BRCA2. Overall, it has been estimated that inherited BRCA1 and BRCA2 mutations account for five to 10 percent of breast cancers and 10 to 15 percent of ovarian cancers among white women in the United States.

Are specific mutations in BRCA1 and BRCA2 more common in certain populations?

Yes. For example, three specific mutations, two in the BRCA1 gene and one in the BRCA2 gene, are the most common mutations found in these genes in the Ashkenazi Jewish population. In one study, 2.3 percent of participants (120 out of 5,318) carried one of these three mutations. This frequency is about five times higher than that found in the general population. It is not known whether the increased frequency of these mutations is responsible for the increased risk of breast cancer in Jewish populations compared with non-Jewish populations.

Other ethnic and geographic populations around the world, such as the Norwegian, Dutch, and Icelandic peoples, also have higher frequencies of specific BRCA1 and BRCA2 mutations.

In addition, limited data indicate that the frequencies of specific BRCA1 and BRCA2 mutations may vary among individual racial and ethnic groups in the United States, including African Americans, Hispanics, Asian Americans, and non-Hispanic whites.

This information about genetic differences between racial and ethnic groups may help health care providers in selecting the most appropriate genetic test(s).

Are genetic tests available to detect BRCA1 and BRCA2 mutations, and how are they performed?

Yes. Several methods are available to test for BRCA1 and BRCA2 mutations. Most of these methods look for changes in BRCA1 and BRCA2 DNA. At least one method looks for changes in the proteins produced by these genes. Frequently, a combination of methods is used.

A blood sample is needed for these tests. The blood is drawn in a laboratory, doctor's office, hospital, or clinic and then sent to a laboratory that specializes in the tests. It usually takes several weeks or longer to get the test results. Individuals who decide to get tested

should check with their health care provider to find out when their test results might be available.

Genetic counseling is generally recommended before and after a genetic test. This counseling should be performed by a health care professional who is experienced in cancer genetics. Genetic counseling usually involves a risk assessment based on the individual's personal and family medical history and discussions about the appropriateness of genetic testing, the specific test(s) that might be used and the technical accuracy of the test(s), the medical implications of a positive or a negative test result, the possibility that a test result might not be informative (an ambiguous result) (see below), the psychological risks and benefits of genetic test results, and the risk of passing a mutation to children.

How do people know if they should consider genetic testing for BRCA1 and BRCA2 mutations?

Currently, there are no standard criteria for recommending or referring someone for BRCA1 or BRCA2 mutation testing.

In a family with a history of breast and/or ovarian cancer, it may be most informative to first test a family member who has breast or ovarian cancer. If that person is found to have a harmful BRCA1 or BRCA2 mutation, then other family members can be tested to see if they also have the mutation.

Regardless, women who have a relative with a harmful BRCA1 or BRCA2 mutation and women who appear to be at increased risk of breast and/or ovarian cancer because of their family history should consider genetic counseling to learn more about their potential risks and about BRCA1 and BRCA2 genetic tests.

The likelihood of a harmful mutation in BRCA1 or BRCA2 is increased with certain familial patterns of cancer. These patterns include the following.

For women who are not of Ashkenazi Jewish descent the patterns are as follows:

- Two first-degree relatives (mother, daughter, or sister) diagnosed with breast cancer, one of whom was diagnosed at age 50 or younger

- Three or more first-degree or second-degree (grandmother or aunt) relatives diagnosed with breast cancer regardless of their age at diagnosis

- A combination of first- and second-degree relatives diagnosed with breast cancer and ovarian cancer (one cancer type per person)

- A first-degree relative with cancer diagnosed in both breasts (bi-lateral breast cancer)

- A combination of two or more first- or second-degree relatives diagnosed with ovarian cancer regardless of age at diagnosis

- A first- or second-degree relative diagnosed with both breast and ovarian cancer regardless of age at diagnosis

- Breast cancer diagnosed in a male relative

For women of Ashkenazi Jewish descent the patterns are as follows:

- Any first-degree relative diagnosed with breast or ovarian cancer

- Two second-degree relatives on the same side of the family diagnosed with breast or ovarian cancer

These family history patterns apply to about two percent of adult women in the general population. Women who have none of these family history patterns have a low probability of having a harmful BRCA1 or BRCA2 mutation.

How much does BRCA1 and BRCA2 mutation testing cost?

The cost for BRCA1 and BRCA2 mutation testing usually ranges from several hundred to several thousand dollars. Insurance policies vary with regard to whether or not the cost of testing is covered. People who are considering BRCA1 and BRCA2 mutation testing may want to find out about their insurance company's policies regarding genetic tests.

What does a positive BRCA1 or BRCA2 test result mean?

A positive test result generally indicates that a person has inherited a known harmful mutation in BRCA1 or BRCA2 and, therefore, has an increased risk of developing certain cancers, as described above. However, a positive test result provides information only about a person's risk of developing cancer. It cannot tell whether an individual will actually develop cancer or when. Not all women who inherit a harmful BRCA1 or BRCA2 mutation will develop breast or ovarian cancer.

A positive genetic test result may have important health and social implications for family members, including future generations.

Unlike most other medical tests, genetic tests can reveal information not only about the person being tested but also about that person's relatives. Both men and women who inherit harmful BRCA1 or BRCA2 mutations, whether they develop cancer themselves or not, may pass the mutations on to their sons and daughters. However, not all children of people who have a harmful mutation will inherit the mutation.

What does a negative BRCA1 or BRCA2 test result mean?

How a negative test result will be interpreted depends on whether or not someone in the tested person's family is known to carry a harmful BRCA1 or BRCA2 mutation. If someone in the family has a known mutation, testing other family members for the same mutation can provide information about their cancer risk. If a person tests negative for a known mutation in his or her family, it is unlikely that they have an inherited susceptibility to cancer associated with BRCA1 or BRCA2. Such a test result is called a "true negative." Having a true negative test result does not mean that a person will not develop cancer; it means that the person's risk of cancer is probably the same as that of people in the general population.

In cases in which a family has a history of breast and/or ovarian cancer and no known mutation in BRCA1 or BRCA2 has been previously identified, a negative test result is not informative. It is not possible to tell whether an individual has a harmful BRCA1 or BRCA2 mutation that was not detected by testing (a "false negative") or whether the result is a true negative. In addition, it is possible for people to have a mutation in a gene other than BRCA1 or BRCA2 that increases their cancer risk but is not detectable by the test(s) used.

What does an ambiguous BRCA1 or BRCA2 test result mean?

If genetic testing shows a change in BRCA1 or BRCA2 that has not been previously associated with cancer in other people, the person's test result may be interpreted as "ambiguous" (uncertain). One study found that 10 percent of women who underwent BRCA1 and BRCA2 mutation testing had this type of ambiguous result.

Because everyone has genetic differences that are not associated with an increased risk of disease, it is sometimes not known whether a specific DNA change affects a person's risk of developing cancer. As more research is conducted and more people are tested for BRCA1 or

BRCA2 changes, scientists will learn more about these changes and cancer risk.

What are the options for a person who has a positive test result?

Several options are available for managing cancer risk in individuals who have a harmful BRCA1 or BRCA2 mutation. However, high-quality data on the effectiveness of these options are limited.

Surveillance: Surveillance means cancer screening, or a way of detecting the disease early. Screening does not, however, change the risk of developing cancer. The goal is to find cancer early, when it may be most treatable.

Surveillance methods for breast cancer may include mammography and clinical breast exams. Studies are currently under way to test the effectiveness of other breast cancer screening methods, such as magnetic resonance imaging (MRI), in women with BRCA1 or BRCA2 mutations. With careful surveillance, many breast cancers will be diagnosed early enough to be successfully treated.

For ovarian cancer, surveillance methods may include transvaginal ultrasound, blood tests for CA–125 antigen, and clinical exams. Surveillance can sometimes find ovarian cancer at an early stage, but it is uncertain whether these methods can help reduce a woman's chance of dying from this disease.

Prophylactic surgery: This type of surgery involves removing as much of the "at-risk" tissue as possible in order to reduce the chance of developing cancer. Bilateral prophylactic mastectomy (removal of healthy breasts) and prophylactic salpingo-oophorectomy (removal of healthy fallopian tubes and ovaries) do not, however, offer a guarantee against developing cancer. Because not all at-risk tissue can be removed by these procedures, some women have developed breast cancer, ovarian cancer, or primary peritoneal carcinomatosis (a type of cancer similar to ovarian cancer) even after prophylactic surgery. In addition, some evidence suggests that the amount of protection salpingo-oophorectomy provides against the development of breast and ovarian cancer may differ between carriers of BRCA1 and BRCA2 mutations.

Risk avoidance: Certain behaviors have been associated with breast and ovarian cancer risk in the general population. Research

115

results on the benefits of modifying individual behaviors to reduce the risk of developing cancer among BRCA1 or BRCA2 mutation carriers are limited.

Chemoprevention: This approach involves the use of natural or synthetic substances to reduce the risk of developing cancer or to reduce the chance that cancer will come back. For example, the drug tamoxifen has been shown in numerous clinical studies to reduce the risk of developing breast cancer by about 50 percent in women who are at increased risk of this disease and to reduce the recurrence of breast cancer in women undergoing treatment for a previously diagnosed breast tumor. As a result, tamoxifen was approved by the U.S. Food and Drug Administration (FDA) as a breast cancer treatment and to reduce the risk of breast cancer development in premenopausal and postmenopausal women who are at increased risk of this disease. Few studies, however, have evaluated the effectiveness of tamoxifen in women with BRCA1 or BRCA2 mutations. Data from three studies suggest that tamoxifen may be able to help lower the risk of breast cancer in BRCA1 and BRCA2 mutation carriers. Two of these studies examined the effectiveness of tamoxifen in helping to reduce the development of cancer in the opposite breast of women undergoing treatment for an initial breast cancer.

Another drug, raloxifene, was shown in a large clinical trial sponsored by the National Cancer Institute (NCI) to reduce the risk of developing invasive breast cancer in postmenopausal women at increased risk of this disease by about the same amount as tamoxifen. As a result, raloxifene was approved by the FDA for breast cancer risk reduction in postmenopausal women. Since tamoxifen and raloxifene inhibit the growth of breast cancer cells in similar ways, raloxifene may be able to help reduce breast cancer risk in postmenopausal BRCA1 and BRCA2 mutation carriers. However, this has not been studied directly.

What are some of the benefits of genetic testing for breast and ovarian cancer risk?

There can be benefits to genetic testing, whether a person receives a positive or a negative result. The potential benefits of a negative result include a sense of relief and the possibility that special preventive checkups, tests, or surgeries may not be needed. A positive test result can bring relief from uncertainty and allow people to make informed decisions about their future, including taking steps to reduce their cancer risk. In addition, many people who have a positive test result

may be able to participate in medical research that could, in the long run, help reduce deaths from breast cancer.

What are some of the risks of genetic testing for breast and ovarian cancer risk?

The direct medical risks, or harms, of genetic testing are very small, but test results may have an effect on a person's emotions, social relationships, finances, and medical choices.

People who receive a positive test result may feel anxious, depressed, or angry. They may choose to undergo preventive measures, such as prophylactic surgery, that have serious long-term implications and whose effectiveness is uncertain.

People who receive a negative test result may experience "survivor guilt," caused by the knowledge that they likely do not have an increased risk of developing a disease that affects one or more loved ones.

Because genetic testing can reveal information about more than one family member, the emotions caused by test results can create tension within families. Test results can also affect personal choices, such as marriage and childbearing. Issues surrounding the privacy and confidentiality of genetic test results are additional potential risks.

What can happen when genetic test results are placed in medical records?

Clinical test results are normally included in a person's medical records. Consequently, individuals considering genetic testing must understand that their results might not be kept private.

Because a person's genetic information is considered health information, it is covered by the Privacy Rule of the Health Information Portability and Accountability Act (HIPAA) of 1996. The Privacy Rule requires that health care providers and others protect the privacy of health information, sets boundaries on the use and release of health records, and empowers individuals to control certain uses and disclosures of their health-related information. Many states also have laws to protect the privacy and limit the release of genetic and other health information.

In 2008, the Genetic Information Nondiscrimination Act (GINA) became Federal law. GINA prohibits discrimination based on genetic information in relation to health insurance and employment, but the law does not cover life insurance, disability insurance, and long-term care insurance. When applying for these types of insurance, people may

be asked to sign forms that give an insurance company permission to access their medical records. The insurance company may take genetic test results into account when making decisions about coverage.

Some physicians keep genetic test results out of medical records. However, even if such results are not included in a person's medical records, information about a person's genetic profile can sometimes be gathered from that person's family medical history.

In general, what factors increase or decrease the chance of developing breast cancer and/or ovarian cancer?

The following factors have been associated with increased or decreased risk of developing breast and/or ovarian cancer in the general population. It is not yet known exactly how these factors influence risk in people with BRCA1 or BRCA2 mutations. In addition, a significant portion of hereditary breast cancers are not associated with BRCA1 or BRCA2 mutations.

Age: The risks of breast and ovarian cancer increase with age. Most breast and ovarian cancers occur in women over the age of 50. Women with harmful BRCA1 or BRCA2 mutations often develop breast or ovarian cancer before age 50.

Family history: Women who have a first-degree relative (mother, sister, or daughter) or other close relative with breast and/or ovarian cancer may be at increased risk of developing these cancers. In addition, women with relatives who have had colon cancer may be at increased risk of developing ovarian cancer.

Medical history: Women who have already had breast cancer are at increased risk of developing breast cancer again, or of developing ovarian cancer.

Hormonal influences: Estrogen is a hormone that is naturally produced by the body and stimulates the normal growth of breast tissue. It is thought that excess estrogen may contribute to breast cancer risk because of its natural role in stimulating breast cell growth. Women who had their first menstrual period before the age of 12 or experienced menopause after age 55 have a slightly increased risk of breast cancer, as do women who had their first child after age 30. Each of these factors increases the amount of time a woman's body is exposed to estrogen. Removal of a woman's ovaries, which are the

main source of estrogen production, reduces the risk of breast cancer. Breast-feeding also reduces breast cancer risk and is thought to exert its effects through hormonal mechanisms.

Birth control pills (oral contraceptives): Most studies have shown a slight increase or no change in risk of breast cancer among women taking birth control pills. In contrast, numerous studies have shown that taking birth control pills decreases a woman's risk of developing ovarian cancer. This protective benefit appears to increase with the duration of oral contraceptive use and persists up to 25 years after discontinuing use. It also appears that the use of birth control pills lowers the risk of ovarian cancer in women who carry harmful BRCA1 or BRCA2 mutations.

Hormone replacement therapy: Doctors may prescribe hormone replacement therapy (HRT) to reduce the discomfort of certain symptoms of menopause, such as hot flashes. However, the results of the Women's Health Initiative (WHI), a large clinical study conducted by the National Heart, Lung, and Blood Institute, part of the National Institutes of Health (NIH), showed that HRT with the hormones estrogen and progestin is associated with harmful side effects, including an increased risk of breast cancer and increased risks of heart attack, blood clots, and stroke. The WHI also showed that HRT with estrogen alone was associated with increased risks of blood clots and stroke, but the effect on breast cancer risk was uncertain. In addition, the WHI showed an increase in ovarian cancer risk among women who received estrogen and progestin HRT, but this finding was not statistically significant. Because of these potential harmful side effects, the FDA has recommended that HRT be used only at the lowest doses for the shortest period of time needed to achieve treatment goals.

No data have been reported to date regarding the effects of HRT on breast cancer risk among women carrying harmful BRCA1 or BRCA2 mutations, and only limited data are available regarding HRT use and ovarian cancer risk among such women. In one study, HRT use did not appear to affect ovarian cancer risk among women with BRCA1 or BRCA2 mutations.

When considering HRT use, both the potential harms and benefits of this type of treatment should be discussed carefully by a woman and her health care provider.

Obesity: Substantial evidence indicates that obesity is associated with an increased risk of breast cancer, especially among postmenopausal

119

women who have not used HRT. Evidence also suggests that obesity is associated with increased mortality (death) from ovarian cancer.

Physical activity: Numerous studies have examined the relationship between physical activity and breast cancer risk, and most of these studies have shown that physical activity, especially strenuous physical activity, is associated with reduced risk. This decrease in risk appears to be more pronounced in premenopausal women and women with lower-than-normal body weight.

Alcohol: There is substantial evidence that alcohol consumption is associated with increased breast cancer risk. However, it is uncertain whether reducing alcohol consumption would decrease breast cancer risk.

Dietary fat: Although early studies suggested a possible association between a high-fat diet and increased breast cancer risk, more recent studies have been inconclusive. In the WHI, a low-fat diet did not help reduce breast cancer risk.

Where can people get more information about genetic testing for cancer risk?

A person who is considering genetic testing should speak with a professional trained in genetics before deciding whether to be tested. These professionals may include doctors, genetic counselors, and other health care workers trained in genetics (such as nurses, psychologists, or social workers).

What research is currently being done to help individuals with harmful BRCA1 or BRCA2 mutations?

Research studies are being conducted to find newer and better ways of detecting, treating, and preventing cancer in BRCA1 and BRCA2 mutation carriers. Additional studies are focused on improving genetic counseling methods and outcomes. Our knowledge in these areas is evolving rapidly.

CHEK2 Gene Carries Risk of Breast Cancer

Summary

Women who carry an abnormal variant of a gene known as CHEK2 are three times more likely to develop breast cancer than women who

do not have the genetic mutation, a large study by Danish researchers has found. Along with BRCA1 and BRCA2, the CHEK2 gene is now confirmed as a risk factor for breast cancer.

Background

Some women who have a strong family history of breast cancer have inherited genetic abnormalities, or mutations, that increase their risk for the disease. The so-called BRCA1 and BRCA2 mutations are the most common genetic abnormalities known to be linked to a high risk for breast cancer. However, BRCA1 and BRCA2 mutations account for fewer than one in 10 breast cancer cases. Families in which no one carries a BRCA1 or BRCA2 mutation may still have a strong history of breast cancer. This suggests that other genetic risks for breast cancer have yet to be identified.

In 2002, researchers showed that a mutation in a gene known as CHEK2 increased risk for breast cancer in women from families with a strong history of the disease. CHEK2 normally produces a protein that helps to prevent tumor cells from growing uncontrollably. The mutated form of the CHEK2 gene fails to do its job.

The authors of the 2002 study estimated that women who carried the CHEK2 mutation were at double the risk for breast cancer. Subsequent studies suggested that the CHEK2 mutation might increase risk for prostate and colorectal cancer, as well. However, many of these studies were small and most were retrospective—that is, researchers' conclusions were based on looking back at what happened to patients in the past. This type of study is generally considered less reliable than a prospective study, in which researchers follow patients forward in time to see what happens to them.

The Study

Researchers in Denmark wanted to confirm whether and to what extent the CHEK2 mutation increased risk for breast, colorectal, and prostate cancer in the general population. They studied 9,231 people who had been monitored for cancer development for an average of 34 years.

The study participants had been interviewed and examined periodically since 1976. Their records contained information about their medical histories, families' disease history, and smoking and alcohol habits. For women, the number of pregnancies and births had been recorded. Participants' DNA was analyzed using blood samples they had given between 1991 and 1994. Researchers found out which participants had

121

been diagnosed with cancer by consulting the Danish Cancer Registry, which records 98 percent of all cancers in Denmark.

In addition, the researchers studied 1,101 women with breast cancer who were recruited at a local hospital. The participants gave blood and completed questionnaires that asked about their medical history, family history of breast cancer, pregnancies and births, use of birth control pills or hormone replacement therapy, and alcohol consumption. These women were compared with 4,665 women who were in the same age range but were cancer free.

Genetic tests were performed on blood samples from all study participants to identify the presence of the CHEK2 mutation. To reduce the chance of incorrect results due to variation in the way the genetic tests were done, all the tests were conducted in the same lab using identical procedures. The researchers then used statistical techniques to estimate cancer risk in both those who had the mutation and those who did not.

The study's senior author is Borge G. Nordestgaard, M.D., of Herlev University Hospital in Herlev, Denmark.

Results

Half of one percent (0.5 percent) of the study participants were found to have the CHEK2 mutation. Women who carried the mutation were 3.2 times more likely to develop breast cancer than those who did not. However, the researchers found no statistically significant increase in risk for colorectal cancer, prostate cancer, or cancer in general among either male or female mutation carriers.

Limitations

Because almost all of the participants in this study were white and of Danish descent, the findings do not shed light on how common the CHEK2 mutation is in people of other races and ethnicities or on whether the mutation confers a similar risk of cancer in other races and ethnic groups.

Comments

This study's results "confirm beyond a doubt" that women who carry the CHEK2 mutation have a two- to threefold elevation in the lifetime risk for breast cancer, says Jeffery P. Struewing, M.D., of the National Cancer Institute's Laboratory of Population Genetics.

The current study is the first prospective study of the cancer risk associated with the CHEK2 mutation, says Struewing. Its findings

and those of earlier studies of the association between the CHEK2 mutation and breast cancer have shown "astonishing consistency," he adds.

Studies to date, which have been conducted in predominantly white populations, show that the CHEK2 mutation occurs in roughly one in every 200 people, Struewing says. This makes it about twice as common as the BRCA1 and BRCA2 mutations, but still relatively uncommon.

On average, a woman with a CHEK2 mutation has about a 20 percent to 30 percent lifetime risk of getting breast cancer, according to Struewing. By contrast, the lifetime risk for a woman with a BRCA1 or BRCA2 mutation averages about 60 percent.

Women from families with a strong history of breast cancer may wish to talk to their doctor or to a genetic counselor about the pros and cons of being tested for breast-cancer susceptibility genes, says Struewing. They may also want to talk to their doctor about steps they can consider taking that may reduce their risk of the disease.

Chapter 10

Breast Cancer Screening

Standard Screening Tests

Tests are used to screen for different types of cancer. Some screening tests are used because they have been shown to be helpful both in finding cancers early and in decreasing the chance of dying from these cancers. Other tests are used because they have been shown to find cancer in some people; however, it has not been proven in clinical trials that use of these tests will decrease the risk of dying from cancer.

Scientists study screening tests to find those with the fewest risks and most benefits. Cancer screening trials also are meant to show whether early detection (finding cancer before it causes symptoms) decreases a person's chance of dying from the disease. For some types of cancer, the chance of recovery is better if the disease is found and treated at an early stage.

Clinical trials that study cancer screening methods are taking place in many parts of the country.

Mammograms and clinical breast exams are two tests are commonly used by health care providers to screen for breast cancer.

Mammogram

A mammogram is an x-ray of the breast. This test may find tumors that are too small to feel. A mammogram may also find ductal

Excerpted from PDQ® Cancer Information Summary. National Cancer Institute; Bethesda, MD. "Breast Cancer Screening (PDQ®): Patient Version." Updated 04/2009. Available at: http://cancer.gov. Accessed July 23, 2009.

carcinoma in situ, abnormal cells in the lining of a breast duct, which may become invasive cancer in some women. The ability of a mammogram to find breast cancer may depend on the size of the tumor, the density of the breast tissue, and the skill of the radiologist.

Clinical Breast Exam (CBE)

A clinical breast exam is an exam of the breast by a doctor or other health professional. The doctor will carefully feel the breasts and under the arms for lumps or anything else that seems unusual.

It is important to know how your breasts usually look and feel. If you feel any lumps or notice any other changes, talk to your doctor.

If a lump or other change is found by mammogram or clinical breast exam, follow-up tests may be needed.

If a lump or anything else that seems abnormal is found using one of these two tests, ultrasound may be used to learn more. Ultrasound is not used by itself as a screening test for breast cancer. This is a procedure in which high-energy sound waves (ultrasound) are bounced off internal tissues or organs and make echoes. The echoes form a picture of body tissues called a sonogram.

Other Screening Tests

Other screening tests are being studied in clinical trials.

MRI (Magnetic Resonance Imaging)

MRI is a procedure that uses a magnet, radio waves, and a computer to make a series of detailed pictures of areas inside the body. This procedure is also called nuclear magnetic resonance imaging (NMRI). MRI does not use any x-rays.

In women with a high-inherited risk of breast cancer, screening trials of MRI breast scans have shown that MRI is more sensitive than mammography for finding breast tumors. It is common for MRI breast scan results to appear abnormal even though no cancer is present. Screening studies of breast MRI in women at high inherited risk are ongoing.

In women at average risk for breast cancer, MRI scans may be done to help with diagnosis. MRI may be used to:

- Study lumps in the breast that remain after surgery or radiation therapy.

- Study breast lumps or enlarged lymph nodes found during a clinical breast exam or a breast self-exam that were not seen on mammography or ultrasound.

- Plan surgery for patients with known breast cancer.

Tissue Sampling

Breast tissue sampling is taking cells from breast tissue to examine under a microscope. Abnormal cells in breast fluid have been linked to an increased risk of breast cancer in some studies. Scientists are studying whether breast tissue sampling can be used to find breast cancer at an early stage or predict the risk of developing breast cancer. Three methods of tissue sampling are under study:

- **Fine-needle aspiration:** A thin needle is inserted into the breast tissue around the areola (darkened area around the nipple) to withdraw cells and fluid.

- **Nipple aspiration:** The use of gentle suction to collect fluid through the nipple. This is done with a device similar to the breast pumps used by nursing women.

- **Ductal lavage:** A hair-size catheter (tube) is inserted into the nipple and a small amount of salt water is released into the duct. The water picks up breast cells and is removed.

Screening clinical trials are taking place in many parts of the country.

Risks of Breast Cancer Screening

Screening tests have risks. Decisions about screening tests can be difficult. Not all screening tests are helpful and most have risks. Before having any screening test, you may want to discuss the test with your doctor. It is important to know the risks of the test and whether it has been proven to reduce the risk of dying from cancer.

The risks of breast cancer screening tests include the following:

Finding breast cancer may not improve health or help a woman live longer. Screening may not help you if you have fast-growing breast cancer or if it has already spread to other places in your body. Also, some breast cancers found on a screening mammogram may never cause symptoms or become life-threatening. When such cancers are found, treatment would not help you live longer and may instead cause

serious treatment-related side effects. At this time, it is not possible to be sure which breast cancers found by screening will cause symptoms and which breast cancers will not.

False-negative test results can occur. Screening test results may appear to be normal even though breast cancer is present. A woman who receives a false-negative test result (one that shows there is no cancer when there really is) may delay seeking medical care even if she has symptoms.

One in five cancers may be missed by mammography. False-negatives occur more often in younger women than in older women because the breast tissue of younger women is more dense. The size of the tumor, the rate of tumor growth, the level of hormones, such as estrogen and progesterone, in the woman's body, and the skill of the radiologist can also affect the chance of a false-negative result.

False-positive test results can occur. Screening test results may appear to be abnormal even though no cancer is present. A false-positive test result (one that shows there is cancer when there really isn't) can cause anxiety and is usually followed by more tests (such as biopsy), which also have risks.

Most abnormal test results turn out not to be cancer. False-positives are more common in younger women, women who have had previous breast biopsies, women with a family history of breast cancer, and women who take hormones, such as estrogen and progesterone. The skill of the doctor also can affect the chance of a false-positive result.

Mammograms expose the breast to radiation. Being exposed to radiation is a risk factor for breast cancer. The risk of developing breast cancer from radiation exposure, such as screening mammograms or x-rays, is greater with higher doses of radiation and in younger women. For women older than 40 years, the benefits of an annual screening mammogram may be greater than the risks from radiation exposure.

The risks and benefits of screening for breast cancer may be different for different groups of people. The benefits of breast cancer screening may vary among age groups.

- In women who have a life expectancy of five years or less, finding and treating early stage breast cancer may reduce their quality of life without helping them live longer.

- In women older than 65 years, the results of a screening test may lead to more diagnostic tests and anxiety while waiting for the test results. Also, the breast cancers found are usually not life-threatening.

- In women 35 years or younger who go to the doctor for breast symptoms, mammogram results may not be helpful in managing their care.

Routine breast cancer screening is advised for women who have had radiation treatment to the chest, especially at a young age. The benefits and risks of mammograms and MRIs for these women are not known. There is no information on the benefits or risks of breast cancer screening in men.

No matter how old you are, if you have risk factors for breast cancer you should ask for medical advice about when to begin having mammograms and how often to be screened.

Chapter 11

Staging and Treating Breast Cancer

Stages of Breast Cancer

After breast cancer has been diagnosed, tests are done to find out if cancer cells have spread within the breast or to other parts of the body.

The process used to find out whether the cancer has spread within the breast or to other parts of the body is called staging. The information gathered from the staging process determines the stage of the disease. It is important to know the stage in order to plan treatment.

There are three ways that cancer spreads in the body:

- **Through tissue:** Cancer invades the surrounding normal tissue.

- **Through the lymph system:** Cancer invades the lymph system and travels through the lymph vessels to other places in the body.

- **Through the blood:** Cancer invades the veins and capillaries and travels through the blood to other places in the body.

When cancer cells break away from the primary (original) tumor and travel through the lymph or blood to other places in the body, another (secondary) tumor may form. This process is called metastasis. The secondary (metastatic) tumor is the same type of cancer as the

Excerpted from PDQ® Cancer Information Summary. National Cancer Institute; Bethesda, MD. "Breast Cancer Treatment (PDQ®): Patient Version." Updated 03/2010. Available at: http://cancer.gov. Accessed May 24, 2010.

primary tumor. For example, if breast cancer spreads to the bones, the cancer cells in the bones are actually breast cancer cells. The disease is metastatic breast cancer, not bone cancer.

The following stages are used for breast cancer:

Stage 0 (Carcinoma in Situ)

There are two types of breast carcinoma in situ.

Ductal carcinoma in situ (DCIS) is a noninvasive condition in which abnormal cells are found in the lining of a breast duct. The abnormal cells have not spread outside the duct to other tissues in the breast. In some cases, DCIS may become invasive cancer and spread to other tissues, although it is not known at this time how to predict which lesions will become invasive.

Lobular carcinoma in situ (LCIS) is a condition in which abnormal cells are found in the lobules of the breast. This condition seldom becomes invasive cancer; however, having lobular carcinoma in situ in one breast increases the risk of developing breast cancer in either breast.

Stage I

- In stage I, cancer has formed. The tumor is 2 centimeters or smaller and has not spread outside the breast.

Stage IIA

- No tumor is found in the breast, but cancer is found in the axillary lymph nodes (the lymph nodes under the arm); or

- The tumor is 2 centimeters or smaller and has spread to the axillary lymph nodes; or

- The tumor is larger than 2 centimeters but not larger than 5 centimeters and has not spread to the axillary lymph nodes.

Stage IIB

In stage IIB, the tumor is one of the following:

- Larger than 2 centimeters but not larger than 5 centimeters and has spread to the axillary lymph nodes; or

- Larger than 5 centimeters but has not spread to the axillary lymph nodes.

Stage IIIA

Stage IIIA is characterized as follows:

- No tumor is found in the breast. Cancer is found in axillary lymph nodes that are attached to each other or to other structures, or cancer may be found in lymph nodes near the breastbone; or

- The tumor is 2 centimeters or smaller. Cancer has spread to axillary lymph nodes that are attached to each other or to other structures, or cancer may have spread to lymph nodes near the breastbone; or

- The tumor is larger than 2 centimeters but not larger than 5 centimeters. Cancer has spread to axillary lymph nodes that are attached to each other or to other structures, or cancer may have spread to lymph nodes near the breastbone; or

- The tumor is larger than 5 centimeters. Cancer has spread to axillary lymph nodes that may be attached to each other or to other structures, or cancer may have spread to lymph nodes near the breastbone.

Stage IIIB

In stage IIIB, the tumor may be any size and cancer has these characteristics:

- Has spread to the chest wall and/or the skin of the breast; and

- May have spread to axillary lymph nodes that may be attached to each other or to other structures, or cancer may have spread to lymph nodes near the breastbone.

Cancer that has spread to the skin of the breast is inflammatory breast cancer.

Stage IIIC

In stage IIIC, there may be no sign of cancer in the breast or the tumor may be any size and may have spread to the chest wall and/or the skin of the breast. Also, cancer has these characteristics:

- Has spread to lymph nodes above or below the collarbone; and

- May have spread to axillary lymph nodes or to lymph nodes near the breastbone.

133

Cancer that has spread to the skin of the breast is inflammatory breast cancer.

Stage IIIC breast cancer is divided into operable and inoperable stage IIIC. In operable stage IIIC, the cancer is found in ten or more axillary lymph nodes; or is found in lymph nodes below the collarbone; or is found in axillary lymph nodes and in lymph nodes near the breastbone.

In inoperable stage IIIC breast cancer, the cancer has spread to the lymph nodes above the collarbone.

Stage IV

In stage IV, the cancer has spread to other organs of the body, most often the bones, lungs, liver, or brain.

Inflammatory Breast Cancer

In inflammatory breast cancer, cancer has spread to the skin of the breast and the breast looks red and swollen and feels warm. The redness and warmth occur because the cancer cells block the lymph vessels in the skin. The skin of the breast may also show the pitted appearance called peau d'orange (like the skin of an orange). There may not be any lumps in the breast that can be felt. Inflammatory breast cancer may be stage IIIB, stage IIIC, or stage IV.

Recurrent Breast Cancer

Recurrent breast cancer is cancer that has recurred (come back) after it has been treated. The cancer may come back in the breast, in the chest wall, or in other parts of the body.

Standard Treatment Options

Different types of treatment are available for patients with breast cancer. Some treatments are standard (the currently used treatment), and some are being tested in clinical trials. Five types of standard treatment are used:

Surgery

Most patients with breast cancer have surgery to remove the cancer from the breast. Some of the lymph nodes under the arm are usually taken out and looked at under a microscope to see if they contain cancer cells.

Breast-conserving surgery, an operation to remove the cancer but not the breast itself, includes the following:

- **Lumpectomy**: Surgery to remove a tumor (lump) and a small amount of normal tissue around it.

- **Partial mastectomy:** Surgery to remove the part of the breast that has cancer and some normal tissue around it. This procedure is also called a segmental mastectomy.

Patients who are treated with breast-conserving surgery may also have some of the lymph nodes under the arm removed for biopsy. This procedure is called lymph node dissection. It may be done at the same time as the breast-conserving surgery or after. Lymph node dissection is done through a separate incision.

Other types of surgery include the following:

- **Total mastectomy:** Surgery to remove the whole breast that has cancer. This procedure is also called a simple mastectomy. Some of the lymph nodes under the arm may be removed for biopsy at the same time as the breast surgery or after. This is done through a separate incision.

- **Modified radical mastectomy:** Surgery to remove the whole breast that has cancer, many of the lymph nodes under the arm, the lining over the chest muscles, and sometimes, part of the chest wall muscles.

- **Radical mastectomy:** Surgery to remove the breast that has cancer, chest wall muscles under the breast, and all of the lymph nodes under the arm. This procedure is sometimes called a Halsted radical mastectomy.

Even if the doctor removes all the cancer that can be seen at the time of the surgery, some patients may be given radiation therapy, chemotherapy, or hormone therapy after surgery to kill any cancer cells that are left. Treatment given after the surgery, to lower the risk that the cancer will come back, is called adjuvant therapy.

If a patient is going to have a mastectomy, breast reconstruction (surgery to rebuild a breast's shape after a mastectomy) may be considered. Breast reconstruction may be done at the time of the mastectomy or at a future time. The reconstructed breast may be made with the patient's own (nonbreast) tissue or by using implants filled with saline or silicone gel.

Radiation Therapy

Radiation therapy is a cancer treatment that uses high-energy x-rays or other types of radiation to kill cancer cells or keep them from growing. There are two types of radiation therapy. External radiation therapy uses a machine outside the body to send radiation toward the cancer. Internal radiation therapy uses a radioactive substance sealed in needles, seeds, wires, or catheters that are placed directly into or near the cancer. The way the radiation therapy is given depends on the type and stage of the cancer being treated.

Chemotherapy

Chemotherapy is a cancer treatment that uses drugs to stop the growth of cancer cells, either by killing the cells or by stopping them from dividing. When chemotherapy is taken by mouth or injected into a vein or muscle, the drugs enter the bloodstream and can reach cancer cells throughout the body (systemic chemotherapy). When chemotherapy is placed directly into the spinal column, an organ, or a body cavity such as the abdomen, the drugs mainly affect cancer cells in those areas (regional chemotherapy). The way the chemotherapy is given depends on the type and stage of the cancer being treated.

Hormone Therapy

Hormone therapy is a cancer treatment that removes hormones or blocks their action and stops cancer cells from growing. Hormones are substances produced by glands in the body and circulated in the bloodstream. Some hormones can cause certain cancers to grow. If tests show that the cancer cells have places where hormones can attach (receptors), drugs, surgery, or radiation therapy is used to reduce the production of hormones or block them from working. The hormone estrogen, which makes some breast cancers grow, is made mainly by the ovaries. Treatment to stop the ovaries from making estrogen is called ovarian ablation.

Hormone therapy with tamoxifen is often given to patients with early stages of breast cancer and those with metastatic breast cancer (cancer that has spread to other parts of the body). Hormone therapy with tamoxifen or estrogens can act on cells all over the body and may increase the chance of developing endometrial cancer. Women taking tamoxifen should have a pelvic exam every year to look for any signs of cancer. Any vaginal bleeding, other than menstrual bleeding, should be reported to a doctor as soon as possible.

Hormone therapy with an aromatase inhibitor is given to some postmenopausal women who have hormone-dependent breast cancer. Hormone-dependent breast cancer needs the hormone estrogen to grow. Aromatase inhibitors decrease the body's estrogen by blocking an enzyme called aromatase from turning androgen into estrogen.

For the treatment of early stage breast cancer, certain aromatase inhibitors may be used as adjuvant therapy instead of tamoxifen or after two or more years of tamoxifen. For the treatment of metastatic breast cancer, aromatase inhibitors are being tested in clinical trials to compare them to hormone therapy with tamoxifen.

Targeted Therapy

Targeted therapy is a type of treatment that uses drugs or other substances to identify and attack specific cancer cells without harming normal cells. Monoclonal antibodies and tyrosine kinase inhibitors are two types of targeted therapies being studied in the treatment of breast cancer.

Monoclonal antibody therapy is a cancer treatment that uses antibodies made in the laboratory, from a single type of immune system cell. These antibodies can identify substances on cancer cells or normal substances that may help cancer cells grow. The antibodies attach to the substances and kill the cancer cells, block their growth, or keep them from spreading. Monoclonal antibodies are given by infusion. They may be used alone or to carry drugs, toxins, or radioactive material directly to cancer cells. Monoclonal antibodies may be used in combination with chemotherapy as adjuvant therapy.

Trastuzumab (Herceptin) is a monoclonal antibody that blocks the effects of the growth factor protein HER2, which sends growth signals to breast cancer cells. About one-fourth of patients with breast cancer have tumors that may be treated with trastuzumab combined with chemotherapy.

Tyrosine kinase inhibitors are targeted therapy drugs that block signals needed for tumors to grow. Tyrosine kinase inhibitors may be used in combination with other anticancer drugs as adjuvant therapy.

Lapatinib is a tyrosine kinase inhibitor that blocks the effects of the HER2 protein and other proteins inside tumor cells. It may be used to treat patients with HER2-positive breast cancer that has progressed following treatment with trastuzumab.

New Types of Treatment Being Tested in Clinical Trials

Patients may want to think about taking part in a clinical trial. For some patients, taking part in a clinical trial may be the best treatment

choice. Clinical trials are part of the cancer research process. Clinical trials are done to find out if new cancer treatments are safe and effective or better than the standard treatment.

Many of today's standard treatments for cancer are based on earlier clinical trials. Patients who take part in a clinical trial may receive the standard treatment or be among the first to receive a new treatment.

Patients who take part in clinical trials also help improve the way cancer will be treated in the future. Even when clinical trials do not lead to effective new treatments, they often answer important questions and help move research forward.

Patients can enter clinical trials before, during, or after starting their cancer treatment. Some clinical trials only include patients who have not yet received treatment. Other trials test treatments for patients whose cancer has not gotten better. There are also clinical trials that test new ways to stop cancer from recurring (coming back) or reduce the side effects of cancer treatment.

Sentinel Lymph Node Biopsy

Sentinel lymph node biopsy is the removal of the sentinel lymph node during surgery. The sentinel lymph node is the first lymph node to receive lymphatic drainage from a tumor. It is the first lymph node the cancer is likely to spread to from the tumor. A radioactive substance and/or blue dye is injected near the tumor. The substance or dye flows through the lymph ducts to the lymph nodes. The first lymph node to receive the substance or dye is removed. A pathologist views the tissue under a microscope to look for cancer cells. If cancer cells are not found, it may not be necessary to remove more lymph nodes. After the sentinel lymph node biopsy, the surgeon removes the tumor (breast-conserving surgery or mastectomy).

High-Dose Chemotherapy with Stem Cell Transplant

High-dose chemotherapy with stem cell transplant is a way of giving high doses of chemotherapy and replacing blood-forming cells destroyed by the cancer treatment. Stem cells (immature blood cells) are removed from the blood or bone marrow of the patient or a donor and are frozen and stored. After the chemotherapy is completed, the stored stem cells are thawed and given back to the patient through an infusion. These reinfused stem cells grow into (and restore) the body's blood cells.

Studies have shown that high-dose chemotherapy followed by stem cell transplant does not work better than standard chemotherapy in the treatment of breast cancer. Doctors have decided that, for now, high-dose chemotherapy should be tested only in clinical trials. Before taking part in such a trial, women should talk with their doctors about the serious side effects, including death, that may be caused by high-dose chemotherapy.

Follow-Up Tests

Some of the tests that were done to diagnose the cancer or to find out the stage of the cancer may be repeated. Some tests will be repeated in order to see how well the treatment is working. Decisions about whether to continue, change, or stop treatment may be based on the results of these tests. This is sometimes called re-staging.

Some of the tests will continue to be done from time to time after treatment has ended. The results of these tests can show if your condition has changed or if the cancer has recurred (come back). These tests are sometimes called follow-up tests or check-ups.

Chapter 12

Breast Cancer Treatment and Pregnancy

Breast cancer is a disease in which malignant (cancer) cells form in the tissues of the breast. Breast cancer is sometimes detected (found) in women who are pregnant or have just given birth. In women who are pregnant or who have just given birth, breast cancer occurs most often between the ages of 32 and 38. Breast cancer occurs about once in every 3,000 pregnancies.

Women who are pregnant, nursing, or have just given birth usually have tender, swollen breasts. This can make small lumps difficult to detect and may lead to delays in diagnosing breast cancer. Because of these delays, cancers are often found at a later stage in these women.

Breast Examination and Prenatal and Postnatal Care

To detect breast cancer, pregnant and nursing women should examine their breasts themselves. Women should also receive clinical breast examinations during their routine prenatal and postnatal examinations.

If an abnormality is found, one or all of the following tests may be used:

- **Ultrasound exam:** A procedure in which high-energy sound waves (ultrasound) are bounced off internal tissues or organs

Excerpted from PDQ® Cancer Information Summary. National Cancer Institute; Bethesda, MD. "Breast Cancer Treatment and Pregnancy (PDQ®): Patient Version." Updated 08/2009. Available at: http://cancer.gov. Accessed May 23, 2010.

and make echoes. The echoes form a picture of body tissues called a sonogram.

- **Mammogram:** An x-ray of the breast. A mammogram can be performed with little risk to the fetus. Mammograms in pregnant women may appear negative even though cancer is present.

- **Biopsy:** The removal of cells or tissues by a pathologist so they can be viewed under a microscope to check for signs of cancer.

Prognosis and Treatment Options

The prognosis (chance of recovery) and treatment options depend on the following:

- The stage of the cancer (whether it is in the breast only or has spread to other places in the body)

- The size of the tumor

- The type of breast cancer

- The age of the fetus

- Whether there are symptoms

- The patient's general health

After breast cancer has been diagnosed, tests are done to find out if cancer cells have spread within the breast or to other parts of the body. The process used to find out if the cancer has spread within the breast or to other parts of the body is called staging. The information gathered from the staging process determines the stage of the disease. It is important to know the stage in order to plan treatment.

Methods used to stage breast cancer can be changed to make them safer for the fetus. Standard methods for giving imaging scans can be adjusted so that the fetus is exposed to less radiation. Tests to measure the level of hormones in the blood may also be used in the staging process.

Different types of treatment are available for patients with breast cancer. Some treatments are standard (the currently used treatment), and some are being tested in clinical trials. A treatment clinical trial is a research study meant to help improve current treatments or obtain information on new treatments for patients with cancer. When clinical trials show that a new treatment is better than the standard treatment, the new treatment may become the standard treatment. Treatment

options for pregnant women depend on the stage of the disease and the age of the fetus.

Three types of standard treatment are used.

Surgery

Most pregnant women with breast cancer have surgery to remove the breast. Some of the lymph nodes under the arm are usually taken out and looked at under a microscope to see if they contain cancer cells. Types of surgery to remove the breast include the following:

- **Simple mastectomy:** A surgical procedure to remove the whole breast that contains cancer. Some of the lymph nodes under the arm may also be removed for biopsy. This procedure is also called a total mastectomy.

- **Modified radical mastectomy:** A surgical procedure to remove the whole breast that has cancer, many of the lymph nodes under the arm, the lining over the chest muscles, and sometimes, part of the chest wall muscles.

Breast-conserving surgery, an operation to remove the cancer but not the breast itself, includes the following:

- **Lumpectomy:** A surgical procedure to remove a tumor (lump) and a small amount of normal tissue around it. Most doctors also take out some of the lymph nodes under the arm.

- **Partial mastectomy:** A surgical procedure to remove the part of the breast that contains cancer and some normal tissue around it. Some of the lymph nodes under the arm may also be removed for biopsy. This procedure is also called a segmental mastectomy.

Even if the doctor removes all of the cancer that can be seen at the time of surgery, the patient may be given radiation therapy, chemotherapy, or hormone therapy after surgery to try to kill any cancer cells that may be left. Treatment given after surgery to increase the chances of a cure is called adjuvant therapy.

Radiation Therapy

Radiation therapy is a cancer treatment that uses high-energy x-rays or other types of radiation to kill cancer cells. There are two types of radiation therapy. External radiation therapy uses a machine

outside the body to send radiation toward the cancer. Internal radiation therapy uses a radioactive substance sealed in needles, seeds, wires, or catheters that are placed directly into or near the cancer. The way the radiation therapy is given depends on the type and stage of the cancer being treated.

Radiation therapy should not be given to pregnant women with early stage (stage I or II) breast cancer because it can harm the fetus. For women with late stage (stage III or IV) breast cancer, it should not be given during the first three months of pregnancy.

Chemotherapy

Chemotherapy is a cancer treatment that uses drugs to stop the growth of cancer cells, either by killing the cells or by stopping the cells from dividing. When chemotherapy is taken by mouth or injected into a vein or muscle, the drugs enter the bloodstream and can reach cancer cells throughout the body (systemic chemotherapy). When chemotherapy is placed directly into the spinal column, an organ, or a body cavity such as the abdomen, the drugs mainly affect cancer cells in those areas (regional chemotherapy). The way the chemotherapy is given depends on the type and stage of the cancer being treated.

Chemotherapy should not be given during the first three months of pregnancy. Chemotherapy given after this time does not usually harm the fetus but may cause early labor and low birth weight.

Hormone Therapy

Hormone therapy is a cancer treatment that removes hormones or blocks their action and stops cancer cells from growing. Hormones are substances produced by glands in the body and circulated in the bloodstream. Some hormones can cause certain cancers to grow. If tests show that the cancer cells have places where hormones can attach (receptors), drugs, surgery, or radiation therapy are used to reduce the production of hormones or block them from working. The effectiveness of hormone therapy, alone or combined with chemotherapy, in treating breast cancer in pregnant women is not yet known.

Pregnancy Termination

Ending the pregnancy does not seem to improve the mother's chance of survival and is not usually a treatment option.

If the cancer must be treated with chemotherapy and radiation therapy, which may harm the fetus, ending the pregnancy is sometimes

considered. This decision may depend on the stage of cancer, the age of the fetus, and the mother's chance of survival.

Treatment Options by Stage

Early Stage Breast Cancer (Stage I and Stage II)

Treatment of early stage breast cancer (stage I and stage II) in pregnant women may be surgery followed by adjuvant therapy as follows:

- Modified radical mastectomy
- Breast-conserving surgery: Lumpectomy, partial mastectomy or segmental mastectomy
- Breast-conserving surgery during pregnancy followed by radiation therapy after the baby is born
- Surgery during pregnancy followed by chemotherapy after the first three months of pregnancy
- Clinical trials of surgery followed by hormone therapy with or without chemotherapy

Late Stage Breast Cancer (Stage III and Stage IV

Treatment of late stage breast cancer (stage III and stage IV) in pregnant women may include the following:

- Radiation therapy
- Chemotherapy

Radiation therapy and chemotherapy should not be given during the first three months of pregnancy

Other Considerations for Pregnancy and Breast Cancer

Lactation (breast milk production) and breast-feeding should be stopped if surgery or chemotherapy is planned.

If surgery is planned, breast-feeding should be stopped to reduce blood flow in the breasts and make them smaller. Breast-feeding should also be stopped if chemotherapy is planned. Many anticancer drugs, especially cyclophosphamide and methotrexate, may occur in high levels in breast milk and may harm the nursing baby. Women receiving chemotherapy should not breast-feed. Stopping lactation does not improve survival of the mother.

Breast cancer does not appear to harm the fetus. Breast cancer cells do not seem to pass from the mother to the fetus.

Pregnancy does not seem to affect the survival of women who have had breast cancer in the past. Some doctors recommend that a woman wait two years after treatment for breast cancer before trying to have a baby, so that any early return of the cancer would be detected. This may affect a woman's decision to become pregnant. The fetus does not seem to be affected if the mother has previously had breast cancer.

The effects of treatment with high-dose chemotherapy and a bone marrow transplant, with or without radiation therapy, on later pregnancies are not known.

Part Three

Gynecologic Cancers

Chapter 13

Cervical Cancer

Chapter Contents

Section 13.1

Understanding Cervical Cancer

Excerpted from "What You Need to Know about Cancer of the Cervix,"
National Cancer Institute (www.cancer.gov), November 20, 2008.

The Cervix and Cancer

The cervix is part of a woman's reproductive system. It's in the pelvis. The cervix is the lower, narrow part of the uterus (womb).

The cervix is a passageway:

- The cervix connects the uterus to the vagina. During a menstrual period, blood flows from the uterus through the cervix into the vagina. The vagina leads to the outside of the body.

- The cervix makes mucus. During sex, mucus helps sperm move from the vagina through the cervix into the uterus.

- During pregnancy, the cervix is tightly closed to help keep the baby inside the uterus. During childbirth, the cervix opens to allow the baby to pass through the vagina.

Growths on the cervix can be benign or malignant. Benign growths are not cancer. They are not as harmful as malignant growths (cancer). Benign growths (polyps, cysts, or genital warts) are rarely a threat to life, and they don't invade the tissues around them. Malignant growths (cervical cancer) may sometimes be a threat to life. They can invade nearby tissues and organs and can spread to other parts of the body.

Cervical cancer begins in cells on the surface of the cervix. Over time, the cervical cancer can invade more deeply into the cervix and nearby tissues. The cancer cells can spread by breaking away from the original (primary) tumor. They enter blood vessels or lymph vessels, which branch into all the tissues of the body. The cancer cells may attach to other tissues and grow to form new tumors that may damage those tissues. The spread of cancer is called metastasis.

150

Cervical Cancer Risk Factors

When you get a diagnosis of cancer, it's natural to wonder what may have caused the disease. Doctors cannot always explain why one woman develops cervical cancer and another does not. However, we do know that a woman with certain risk factors may be more likely than others to develop cervical cancer. A risk factor is something that may increase the chance of developing a disease.

Studies have found a number of factors that may increase the risk of cervical cancer. For example, infection with HPV (human papillomavirus) is the main cause of cervical cancer. HPV infection and other risk factors may act together to increase the risk even more:

- **HPV infection:** HPV is the cause of nearly all cervical cancers. HPV is a group of viruses that can infect the cervix. An HPV infection that doesn't go away can cause cervical cancer in some women. HPV infections are very common. These viruses are passed from person to person through sexual contact. Most adults have been infected with HPV at some time in their lives, but most infections clear up on their own. Some types of HPV

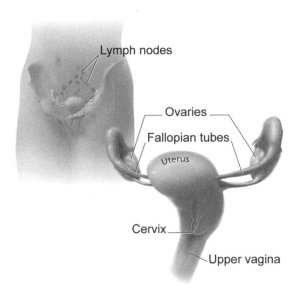

Figure 13.1. *The cervix and nearby organs. (Source: Don Bliss, National Cancer Institute)*

can cause changes to cells in the cervix. If these changes are found early, cervical cancer can be prevented by removing or killing the changed cells before they can become cancer cells. A vaccine for females aged 9–26 protects against two types of HPV infection that cause cervical cancer.

- **Lack of regular Pap tests:** Cervical cancer is more common among women who don't have regular Pap tests. The Pap test helps doctors find abnormal cells. Removing or killing the abnormal cells usually prevents cervical cancer.

- **Smoking:** Among women who are infected with HPV, smoking cigarettes slightly increases the risk of cervical cancer.

- **Weakened immune system** (the body's natural defense system): Infection with HIV (the virus that causes AIDS) or taking drugs that suppress the immune system increases the risk of cervical cancer.

- **Sexual history:** Women who have had many sexual partners have a higher risk of developing cervical cancer. Also, a woman who has had sex with a man who has had many sexual partners may be at higher risk of developing cervical cancer. In both cases, the risk of developing cervical cancer is higher because these women have a higher risk of HPV infection.

- **Using birth control pills for a long time:** Using birth control pills for a long time (five or more years) may slightly increase the risk of cervical cancer among women with HPV infection. However, the risk decreases quickly when women stop using birth control pills.

- **Having many children:** Studies suggest that giving birth to many children (five or more) may slightly increase the risk of cervical cancer among women with HPV infection.

- **DES (diethylstilbestrol):** DES may increase the risk of a rare form of cervical cancer in daughters exposed to this drug before birth. DES was given to some pregnant women in the United States between about 1940 and 1971. (It is no longer given to pregnant women.)

Having an HPV infection or other risk factors does not mean that a woman will develop cervical cancer. Most women who have risk factors for cervical cancer never develop it.

Symptoms

Early cervical cancers usually don't cause symptoms. When the cancer grows larger, women may notice one or more of these symptoms:

- Abnormal vaginal bleeding
- Bleeding that occurs between regular menstrual periods
- Bleeding after sexual intercourse, douching, or a pelvic exam
- Menstrual periods that last longer and are heavier than before
- Bleeding after going through menopause
- Increased vaginal discharge
- Pelvic pain
- Pain during sex

Infections or other health problems may also cause these symptoms. Only a doctor can tell for sure. A woman with any of these symptoms should tell her doctor so that problems can be diagnosed and treated as early as possible.

Detecting Cervical Cancer

Doctors recommend that women help reduce their risk of cervical cancer by having regular Pap tests. A Pap test (sometimes called Pap smear or cervical smear) is a simple test used to look at cervical cells. Pap tests can find cervical cancer or abnormal cells that can lead to cervical cancer.

Finding and treating abnormal cells can prevent most cervical cancer. Also, the Pap test can help find cancer early, when treatment is more likely to be effective.

For most women, the Pap test is not painful. It's done in a doctor's office or clinic during a pelvic exam. The doctor or nurse scrapes a sample of cells from the cervix. A lab checks the cells under a microscope for cell changes. Most often, abnormal cells found by a Pap test are not cancerous. The same sample of cells may be tested for HPV infection.

Section 13.2

How Does Your Doctor Know You Have Cervical Cancer?

If you're having symptoms that are like those of cervical cancer, your doctor will want to know why. Your doctor will ask some questions. You'll probably talk about these issues:

- Medical history

- Smoking history

- Family history of cancer

- How old you were when you first had sexual intercourse

- If you have had unprotected sex

- Other risk factors such as a history of genital warts or human papillomavirus (HPV) infection

And to learn more about your symptoms, your doctor will do a pelvic exam and may do other tests.

Many women don't have symptoms of cervical cancer. Sometimes your doctor may first see signs of cancer during a pelvic exam or a Pap test.

What a Doctor Learns from a Pelvic Exam

Your doctor or healthcare provider does a pelvic exam in the office. This exam is recommended as a regular screening for women. For it, you'll remove your clothes from the waist down and put on a medical gown. You lie on your back on an exam table and bend your knees. You place your feet in supports called stirrups at the end of the table. This position allows the doctor to look at or feel your uterus, vagina, ovaries,

fallopian tubes, bladder, and rectum. The doctor places a plastic or metal tool called a speculum inside your vagina to widen it. This lets the doctor see the upper portion of your vagina and your cervix. After removing the speculum, the doctor inserts two or three gloved fingers into your vagina and uses his or her other hand to press on your abdomen. This is to feel for lumps or anything unusual.

You may also have a Pap test and HPV test during a pelvic exam.

Some cervical cancers may be found during a pelvic exam. While your doctor cannot see precancerous changes such as dysplasia, he or she can see some invasive cancers during an exam. If the doctor or nurse notices something suspicious during the pelvic exam, additional tests can help determine whether you have cervical cancer.

What Your Doctor Learns from a Pap Test

A Pap test is the standard way to see if there are any cell changes that cause concern. You should see your doctor once a year for a regular Pap test if you are sexually active or over the age of 18. This test can help find cervical cancer or problems before they become cancer. The Pap test is simple and relatively painless. You can have it right in your healthcare provider's office. You should not have this test done during your period. The best time to have a Pap test is 10 to 20 days after the first day of your last period.

A Pap test may feel uncomfortable, but it should not hurt, and it takes just seconds. The doctor uses a tool called a speculum to widen your vagina and examine the upper part of your vagina and cervix, which is the area that connects your vagina to your uterus. The doctor then uses a small, soft brush to collect cells from the cervix and vagina. A specialized doctor called a pathologist looks at the cells under a microscope to check for cancer.

There are two types of Pap tests. The difference between them has to do with how the cells are checked after they are taken from your cervix. There is not a difference in how the cells are removed from you.

- With the regular method, the cell sample gets put on a slide and checked in a lab.

- With the newer liquid-based test, the doctor mixes a special liquid with the cells. This helps to preserve the cells for testing so that they can be seen and checked in the lab.

Studies show that the newer test is more successful in finding precancerous cells.

You should avoid these things before your Pap test.

- Do not douche for at least two days (48 hours).

- Do not have sex for two days (48 hours).

- Do not use a tampon for two days (48 hours).

- Do not use any kind of vaginal products or medicines for two days (48 hours).

Ask when you can expect results and how you will receive them. For instance, will you receive results by telephone or in the mail? Knowing how long you will have to wait for results may help you feel less anxious.

Why Your Doctor Does an HPV Test

If your Pap test shows that abnormal cells may be present, your doctor may do a HPV test. This test looks at the abnormal cells to see if HPV is present. Some types of HPV increase the risk of cervical cancer. The HPV test can be done along with the regular Pap test for women over age 30. The combined test is not used for women under 30 years old because in most women under 30 who have HPV, the virus is very common, but will go away before it causes any cell changes or symptoms. Your healthcare provider may also perform an HPV test if you have certain Pap abnormalities to determine if you require more testing. The preparation for the HPV test is the same as for a Pap test. Avoid sex, douching, tampon use, or any kind of vaginal products or medicines for two days before the test.

How Your Doctor Uses Colposcopy

If your doctor finds something suspicious during the pelvic exam or Pap test, he or she may decide to do a colposcopy. This test helps find abnormal areas in the cervix. This minor procedure can be done in your doctor's office. You lie in the same position as for a pelvic exam, on your back with your knees up and feet in stirrups. The doctor inserts a tool called a speculum to widen your vagina. The doctor or nurse puts a vinegar-like solution (3% to 5% acetic acid) on your cervix. This helps highlight abnormal areas. Next, your doctor places a special microscope called a colposcope at the opening of your vagina to magnify the surface of the cervix up to 40 times its normal size. You may have a biopsy during a colposcopy. This involves removing tissue to be examined under a microscope. It may pinch some.

Depending on the results of these tests, your doctor may need to do a biopsy.

Tests That Help Evaluate Cervical Cancer

Your doctor took a biopsy from your cervix to know that you have cancer. Your doctor may request more tests to learn more about your type of cancer and its specific location to help decide on the treatment that is likely to be most effective for you.

Your doctor will probably order imaging tests. These tests use machines that allow him or her to see inside your body and find the areas that have cancer. Most women need more than one test to find out their stage of cervical cancer. The tests will also help determine the best treatment for you. You'll probably have a few weeks to make decisions about your treatment.

Here are some of the tests that may be used for cervical cancer. Your doctor will likely only do the first three if you have a large tumor.

- **Pelvic exam under general anesthesia:** If you have a large tumor, your doctor may need to take a closer look at your cervix and check other areas, such as your bladder and rectum, to see if the cancer has spread. To do this, your doctor will put you to sleep with a general anesthesia. Then he or she will do one or both of these tests.

- **Proctoscopy:** To see if the cancer has spread to the rectum and the bottom part of the large intestine, the doctor uses a special instrument called a sigmoidoscope. For this test, you undress from the waist down and put on a hospital gown. You lie on your left side on the exam table. You pull your knees up toward your chest. The doctor gently inserts the sigmoidoscope through your rectum and into your large intestine. Air blows through the scope to allow for better viewing. The air may cause cramps. You may feel like you need to take a bowel movement. The doctor can look for abnormal areas and take biopsies during this procedure. After the test, you will expel the air by passing gas.

- **Cystoscopy:** This test lets the doctor see if the cancer has spread to your bladder. For it, the doctor looks at the inside of your bladder with a special instrument called a cystoscope. You lie on your back with your knees up and slightly apart. The doctor or nurse cleans your urethra (the opening where you urinate from) and applies some numbing medication. Or you may have general anesthesia so you fall to sleep and don't feel anything.

The doctor inserts the cystoscope through your urethra and up into your bladder. Water or saline solution flows through the scope into your bladder. This stretches the bladder wall, giving the doctor a better view. You may have some discomfort or feel an urge to urinate. If needed, the doctor can take a small sample of tissue to check for cancer. The whole test takes between five and 20 minutes. You will likely need a ride home after the test. You may feel a burning sensation when you urinate for a few days after the test.

- **Chest x-ray:** Doctors use this test to find out if the cancer has spread to your lungs. Unless the cancer is very advanced, it is not likely that the cancer has spread here. For the test, you stand in front of an x-ray scanner and hold your breath as the technician takes the picture. The test does not hurt, but the x-ray plate may feel cold against your skin.

- **Computed tomography (CT) scan:** The doctor may order a CT scan to see if the cancer has spread to lymph nodes or to other internal organs such as your liver or lungs. Unfortunately, CT scans have not been helpful in finding smaller amounts of cancer in the pelvic lymph nodes. A CT scan uses x-rays to take pictures of your body from many angles. These special x-rays are much more sensitive than a typical x-ray. To have the test, you lie still on a table as it gradually slides through the center of the CT scanner. Then the scanner directs a continuous beam of x-rays at your pelvis. A computer uses the data from the x-rays to create many pictures of your pelvis, which can be used together to create a three-dimensional picture. A CT scan is painless and noninvasive. You may be asked to hold your breath one or more times during the scan. In some cases, you may be asked to drink a contrast dye four to six hours before the scan. And you may be asked not to eat anything in the time between drinking the contrast dye and the scan. The contrast dye will gradually pass through your system and exit through your bowel movements.

- **Magnetic resonance imaging (MRI):** MRIs are used to find if cancer has spread. This is another method of staging cervical cancer. MRIs use radio waves and magnets to create images of your body. For this test, you lie still on a table as it passes through a tubelike scanner. The scanner directs a continuous beam of small amounts of radiofrequency radiation at the area being examined. A computer uses the data from the radio waves to create a three-dimensional picture of the inside of your body.

You may need more than one set of images. Each one may take two to 15 minutes, so the whole scan may take an hour or more. This test is painless and noninvasive. Ask for earplugs if they aren't offered since there is a loud thumping noise during the scan. If you're claustrophobic, you may receive a sedative before having this test.

- **Intravenous pyelogram (IVP):** This test allows your doctor to see if cancer has spread to the urinary tract. An IVP is an x-ray of your kidneys, bladder, and uterus, which are the tubes that carry urine from the kidneys down to the bladder. You will need to urinate before the exam. For this test, you lie flat on an exam table. After the nurse or doctor injects dye into a vein, a series of x-rays are taken at different intervals. You must stay still during the test. The test can take up to an hour. You may not need IVP if you've had a CT scan.

- **Positron-emission tomography (PET) scan:** This test shows whether the cancer has spread. The first step is for a doctor or nurse to inject a small amount of radioactive sugar into your vein. After about an hour, you lie down on an x-ray table that passes through a scanner. The scanner creates pictures that show where the sugar has collected in your body. Cancer cells use more sugar than normal cells. These imaging tests can help stage the cancer.

How Your Doctor Uses Biopsies to Diagnose Cervical Cancer

If your Pap test results show potential problems, or if your doctor feels something during a pelvic exam, you may need a biopsy. For it, your doctor removes a small amount of tissue from your cervix. Then a pathologist looks at it under a microscope to check for cancer cells. Every suspected cervical abnormality should be biopsied, even if a doctor cannot see it.

These are the different types of biopsies for diagnosing cervical precancers and cancer.

- **Colposcopic biopsy:** To take this biopsy, the doctor uses a special microscope called a colposcope. The doctor places this at the opening of your vagina. It magnifies the cervix up to 40 times. Then, the doctor removes a small amount of tissue from the abnormal area on your cervix. A colposcopy can't see cells high up in the cervix, so the doctor usually does an endocervical curettage (ECC) at the same time.

- **Endocervical curettage (ECC):** With this biopsy, the doctor scrapes tissue from the area between the outer part of the cervix and the inner part of the uterus. A pathologist looks at the removed cells to check for cancer.

- **Conization:** This test is also called a cone biopsy. The doctor does it to look at cells that are deeper in the cervix. The doctor uses a knife or electricity to remove a cone-shaped sample of tissue. Then a pathologist looks at the tissue to see if abnormal cells exist. If the doctor uses a knife, you'll have the biopsy done in the hospital, while you're sedated or asleep from general anesthesia. If your doctor uses a wire and electricity, it's called a loop excision (LEEP). You may have this kind of biopsy in the doctor's office. First, you'll have medicine put into the cervix to numb it.

- **Endometrial biopsy (EMB):** Sometimes, a doctor cannot determine whether abnormal cells exist in the cervix or in the internal lining of the uterus, called the endometrium. If the doctor believes the abnormal cells might be coming from the endometrium, he or she may perform an EMB. For it, a doctor scrapes cells from the lining of the uterus until he or she finds out where the problem exists. This test can be done at the doctor's office or in the hospital. No anesthesia is needed.

Some women may experience vaginal bleeding or cramps after these tests. This usually does not last long.

If the biopsy shows you have cancer, your doctor may order more tests, such as a computed tomography (CT scan). The results of all the tests determine the stage, which is the degree of spread, of the cancer. With this knowledge, your healthcare team designs the best treatment for you. Find out how your doctor plans on letting you know about your test results. And let your doctor know if there is a way you would like to be told about the results.

Questions to Ask Your Doctor about Cervical Biopsies

It is important that you take the time to gather as much information as possible. Below is a list of questions about biopsies you can talk about with your doctor.

- What type of biopsy will I have?

- Why do I need a biopsy?

- How long will it take?

- Will you use any numbing (anesthetic) medicine?

- Will I be awake during the biopsy?

- Will it hurt?

- How will I feel after it is over?

- How will I care for myself after the procedure?

- What are the side effects of a biopsy?

- How soon will I know the results?

- If I do have cancer, who will talk with me about treatment? When?

Advances in Diagnosing Cervical Cancer

Researchers continue to look into new and improved methods for diagnosing cervical cancer. Doctors use positron-emission tomography (PET) scans to take pictures of body functions such as blood flow. A review of several PET scan studies showed that the scans can find cervical cancer that has spread to the lymph nodes. This could help women avoid surgery to remove these nodes.

A study comparing CT scans to MRI scans is also underway. The goal of this study is to find out which imaging method better measures the size, extent, and location of cervical cancer before surgery. Results are expected soon.

Section 13.3

Staging and Treating Cervical Cancer

Excerpted from PDQ® Cancer Information Summary. National Cancer Institute; Bethesda, MD. "Cervical Cancer Treatment (PDQ®): Patient Version." Updated 4/2010. Available at: http://cancer.gov. Accessed May 23, 2010.

Stages of Cervical Cancer

After cervical cancer has been diagnosed, tests are done to find out if cancer cells have spread within the cervix or to other parts of the body.

The process used to find out if cancer has spread within the cervix or to other parts of the body is called staging. The information gathered from the staging process determines the stage of the disease. It is important to know the stage in order to plan treatment.

There are three ways that cancer spreads in the body:

- **Through tissue:** Cancer invades the surrounding normal tissue.

- **Through the lymph system:** Cancer invades the lymph system and travels through the lymph vessels to other places in the body.

- **Through the blood:** Cancer invades the veins and capillaries and travels through the blood to other places in the body.

When cancer cells break away from the primary (original) tumor and travel through the lymph or blood to other places in the body, another (secondary) tumor may form. This process is called metastasis. The secondary (metastatic) tumor is the same type of cancer as the primary tumor. The following stages are used for cervical cancer:

Stage 0 (Carcinoma in Situ)

In stage 0, abnormal cells are found in the innermost lining of the cervix. These abnormal cells may become cancer and spread into nearby normal tissue. Stage 0 is also called carcinoma in situ.

Stage I

In stage I, cancer has formed and is found in the cervix only. Stage I is divided into stages IA and IB, based on the amount of cancer that is found. For the purpose of understanding the sizes given, it may help to compare them to familiar objects. A sharp pencil point is about 1 mm, a new crayon point is about 2 mm, and a new pencil eraser is about 5 mm.

- **Stage IA:** A very small amount of cancer that can only be seen with a microscope is found in the tissues of the cervix. Stage IA is divided into stages IA1 and IA2, based on the size of the tumor. In stage IA1, the cancer is not more than 3 millimeters deep and not more than 7 millimeters wide. In stage IA2, the cancer is more than 3 but not more than 5 millimeters deep, and not more than 7 millimeters wide.

- **Stage IB:** In stage IB, cancer can only be seen with a microscope and is more than 5 millimeters deep or more than 7 millimeters wide, or can be seen without a microscope. Cancer that can be seen without a microscope is divided into stages IB1 and IB2, based on the size of the tumor. In stage IB1, the cancer can be seen without a microscope and is not larger than 4 centimeters. In stage IB2, the cancer can be seen without a microscope and is larger than 4 centimeters.

Stage II

In stage II, cancer has spread beyond the cervix but not to the pelvic wall (the tissues that line the part of the body between the hips) or to the lower third of the vagina. Stage II is divided into stages IIA and IIB, based on how far the cancer has spread.

- **Stage IIA:** Cancer has spread beyond the cervix to the upper two thirds of the vagina but not to tissues around the uterus.

- **Stage IIB:** Cancer has spread beyond the cervix to the upper two thirds of the vagina and to the tissues around the uterus.

Stage III

In stage III, cancer has spread to the lower third of the vagina, may have spread to the pelvic wall, and/or has caused the kidney to stop working. Stage III is divided into stages IIIA and IIIB, based on how far the cancer has spread.

- **Stage IIIA:** Cancer has spread to the lower third of the vagina but not to the pelvic wall.

- **Stage IIIB:** Cancer has spread to the pelvic wall and/or the tumor has become large enough to block the ureters (the tubes that connect the kidneys to the bladder). This blockage can cause the kidneys to enlarge or stop working. Cancer cells may also have spread to lymph nodes in the pelvis.

Stage IV

In stage IV, cancer has spread to the bladder, rectum, or other parts of the body. Stage IV is divided into stages IVA and IVB, based on where the cancer is found.

- **Stage IVA:** Cancer has spread to the bladder or rectal wall and may have spread to lymph nodes in the pelvis.

- **Stage IVB:** Cancer has spread beyond the pelvis and pelvic lymph nodes to other places in the body, such as the abdomen, liver, intestinal tract, or lungs.

Recurrent Cervical Cancer

Recurrent cervical cancer is cancer that has recurred (come back) after it has been treated. The cancer may come back in the cervix or in other parts of the body.

Treatment Options

Different types of treatment are available for patients with cervical cancer. Some treatments are standard (the currently used treatment), and some are being tested in clinical trials. A treatment clinical trial is a research study meant to help improve current treatments or obtain information on new treatments for patients with cancer. When clinical trials show that a new treatment is better than the standard treatment, the new treatment may become the standard treatment. Patients may want to think about taking part in a clinical trial. Some clinical trials are open only to patients who have not started treatment.

Three types of standard treatment are used for cervical cancer: surgery, radiation therapy, and chemotherapy.

Surgery

Surgery (removing the cancer in an operation) is sometimes used to treat cervical cancer. The following surgical procedures may be used:

- **Conization:** A procedure to remove a cone-shaped piece of tissue from the cervix and cervical canal. A pathologist views the tissue under a microscope to look for cancer cells. Conization may be used to diagnose or treat a cervical condition. This procedure is also called a cone biopsy.

- **Total hysterectomy:** Surgery to remove the uterus, including the cervix. If the uterus and cervix are taken out through the vagina, the operation is called a vaginal hysterectomy. If the uterus and cervix are taken out through a large incision (cut) in the abdomen, the operation is called a total abdominal hysterectomy. If the uterus and cervix are taken out through a small incision in the abdomen using a laparoscope, the operation is called a total laparoscopic hysterectomy.

- **Radical hysterectomy:** Surgery to remove the uterus, cervix, part of the vagina, and a wide area of ligaments and tissues around these organs. The ovaries, fallopian tubes, or nearby lymph nodes may also be removed.

- **Modified radical hysterectomy:** Surgery to remove the uterus, cervix, upper part of the vagina, and ligaments and tissues that closely surround these organs. Nearby lymph nodes may also be removed. In this type of surgery, not as many tissues and/or organs are removed as in a radical hysterectomy.

- **Bilateral salpingo-oophorectomy:** Surgery to remove both ovaries and both fallopian tubes.

- **Pelvic exenteration:** Surgery to remove the lower colon, rectum, and bladder. In women, the cervix, vagina, ovaries, and nearby lymph nodes are also removed. Artificial openings (stoma) are made for urine and stool to flow from the body to a collection bag. Plastic surgery may be needed to make an artificial vagina after this operation.

- **Cryosurgery:** A treatment that uses an instrument to freeze and destroy abnormal tissue, such as carcinoma in situ. This type of treatment is also called cryotherapy.

- **Laser surgery:** A surgical procedure that uses a laser beam (a narrow beam of intense light) as a knife to make bloodless cuts in tissue or to remove a surface lesion such as a tumor.

- **Loop electrosurgical excision procedure (LEEP):** A treatment that uses electrical current passed through a thin wire loop as a knife to remove abnormal tissue or cancer.

Radiation Therapy

Radiation therapy is a cancer treatment that uses high-energy x-rays or other types of radiation to kill cancer cells or keep them from growing. There are two types of radiation therapy. External radiation therapy uses a machine outside the body to send radiation toward the cancer. Internal radiation therapy uses a radioactive substance sealed in needles, seeds, wires, or catheters that are placed directly into or near the cancer. The way the radiation therapy is given depends on the type and stage of the cancer being treated.

Chemotherapy

Chemotherapy is a cancer treatment that uses drugs to stop the growth of cancer cells, either by killing the cells or by stopping them from dividing. When chemotherapy is taken by mouth or injected into a vein or muscle, the drugs enter the bloodstream and can reach cancer cells throughout the body (systemic chemotherapy). When chemotherapy is placed directly into the spinal column, an organ, or a body cavity such as the abdomen, the drugs mainly affect cancer cells in those areas (regional chemotherapy). The way the chemotherapy is given depends on the type and stage of the cancer being treated.

Follow-Up Tests

Some of the tests that were done to diagnose the cancer or to find out the stage of the cancer may be repeated. Some tests will be repeated in order to see how well the treatment is working. Decisions about whether to continue, change, or stop treatment may be based on the results of these tests. This is sometimes called re-staging.

Some of the tests will continue to be done from time to time after treatment has ended. The results of these tests can show if your condition has changed or if the cancer has recurred (come back). These tests are sometimes called follow-up tests or check-ups.

Chapter 14

Endometrial Cancer

Chapter Contents

Section 14.1

Understanding Endometrial Cancer

Excerpted from PDQ® Cancer Information Summary. National Cancer Institute; Bethesda, MD. "Endometrial Cancer Prevention (PDQ®): Patient Version." Updated 05/2009. Available at: http://cancer.gov. Accessed July 23, 2009.

Endometrial cancer is the most common invasive cancer of the female reproductive system. It is a disease in which malignant (cancer) cells form in the tissues of the endometrium. The endometrium is the lining of the uterus. The uterus is part of the female reproductive system. It is a hollow, pear-shaped, muscular organ in the pelvis, where a fetus grows.

Cancer of the endometrium is different from cancer of the muscle of the uterus, which is called sarcoma of the uterus.

Endometrial cancer usually occurs in women after menopause and affects more white women than black women. Black women diagnosed with endometrial cancer are more likely to have more advanced disease at diagnosis and are more likely to die from endometrial cancer than white women.

Endometrial Cancer Prevention

Avoiding risk factors and increasing protective factors may help prevent cancer. The following risk factors may increase the risk of endometrial cancer:

- Estrogen

- Tamoxifen

- Inherited risk

- Polycystic ovary syndrome

- Body fat

The following protective factors may decrease the risk of endometrial cancer:

- Combination oral contraceptives
- Physical activity
- Pregnancy and breastfeeding
- Diet

Cancer prevention clinical trials are used to study ways to prevent cancer. New ways to prevent endometrial cancer are being studied.

Avoiding risk factors and increasing protective factors may help prevent cancer. Avoiding cancer risk factors such as smoking, being overweight, and lack of exercise may help prevent certain cancers. Increasing protective factors such as quitting smoking, eating a healthy diet, and exercising may also help prevent some cancers. Talk to your doctor or other health care professional about how you might lower your risk of cancer.

Risk Factors

The following risk factors may increase the risk of endometrial cancer:

Estrogen

Estrogen is a hormone made by the body. It helps the body develop and maintain female sex characteristics. Estrogen can affect the growth of some cancers, including endometrial cancer. A woman's risk of developing endometrial cancer is increased by being exposed to estrogen in the following ways:

Estrogen-only hormone replacement therapy: Estrogen may be given to replace the estrogen no longer produced by the ovaries in postmenopausal women or women whose ovaries have been removed. This is called hormone replacement therapy (HRT), or hormone therapy (HT). The use of hormone replacement therapy that contains only estrogen increases the risk of endometrial cancer. For this reason, estrogen therapy alone is usually prescribed only for women who do not have a uterus.

When estrogen is combined with progestin (another hormone), it is called combination estrogen-progestin replacement therapy. For postmenopausal women, taking estrogen in combination with progestin does not increase the risk of endometrial cancer.

Early menstruation: Beginning to have menstrual periods at an early age increases the number of years the body is exposed to estrogen and increases a woman's risk of endometrial cancer.

Late menopause: Women who reach menopause at an older age are exposed to estrogen for a longer time and have an increased risk of endometrial cancer.

Never being pregnant: Because estrogen levels are lower during pregnancy, women who have never been pregnant are exposed to estrogen for a longer time than women who have been pregnant. This increases the risk of endometrial cancer.

Tamoxifen

Tamoxifen is one of a group of drugs called selective estrogen receptor modulators, or SERMs. Tamoxifen acts like estrogen on some tissues in the body, such as the uterus, but blocks the effects of estrogen on other tissues, such as the breast. When tamoxifen is used to prevent breast cancer in women who are at high risk for the disease, it increases the risk of endometrial cancer. This risk is greater in postmenopausal women.

Raloxifene is a SERM that is used to prevent bone weakness in postmenopausal women. It does not have estrogen-like effects on the uterus and has not been shown to increase the risk of endometrial cancer. Other SERMs are being studied in clinical trials.

Inherited Risk

Hereditary nonpolyposis colon cancer (HNPCC) syndrome is an inherited disorder caused by changes in certain genes. Women who have HNPCC syndrome have a much higher risk of developing endometrial cancer than women who do not have HNPCC syndrome.

Polycystic Ovary Syndrome

Women who have polycystic ovary syndrome (a disorder of the hormones made by the ovaries) have an increased risk of endometrial cancer.

Body Fat

Obesity increases the risk of endometrial cancer. This may be because obesity is related to other risk factors such as estrogen levels,

polycystic ovary syndrome, lack of physical activity, and a diet that is high in saturated fats. It is not known if losing weight decreases the risk of endometrial cancer.

Protective Factors

The following protective factors may decrease risk of endometrial cancer:

- **Combination oral contraceptives:** Taking contraceptives that combine estrogen and progestin (combination oral contraceptives) decreases the risk of endometrial cancer. The protective effect of combination oral contraceptives increases with the length of time they are used, and can last for many years after oral contraceptive use has been stopped.

- **Physical activity:** Physical activity may lower the risk of endometrial cancer.

- **Pregnancy and breast-feeding:** Estrogen levels are lower during pregnancy and when breast-feeding. Being pregnant and/ or breast-feeding may lower the risk of endometrial cancer.

- **Diet:** A diet low in saturated fats and high in fruits and vegetables may lower the risk of endometrial cancer. The risk may also be lowered when soy -based foods are a regular part of the diet.

Section 14.2

Endometrial Cancer Screening

Excerpted from PDQ® Cancer Information Summary. National Cancer Institute; Bethesda, MD. "Endometrial Cancer Screening (PDQ®): Patient Version." Updated 06/2009. Available at: http://cancer.gov. Accessed July 23, 2009.

Tests are used to screen for different types of cancer. Some screening tests are used because they have been shown to be helpful both in finding cancers early and decreasing the chance of dying from these cancers. Other tests are used because they have been shown to find cancer in some people; however, it has not been proven in clinical trials that use of these tests will decrease the risk of dying from cancer.

Scientists study screening tests to find those with the fewest risks and most benefits. Cancer screening trials also are meant to show whether early detection (finding cancer before it causes symptoms) decreases a person's chance of dying from the disease. For some types of cancer, finding and treating the disease at an early stage may result in a better chance of recovery.

Endometrial cancer is usually found early. Endometrial cancer usually causes symptoms (such as vaginal bleeding) and is found at an early stage, when there is a good chance of recovery. There is no standard or routine screening test for endometrial cancer.

Screening for endometrial cancer is under study and there are screening clinical trials taking place in many parts of the country. Tests that may detect (find) endometrial cancer are being studied.

Pap Test

A Pap test is a procedure to collect cells from the surface of the cervix and vagina. A piece of cotton, a brush, or a small wooden stick is used to gently scrape cells from the cervix and vagina. The cells are viewed under a microscope to find out if they are abnormal. This procedure is also called a Pap smear.

Pap tests are not used to screen for endometrial cancer; however, Pap test results sometimes show signs of an abnormal endometrium (lining of the uterus). Follow-up tests may detect endometrial cancer.

Transvaginal Ultrasound

It has not been proven that screening by transvaginal ultrasound (TVU) lowers the number of deaths caused by endometrial cancer.

Transvaginal ultrasound (TVU) is a procedure used to examine the vagina, uterus, fallopian tubes, and bladder. It is also called endovaginal ultrasound. An ultrasound transducer (probe) is inserted into the vagina and used to bounce high-energy sound waves (ultrasound) off internal tissues or organs and make echoes. The echoes form a picture of body tissues called a sonogram. The doctor can identify tumors by looking at the sonogram.

TVU is commonly used to examine women who have abnormal vaginal bleeding. For women who have or are at risk for hereditary non-polyposis colon cancer, experts suggest yearly screening with transvaginal ultrasound, beginning as early as age 25.

Endometrial Sampling

It has not been proven that screening by endometrial sampling (biopsy) lowers the number of deaths caused by endometrial cancer.

Endometrial sampling is the removal of tissue from the endometrium by inserting a brush, curette, or thin, flexible tube through the cervix and into the uterus. The tool is used to gently scrape a small amount of tissue from the endometrium and then remove the tissue samples. A pathologist views the tissue under a microscope to look for cancer cells.

Endometrial sampling is commonly used to examine women who have abnormal vaginal bleeding. If you have abnormal vaginal bleeding, check with your doctor.

Section 14.3

Staging and Treating Endometrial Cancer

Excerpted from PDQ® Cancer Information Summary. National Cancer Institute; Bethesda, MD. "Endometrial Cancer Treatment PDQ®): Patient Version." Updated 10/2009. Available at: http://cancer.gov. Accessed May 24, 2010.

Diagnosing Endometrial Cancer

Possible signs of endometrial cancer include unusual vaginal discharge or pain in the pelvis. These and other symptoms may be caused by endometrial cancer. Other conditions may cause the same symptoms. A doctor should be consulted if any of the following problems occur:

- Bleeding or discharge not related to menstruation (periods)

- Difficult or painful urination

- Pain during sexual intercourse

- Pain in the pelvic area

Tests that examine the endometrium are used to detect (find) and diagnose endometrial cancer.

Because endometrial cancer begins inside the uterus, it does not usually show up in the results of a Pap test. For this reason, a sample of endometrial tissue must be removed and examined under a microscope to look for cancer cells. One of the following procedures may be used:

Endometrial biopsy: The removal of tissue from the endometrium (inner lining of the uterus) by inserting a thin, flexible tube through the cervix and into the uterus. The tube is used to gently scrape a small amount of tissue from the endometrium and then remove the tissue samples. A pathologist views the tissue under a microscope to look for cancer cells.

Dilatation and curettage: Surgery to remove samples of tissue or the inner lining of the uterus. The cervix is dilated and a curette (spoon-shaped instrument) is inserted into the uterus to remove tissue. Tissue samples may be taken and checked under a microscope for signs of disease. This procedure is also called a D&C.

Prognosis

The prognosis (chance of recovery) and treatment options depend on the following:

- The stage of the cancer (whether it is in the endometrium only, involves the whole uterus, or has spread to other places in the body).

- How the cancer cells look under a microscope.

- Whether the cancer cells are affected by progesterone.

Endometrial cancer is highly curable.

Stages of Endometrial Cancer

After endometrial cancer has been diagnosed, tests are done to find out if cancer cells have spread within the uterus or to other parts of the body.

The process used to find out whether the cancer has spread within the uterus or to other parts of the body is called staging. The information gathered from the staging process determines the stage of the disease. It is important to know the stage in order to plan treatment. Certain tests and procedures are used in the staging process. A hysterectomy (an operation in which the uterus is removed) will usually be done to help find out how far the cancer has spread. The following stages are used for endometrial cancer.

Stage I

In stage I, cancer is found in the uterus only. Stage I is divided into stages IA, IB, and IC, based on how far the cancer has spread.

- **Stage IA:** Cancer is in the endometrium only.

- **Stage IB:** Cancer has spread into the inner half of the myometrium (muscle layer of the uterus).

- **Stage IC:** Cancer has spread into the outer half of the myometrium.

Stage II

In stage II, cancer has spread from the uterus to the cervix, but has not spread outside the uterus. Stage II is divided into stages IIA and IIB, based on how far the cancer has spread into the cervix.

- **Stage IIA:** Cancer has spread to the glands where the cervix and uterus meet.

- **Stage IIB:** Cancer has spread into the connective tissue of the cervix.

Stage III

In stage III, cancer has spread beyond the uterus and cervix, but has not spread beyond the pelvis. Stage III is divided into stages IIIA, IIIB, and IIIC, based on how far the cancer has spread within the pelvis.

- **Stage IIIA:** Cancer has spread to one or more of the following: the outermost layer of the uterus; or tissue just beyond the uterus; or the peritoneum.

- **Stage IIIB:** Cancer has spread beyond the uterus and cervix, into the vagina.

- **Stage IIIC:** Cancer has spread to lymph nodes near the uterus.

Stage IV

In stage IV, cancer has spread beyond the pelvis. Stage IV is divided into stages IVA and IVB, based on how far the cancer has spread.

- **Stage IVA:** Cancer has spread to the bladder and/or bowel wall.

- **Stage IVB:** Cancer has spread to other parts of the body beyond the pelvis, including lymph nodes in the abdomen and/or groin.

Recurrent Endometrial Cancer

Recurrent endometrial cancer is cancer that has recurred (come back) after it has been treated. The cancer may come back in the pelvis, in lymph nodes in the abdomen, or in other parts of the body.

Treatment Option Overview

Different types of treatment are available for patients with endometrial cancer. Some treatments are standard (the currently used treatment), and some are being tested in clinical trials. Three types of standard treatment are used:

Surgery

Surgery (removing the cancer in an operation) is the most common treatment for endometrial cancer. The following surgical procedures may be used:

- **Total hysterectomy:** Surgery to remove the uterus, including the cervix. If the uterus and cervix are taken out through the vagina, the operation is called a vaginal hysterectomy. If the uterus and cervix are taken out through a large incision (cut) in the abdomen, the operation is called a total abdominal hysterectomy. If the uterus and cervix are taken out through a small incision (cut) in the abdomen using a laparoscope, the operation is called a total laparoscopic hysterectomy.

- **Bilateral salpingo-oophorectomy:** Surgery to remove both ovaries and both fallopian tubes.

- **Radical hysterectomy:** Surgery to remove the uterus, cervix, and part of the vagina. The ovaries, fallopian tubes, or nearby lymph nodes may also be removed.

Even if the doctor removes all the cancer that can be seen at the time of the surgery, some patients may be given radiation therapy or hormone treatment after surgery to kill any cancer cells that are left. Treatment given after the surgery, to lower the risk that the cancer will come back, is called adjuvant therapy.

Radiation Therapy

Radiation therapy is a cancer treatment that uses high-energy x-rays or other types of radiation to kill cancer cells or keep them from growing. There are two types of radiation therapy. External radiation therapy uses a machine outside the body to send radiation toward the cancer. Internal radiation therapy uses a radioactive substance sealed in needles, seeds, wires, or catheters that are placed directly into or

near the cancer. The way the radiation therapy is given depends on the type and stage of the cancer being treated.

Hormone Therapy

Hormone therapy is a cancer treatment that removes hormones or blocks their action and stops cancer cells from growing. Hormones are substances made by glands in the body and circulated in the bloodstream. Some hormones can cause certain cancers to grow. If tests show that the cancer cells have places where hormones can attach (receptors), drugs, surgery, or radiation therapy are used to reduce the production of hormones or block them from working.

Clinical Trials

For some patients, taking part in a clinical trial may be the best treatment choice. Clinical trials are part of the cancer research process. Clinical trials are done to find out if new cancer treatments are safe and effective or better than the standard treatment.

Many of today's standard treatments for cancer are based on earlier clinical trials. Patients who take part in a clinical trial may receive the standard treatment or be among the first to receive a new treatment.

Patients who take part in clinical trials also help improve the way cancer will be treated in the future. Even when clinical trials do not lead to effective new treatments, they often answer important questions and help move research forward.

Some clinical trials only include patients who have not yet received treatment. Other trials test treatments for patients whose cancer has not gotten better. There are also clinical trials that test new ways to stop cancer from recurring (coming back) or reduce the side effects of cancer treatment. Clinical trials are taking place in many parts of the country.

Chemotherapy

Chemotherapy is currently being tested as a treatment for endometrial cancer. Chemotherapy is a cancer treatment that uses drugs to stop the growth of cancer cells, either by killing the cells or by stopping the cells from dividing. When chemotherapy is taken by mouth or injected into a vein or muscle, the drugs enter the bloodstream and can reach cancer cells throughout the body (systemic chemotherapy). When

chemotherapy is placed directly into the spinal column, an organ, or a body cavity such as the abdomen, the drugs mainly affect cancer cells in those areas (regional chemotherapy). The way the chemotherapy is given depends on the type and stage of the cancer being treated.

Follow-Up Tests

Follow-up tests may be needed. Some of the tests that were done to diagnose the cancer or to find out the stage of the cancer may be repeated. Some tests will be repeated in order to see how well the treatment is working. Decisions about whether to continue, change, or stop treatment may be based on the results of these tests. This is sometimes called re-staging.

Some of the tests will continue to be done from time to time after treatment has ended. The results of these tests can show if your condition has changed or if the cancer has recurred (come back). These tests are sometimes called follow-up tests or check-ups.

Chapter 15

Gestational Trophoblastic Tumors

Description

Gestational trophoblastic tumor, a rare cancer in women, is a disease in which cancer (malignant) cells grow in the tissues that are formed following conception (the joining of sperm and egg). Gestational trophoblastic tumors start inside the uterus, the hollow, muscular, pear-shaped organ where a baby grows. This type of cancer occurs in women during the years when they are able to have children. There are two types of gestational trophoblastic tumors: hydatidiform mole and choriocarcinoma.

If a patient has a hydatidiform mole (also called a molar pregnancy), the sperm and egg cells have joined without the development of a baby in the uterus. Instead, the tissue that is formed resembles grape-like cysts. Hydatidiform mole does not spread outside of the uterus to other parts of the body.

If a patient has a choriocarcinoma, the tumor may have started from a hydatidiform mole or from tissue that remains in the uterus following an abortion or delivery of a baby. Choriocarcinoma can spread from the uterus to other parts of the body. A very rare type of gestational trophoblastic tumor starts in the uterus where the placenta was attached. This type of cancer is called placental-site trophoblastic disease.

PDQ® Cancer Information Summary. National Cancer Institute; Bethesda, MD. "Gestational Trophoblastic Tumors Treatment (PDQ®): Patient Version." Updated 06/2008. Available at: http://cancer.gov. Accessed July 23, 2009.

Gestational trophoblastic tumor is not always easy to find. In its early stages, it may look like a normal pregnancy. A doctor should be seen if the there is vaginal bleeding (not menstrual bleeding) and if a woman is pregnant and the baby hasn't moved at the expected time.

If there are symptoms, a doctor may use several tests to see if the patient has a gestational trophoblastic tumor. An internal (pelvic) examination is usually the first of these tests. The doctor will feel for any lumps or strange feeling in the shape or size of the uterus. The doctor may then do an ultrasound, a test that uses sound waves to find tumors. A blood test will also be done to look for high levels of a hormone called beta-HCG (beta human chorionic gonadotropin) which is present during normal pregnancy. If a woman is not pregnant and HCG is in the blood, it can be a sign of gestational trophoblastic tumor.

The chance of recovery (prognosis) and choice of treatment depend on the type of gestational trophoblastic tumor, whether it has spread to other places, and the patient's general state of health.

Stages of Gestational Trophoblastic Tumors

Once gestational trophoblastic tumor has been found, more tests will be done to find out if the cancer has spread from inside the uterus to other parts of the body. This process of finding out the extent of potential spread is called staging. Treatment of gestational trophoblastic tumor depends on the stage of the disease and the patient's age and general health. The following stages are used for gestational trophoblastic tumor:

- **Hydatidiform mole:** Cancer is found only in the space inside the uterus. If the cancer is found in the muscle of the uterus, it is called an invasive mole (choriocarcinoma destruens).

- **Placental-site gestational trophoblastic tumors:** Cancer is found in the place where the placenta was attached and in the muscle of the uterus.

- **Nonmetastatic:** Cancer cells have grown inside the uterus from tissue remaining following treatment of a hydatidiform mole or following an abortion or delivery of a baby. Cancer has not spread outside the uterus.

In addition to the above stages, other stages may be identified. In metastatic cancer, cancer cells have grown inside the uterus from tissue remaining following treatment of a hydatidiform mole or following an abortion or delivery of a baby. The cancer has spread from the

uterus to other parts of the body. Metastatic gestational trophoblastic tumors are considered good prognosis or poor prognosis.

- **Metastatic, good prognosis:** Metastatic gestational tropho-blastic tumor is considered good prognosis if all of the following are true: The last pregnancy was less than four months ago; the level of beta-HCG in the blood is low; cancer has not spread to the liver or brain; and the patient has not received chemotherapy earlier.

- **Metastatic, poor prognosis:** Metastatic gestational tropho-blastic tumor is considered poor prognosis if any the following are true: The last pregnancy was more than four months ago; the level of beta-HCG in the blood is high; cancer has spread to the liver or brain; the patient received chemotherapy earlier and the cancer did not go away; or the tumor began after the completion of a normal pregnancy.

In addition, gestational trophoblastic tumor may be described as recurrent. Recurrent disease means that the cancer has come back (recurred) after it has been treated. It may come back in the uterus or in another part of the body.

Treatment Options

Different types of treatment are available for patients with gesta-tional trophoblastic tumor. Some treatments are standard (the cur-rently used treatment), and some are being tested in clinical trials. Two kinds of standard treatment are used: surgery (taking out the cancer) and chemotherapy (using drugs to kill cancer cells). Radiation therapy (using high-energy x-rays to kill cancer cells) may be used in certain cases to treat cancer that has spread to other parts of the body.

The doctor may take out the cancer using one of the following op-erations:

- Dilation and curettage (D&C) with suction evacuation is stretching the opening of the uterus (the cervix) and removing the material inside the uterus with a small vacuum-like device. The walls of the uterus are then scraped gently to remove any material that may remain in the uterus. This is used only for molar pregnancies.

- Hysterectomy is an operation to take out the uterus. The ovaries usually are not removed in the treatment of this disease.

Chemotherapy uses drugs to kill cancer cells. It may be taken by pill or put into the body by a needle in a vein or muscle. It is called a systemic treatment because the drugs enter the bloodstream, travel through the body, and can kill cancer cells outside the uterus. Chemotherapy may be given before or after surgery or alone.

Radiation therapy uses high-energy x-rays to kill cancer cells and shrink tumors. Radiation may come from a machine outside the body (external-beam radiation therapy) or from putting materials that produce radiation (radioisotopes) through thin plastic tubes into the area where the cancer cells are found (internal radiation).

Clinical Trials

For some patients, taking part in a clinical trial may be the best treatment choice. Clinical trials are part of the cancer research process. Clinical trials are done to find out if new cancer treatments are safe and effective or better than the standard treatment.

Many of today's standard treatments for cancer are based on earlier clinical trials. Patients who take part in a clinical trial may receive the standard treatment or be among the first to receive a new treatment.

Patients who take part in clinical trials also help improve the way cancer will be treated in the future. Even when clinical trials do not lead to effective new treatments, they often answer important questions and help move research forward.

Some clinical trials only include patients who have not yet received treatment. Other trials test treatments for patients whose cancer has not gotten better. There are also clinical trials that test new ways to stop cancer from recurring (coming back) or reduce the side effects of cancer treatment.

Hydatidiform Mole

Treatment may be one of the following:

- Removal of the mole using dilation and curettage (D&C) and suction evacuation

- Surgery to remove the uterus (hysterectomy)

Following surgery, the doctor will follow the patient closely with regular blood tests to make sure the level of beta-HCG in the blood falls to normal levels. If the blood level of beta-HCG increases or does not go down to normal, more tests will be done to see whether the tumor

has spread. Treatment will then depend on whether the patient has nonmetastatic disease or metastatic disease.

Placental-Site Gestational Trophoblastic Tumors

Treatment will probably be surgery to remove the uterus (hysterectomy).

Nonmetastatic Gestational Trophoblastic Tumors

Treatment may be one of the following:

- Chemotherapy
- Surgery to remove the uterus (hysterectomy) if the patient no longer wishes to have children

Good Prognosis Metastatic Gestational Trophoblastic Tumors

Treatment may be one of the following:

- Chemotherapy
- Surgery to remove the uterus (hysterectomy) followed by chemotherapy
- Chemotherapy followed by hysterectomy if cancer remains following chemotherapy

Poor Prognosis Metastatic Gestational Trophoblastic Tumors

Treatment will probably be chemotherapy. Radiation therapy may also be given to places where the cancer has spread, such as the brain.

Recurrent Gestational Trophoblastic Tumors

Treatment will probably be chemotherapy.

Chapter 16

Ovarian Cancer

Chapter Contents

Section 16.1

What You Need to Know About Ovarian Cancer

Excerpted from "What You Need to Know About Ovarian Cancer,"
National Cancer Institute (www.cancer.gov), 2006.

The Ovaries

The ovaries are part of a woman's reproductive system. They are in
the pelvis. Each ovary is about the size of an almond.

The ovaries make the female hormones—estrogen and progesterone. They also release eggs. An egg travels from an ovary through a
fallopian tube to the womb (uterus).

When a woman goes through her "change of life" (menopause), her
ovaries stop releasing eggs and make far lower levels of hormones.

Benign and Malignant Cysts

An ovarian cyst may be found on the surface of an ovary or inside
it. A cyst contains fluid. Sometimes it contains solid tissue too. Most
ovarian cysts are benign (not cancer).

Most ovarian cysts go away with time. Sometimes, a doctor will find
a cyst that does not go away or that gets larger. The doctor may order
tests to make sure that the cyst is not cancer.

Ovarian Cancer

Ovarian cancer can invade, shed, or spread to other organs:

- **Invade:** A malignant ovarian tumor can grow and invade organs
  next to the ovaries, such as the fallopian tubes and uterus.

- **Shed:** Cancer cells can shed (break off) from the main ovarian tumor. Shedding into the abdomen may lead to new tumors
  forming on the surface of nearby organs and tissues. The doctor
  may call these seeds or implants.

- **Spread:** Cancer cells can spread through the lymphatic system
  to lymph nodes in the pelvis, abdomen, and chest. Cancer cells

may also spread through the bloodstream to organs such as the liver and lungs.

When cancer spreads from its original place to another part of the body, the new tumor has the same kind of abnormal cells and the same name as the original tumor. For example, if ovarian cancer spreads to the liver, the cancer cells in the liver are actually ovarian cancer cells. The disease is metastatic ovarian cancer, not liver cancer. For that reason, it is treated as ovarian cancer, not liver cancer. Doctors call the new tumor "distant" or metastatic disease.

Risk Factors

Doctors cannot always explain why one woman develops ovarian cancer and another does not. However, we do know that women with certain risk factors may be more likely than others to develop ovarian cancer. A risk factor is something that may increase the chance of developing a disease. Studies have found the following risk factors for ovarian cancer:

- **Family history of cancer:** Women who have a mother, daughter, or sister with ovarian cancer have an increased risk of the disease. Also, women with a family history of cancer of the breast, uterus, colon, or rectum may also have an increased risk of ovarian cancer. If several women in a family have ovarian or breast cancer, especially at a young age, this is considered a strong family history. If you have a strong family history of ovarian or breast cancer, you may wish to talk to a genetic counselor. The counselor may suggest genetic testing for you and the women in your family. Genetic tests can sometimes show the presence of specific gene changes that increase the risk of ovarian cancer.

- **Personal history of cancer:** Women who have had cancer of the breast, uterus, colon, or rectum have a higher risk of ovarian cancer.

- **Age over 55:** Most women are over age 55 when diagnosed with ovarian cancer.

- **Never pregnant:** Older women who have never been pregnant have an increased risk of ovarian cancer.

- **Menopausal hormone therapy:** Some studies have suggested that women who take estrogen by itself (estrogen without progesterone) for ten or more years may have an increased risk of ovarian cancer.

Scientists have also studied whether taking certain fertility drugs, using talcum powder, or being obese are risk factors. It is not clear whether these are risk factors, but if they are, they are not strong risk factors.

Having a risk factor does not mean that a woman will get ovarian cancer. Most women who have risk factors do not get ovarian cancer. On the other hand, women who do get the disease often have no known risk factors, except for growing older. Women who think they may be at risk of ovarian cancer should talk with their doctor.

Symptoms

Early ovarian cancer may not cause obvious symptoms. But, as the cancer grows, symptoms may include the following:

- Pressure or pain in the abdomen, pelvis, back, or legs
- A swollen or bloated abdomen
- Nausea, indigestion, gas, constipation, or diarrhea
- Feeling very tired all the time

Less common symptoms include:

- Shortness of breath
- Feeling the need to urinate often
- Unusual vaginal bleeding (heavy periods, or bleeding after menopause)

Most often these symptoms are not due to cancer, but only a doctor can tell for sure. Any woman with these symptoms should tell her doctor.

Diagnosis

If you have a symptom that suggests ovarian cancer, your doctor must find out whether it is due to cancer or to some other cause. Your doctor may ask about your personal and family medical history.

You may have one or more of the following tests. Your doctor can explain more about each test:

- **Physical exam:** Your doctor checks general signs of health. Your doctor may press on your abdomen to check for tumors or an abnormal buildup of fluid (ascites). A sample of fluid can be taken to look for ovarian cancer cells.
- **Pelvic exam:** Your doctor feels the ovaries and nearby organs for lumps or other changes in their shape or size. A Pap test is

part of a normal pelvic exam, but it is not used to collect ovarian cells. The Pap test detects cervical cancer. The Pap test is not used to diagnose ovarian cancer.

- **Blood tests:** Your doctor may order blood tests. The lab may check the level of several substances, including CA-125. CA-125 is a substance found on the surface of ovarian cancer cells and on some normal tissues. A high CA-125 level could be a sign of cancer or other conditions. The CA-125 test is not used alone to diagnose ovarian cancer. This test is approved by the Food and Drug Administration for monitoring a woman's response to ovarian cancer treatment and for detecting its return after treatment.

- **Ultrasound:** The ultrasound device uses sound waves that people cannot hear. The device aims sound waves at organs inside the pelvis. The waves bounce off the organs. A computer creates a picture from the echoes. The picture may show an ovarian tumor. For a better view of the ovaries, the device may be inserted into the vagina (transvaginal ultrasound).

- **Biopsy:** A biopsy is the removal of tissue or fluid to look for cancer cells. Based on the results of the blood tests and ultrasound, your doctor may suggest surgery (a laparotomy) to remove tissue and fluid from the pelvis and abdomen. Surgery is usually needed to diagnose ovarian cancer.

Laparoscopy

Although most women have a laparotomy for diagnosis, some women have a procedure known as laparoscopy. The doctor inserts a thin, lighted tube (a laparoscope) through a small incision in the abdomen. Laparoscopy may be used to remove a small, benign cyst or an early ovarian cancer. It may also be used to learn whether cancer has spread.

A pathologist uses a microscope to look for cancer cells in the tissue or fluid. If ovarian cancer cells are found, the pathologist describes the grade of the cells. Grades 1, 2, and 3 describe how abnormal the cancer cells look. Grade 1 cancer cells are not as likely as to grow and spread as Grade 3 cells.

Staging

To plan the best treatment, your doctor needs to know the grade of the tumor and the extent (stage) of the disease. The stage is based on whether the tumor has invaded nearby tissues, whether the cancer has spread, and if so, to what parts of the body. Usually, surgery is needed

before staging can be complete. The surgeon takes many samples of tissue from the pelvis and abdomen to look for cancer.

Your doctor may order tests to find out whether the cancer has spread:

- **CT scan:** Doctors often use CT scans to make pictures of organs and tissues in the pelvis or abdomen. An x-ray machine linked to a computer takes several pictures. You may receive contrast material by mouth and by injection into your arm or hand. The contrast material helps the organs or tissues show up more clearly. Abdominal fluid or a tumor may show up on the CT scan.

- **Chest x-ray:** X-rays of the chest can show tumors or fluid.

- **Barium enema x-ray:** Your doctor may order a series of x-rays of the lower intestine. You are given an enema with a barium solution. The barium outlines the intestine on the x-rays. Areas blocked by cancer may show up on the x-rays.

- **Colonoscopy:** Your doctor inserts a long, lighted tube into the rectum and colon. This exam can help tell if cancer has spread to the colon or rectum.

These are the stages of ovarian cancer:

- **Stage I:** Cancer cells are found in one or both ovaries. Cancer cells may be found on the surface of the ovaries or in fluid collected from the abdomen.

- **Stage II:** Cancer cells have spread from one or both ovaries to other tissues in the pelvis. Cancer cells are found on the fallopian tubes, the uterus, or other tissues in the pelvis. Cancer cells may be found in fluid collected from the abdomen.

- **Stage III:** Cancer cells have spread to tissues outside the pelvis or to the regional lymph nodes. Cancer cells may be found on the outside of the liver.

- **Stage IV:** Cancer cells have spread to tissues outside the abdomen and pelvis. Cancer cells may be found inside the liver, in the lungs, or in other organs.

Treatment

Many women with ovarian cancer want to take an active part in making decisions about their medical care. It is natural to want to

learn all you can about your disease and treatment choices. Knowing more about ovarian cancer helps many women cope.

Shock and stress after the diagnosis can make it hard to think of everything you want to ask your doctor. It often helps to make a list of questions before an appointment. To help remember what your doctor says, you may take notes or ask whether you may use a tape recorder. You may also want to have a family member or friend with you when you talk to your doctor- to take part in the discussion, to take notes, or just to listen.

You do not need to ask all your questions at once. You will have other chances to ask your doctor or nurse to explain things that are not clear and to ask for more details.

Your doctor may refer you to a gynecologic oncologist, a surgeon who specializes in treating ovarian cancer. Or you may ask for a referral. Other types of doctors who help treat women with ovarian cancer include gynecologists, medical oncologists, and radiation oncologists. You may have a team of doctors and nurses.

Getting a Second Opinion

Before starting treatment, you might want a second opinion about your diagnosis and treatment plan. Many insurance companies cover a second opinion if you or your doctor requests it.

It may take some time and effort to gather medical records and arrange to see another doctor. In most cases, a brief delay in starting treatment will not make treatment less effective. To make sure, you should discuss this delay with your doctor. Sometimes women with ovarian cancer need treatment right away.

Treatment Methods

Your doctor can describe your treatment choices and the expected results. Most women have surgery and chemotherapy. Rarely, radiation therapy is used.

Cancer treatment can affect cancer cells in the pelvis, in the abdomen, or throughout the body:

- **Local therapy:** Surgery and radiation therapy are local therapies. They remove or destroy ovarian cancer in the pelvis. When ovarian cancer has spread to other parts of the body, local therapy may be used to control the disease in those specific areas.

- **Intraperitoneal chemotherapy:** Chemotherapy can be given directly into the abdomen and pelvis through a thin tube. The drugs destroy or control cancer in the abdomen and pelvis.

- **Systemic chemotherapy:** When chemotherapy is taken by mouth or injected into a vein, the drugs enter the bloodstream and destroy or control cancer throughout the body.

You may want to know how treatment may change your normal activities. You and your doctor can work together to develop a treatment plan that meets your medical and personal needs.

Because cancer treatments often damage healthy cells and tissues, side effects are common. Side effects depend mainly on the type and extent of the treatment. Side effects may not be the same for each woman, and they may change from one treatment session to the next. Before treatment starts, your health care team will explain possible side effects and suggest ways to help you manage them.

You may want to talk to your doctor about taking part in a clinical trial, a research study of new treatment methods. Clinical trials are an important option for women with all stages of ovarian cancer.

Surgery

The surgeon makes a long cut in the wall of the abdomen. This type of surgery is called a laparotomy. If ovarian cancer is found, the surgeon removes these tissues:

- Both ovaries and fallopian tubes (salpingo-oophorectomy)

- The uterus (hysterectomy)

- The omentum (the thin, fatty pad of tissue that covers the intestines)

- Nearby lymph nodes

- Samples of tissue from the pelvis and abdomen

If the cancer has spread, the surgeon removes as much cancer as possible. This is called "debulking" surgery.

If you have early Stage I ovarian cancer, the extent of surgery may depend on whether you want to get pregnant and have children. Some women with very early ovarian cancer may decide with their doctor to have only one ovary, one fallopian tube, and the omentum removed.

You may be uncomfortable for the first few days after surgery. Medicine can help control your pain. Before surgery, you should discuss the plan for pain relief with your doctor or nurse. After surgery, your doctor can adjust the plan if you need more pain relief.

The time it takes to heal after surgery is different for each woman. You will spend several days in the hospital. It may be several weeks before you return to normal activities.

If you haven't gone through menopause yet, surgery may cause hot flashes, vaginal dryness, and night sweats. These symptoms are caused by the sudden loss of female hormones. Talk with your doctor or nurse about your symptoms so that you can develop a treatment plan together. There are drugs and lifestyle changes that can help, and most symptoms go away or lessen with time.

Chemotherapy

Chemotherapy uses anticancer drugs to kill cancer cells. Most women have chemotherapy for ovarian cancer after surgery. Some women have chemotherapy before surgery. Usually, more than one drug is given. Drugs for ovarian cancer can be given in different ways:

- **By vein (IV):** The drugs can be given through a thin tube inserted into a vein.

- **By vein and directly into the abdomen:** Some women get IV chemotherapy along with intraperitoneal (IP) chemotherapy. For IP chemotherapy, the drugs are given through a thin tube inserted into the abdomen.

- **By mouth:** Some drugs for ovarian cancer can be given by mouth.

Chemotherapy is given in cycles. Each treatment period is followed by a rest period. The length of the rest period and the number of cycles depend on the anticancer drugs used.

You may have your treatment in a clinic, at the doctor's office, or at home. Some women may need to stay in the hospital during treatment.

The side effects of chemotherapy depend mainly on which drugs are given and how much. The drugs can harm normal cells that divide rapidly:

- **Blood cells:** These cells fight infection, help blood to clot, and carry oxygen to all parts of your body. When drugs affect your blood cells, you are more likely to get infections, bruise or bleed easily, and feel very weak and tired. Your health care team checks you for low levels of blood cells. If blood tests show low levels, your health care team can suggest medicines that can help your body make new blood cells.

- **Cells in hair roots:** Some drugs can cause hair loss. Your hair will grow back, but it may be somewhat different in color and texture.

- **Cells that line the digestive tract:** Some drugs can cause poor appetite, nausea and vomiting, diarrhea, or mouth and lip sores. Ask your health care team about medicines that help with these problems.

Some drugs used to treat ovarian cancer can cause hearing loss, kidney damage, joint pain, and tingling or numbness in the hands or feet. Most of these side effects usually go away after treatment ends.

Radiation Therapy

Radiation therapy (also called radiotherapy) uses high-energy rays to kill cancer cells. A large machine directs radiation at the body.

Radiation therapy is rarely used in the initial treatment of ovarian cancer, but it may be used to relieve pain and other problems caused by the disease. The treatment is given at a hospital or clinic. Each treatment takes only a few minutes.

Side effects depend mainly on the amount of radiation given and the part of your body that is treated. Radiation therapy to your abdomen and pelvis may cause nausea, vomiting, diarrhea, or bloody stools. Also, your skin in the treated area may become red, dry, and tender. Although the side effects can be distressing, your doctor can usually treat or control them. Also, they gradually go away after treatment ends.

Supportive Care

Ovarian cancer and its treatment can lead to other health problems. You may receive supportive care to prevent or control these problems and to improve your comfort and quality of life. Your health care team can help you with the following problems:

- **Pain:** Your doctor or a specialist in pain control can suggest ways to relieve or reduce pain.

- **Swollen abdomen (from abnormal fluid buildup called ascites):** The swelling can be uncomfortable. Your health care team can remove the fluid whenever it builds up.

- **Blocked intestine**: Cancer can block the intestine. Your doctor may be able to open the blockage with surgery.

- **Swollen legs (from lymphedema):** Swollen legs can be uncomfortable and hard to bend. You may find exercises, massages, or compression bandages helpful. Physical therapists trained to manage lymphedema can also help.

- **Shortness of breath:** Advanced cancer can cause fluid to collect around the lungs. The fluid can make it hard to breathe. Your health care team can remove the fluid whenever it builds up.

- **Sadness:** It is normal to feel sad after a diagnosis of a serious illness. Some people find it helpful to talk about their feelings.

Section 16.2

Ovarian Germ Cell Tumors

Excerpted from PDQ® Cancer Information Summary. National Cancer Institute; Bethesda, MD. "Ovarian Germ Cell Tumors Treatment (PDQ®): Patient Version." Updated 01/2010. Available at: http://cancer.gov. Accessed May 15, 2010.

Ovarian germ cell tumor is a disease in which malignant (cancer) cells form in the germ (egg) cells of the ovary. Germ cell tumors begin in the reproductive cells (egg or sperm) of the body. Ovarian germ cell tumors usually occur in teenage girls or young women and most often affect just one ovary.

Ovarian germ cell tumor is a general name that is used to describe several different types of cancer. The most common ovarian germ cell tumor is called dysgerminoma.

Possible signs of ovarian germ cell tumor are swelling of the abdomen or vaginal bleeding after menopause.

Ovarian germ cell tumors can be difficult to diagnose (find) early. Often there are no symptoms in the early stages, but tumors may be found during regular gynecologic examinations (checkups). A woman who has swelling of the abdomen without weight gain in other places should see a doctor. A woman who no longer has menstrual periods (who has gone through menopause) should also see a doctor if she has bleeding from the vagina.

Tests that examine the ovaries, pelvic area, blood, and ovarian tissue are used to detect (find) and diagnose ovarian germ cell tumor. Ovarian germ cell tumors are generally curable if found and treated early.

Staging Ovarian Germ Cell Tumors

After ovarian germ cell tumor has been diagnosed, tests are done to find out if cancer cells have spread within the ovary or to other parts of the body.

Many of the tests used to diagnose ovarian germ cell tumor are also used to determine the stage of the disease. Unless a doctor is sure the cancer has spread from the ovaries to other parts of the body, surgery is required to determine the stage of cancer in an operation called a laparotomy. The doctor must cut into the abdomen and carefully look at all the organs to see if they contain cancer. The doctor will cut out small pieces of tissue and look at them under a microscope to see whether they contain cancer. The doctor may also wash the abdominal cavity with fluid and then look at the fluid under a microscope to see if it contains cancer cells. Usually the doctor will remove the cancer and other organs that contain cancer during the laparotomy.

After ovarian germ cell tumor has been diagnosed, tests are done to find out if cancer cells have spread within the ovary or to other parts of the body. The following stages are used for ovarian germ cell tumors:

Stage I

In stage I, cancer is found in one or both of the ovaries and has not spread. Stage I is divided into stage IA, stage IB, and stage IC.

- **Stage IA:** Cancer is found in a single ovary.

- **Stage IB:** Cancer is found in both ovaries.

- **Stage IC:** Cancer is found in one or both ovaries and one of the following is true: cancer is found on the outside surface of one or both ovaries; or the capsule (outer covering) of the tumor has ruptured (broken open); or cancer cells are found in the fluid of the peritoneal cavity (the body cavity that contains most of the organs in the abdomen) or in washings of the peritoneum (tissue lining the peritoneal cavity).

Stage II

In stage II, cancer is found in one or both ovaries and has spread into other areas of the pelvis. Stage II is divided into stage IIA, stage IIB, and stage IIC.

- **Stage IIA:** Cancer has spread to the uterus and/or the fallopian tubes (the long slender tubes through which eggs pass from the ovaries to the uterus).

- **Stage IIB:** Cancer has spread to other tissue within the pelvis.

- **Stage IIC:** Cancer has spread to the uterus and/or fallopian tubes and/or other tissue within the pelvis and cancer cells are found in the fluid of the peritoneal cavity (the body cavity that contains most of the organs in the abdomen) or in washings of the peritoneum (tissue lining the peritoneal cavity).

Stage III

In stage III, cancer is found in one or both ovaries and has spread to other parts of the abdomen. Stage III is divided into stage IIIA, stage IIIB, and stage IIIC as follows:

- **Stage IIIA:** The tumor is found only in the pelvis, but cancer cells have spread to the surface of the peritoneum (tissue that lines the abdominal wall and covers most of the organs in the abdomen).

- **Stage IIIB:** Cancer has spread to the peritoneum but is 2 centimeters or smaller in diameter.

- **Stage IIIC:** Cancer has spread to the peritoneum and is larger than 2 centimeters in diameter and/or has spread to lymph nodes in the abdomen.

Cancer that has spread to the surface of the liver is also considered stage III disease.

Stage IV

In stage IV, cancer is found in one or both ovaries and has metastasized (spread) beyond the abdomen to other parts of the body. Cancer that has spread to tissues in the liver is also considered stage IV disease.

Recurrent Ovarian Germ Cell Tumors

Recurrent ovarian germ cell tumor is cancer that has recurred (come back) after it has been treated. The cancer may come back in the other ovary or in other parts of the body.

Standard Treatments for Ovarian Germ Cell Tumors

Different types of treatment are available for patients with ovarian germ cell tumor. Some treatments are standard (the currently used treatment), and some are being tested in clinical trials. Three types of standard treatment are used.

Surgery

Surgery is the most common treatment of ovarian germ cell tumor. A doctor may take out the cancer using one of the following types of surgery:

- **Unilateral salpingo-oophorectomy:** A surgical procedure to remove one ovary and one fallopian tube.

- **Total hysterectomy:** A surgical procedure to remove the uterus, including the cervix. If the uterus and cervix are taken out through the vagina, the operation is called a vaginal hysterectomy. If the uterus and cervix are taken out through a large incision (cut) in the abdomen, the operation is called a total abdominal hysterectomy. If the uterus and cervix are taken out through a small incision (cut) in the abdomen using a laparoscope, the operation is called a total laparoscopic hysterectomy.

- **Bilateral salpingo-oophorectomy:** A surgical procedure to remove both ovaries and both fallopian tubes.

- **Tumor debulking:** A surgical procedure in which as much of the tumor as possible is removed. Some tumors may not be able to be completely removed.

Chemotherapy and Radiation Therapy

Chemotherapy is a cancer treatment that uses drugs to stop the growth of cancer cells, either by killing the cells or by stopping the cells from dividing. Radiation therapy is a cancer treatment that uses high-energy x-rays or other types of radiation to kill cancer cells.

Even if the doctor removes all the cancer that can be seen at the time of the operation, some patients may be offered chemotherapy or radiation after surgery to kill any cancer cells that are left. Treatment given after the surgery, to lower the risk that the cancer will come back, is called adjuvant therapy.

Following radiation or chemotherapy, an operation called a second-look laparotomy is sometimes done. This is similar to the laparotomy

that is done to determine the stage of the cancer. During the second-look operation, the doctor will take samples of lymph nodes and other tissues in the abdomen to see if any cancer is left.

New Treatments for Ovarian Germ Cell Tumors

Patients who take part in clinical trials also help improve the way cancer will be treated in the future. Even when clinical trials do not lead to effective new treatments, they often answer important questions and help move research forward. The following treatments are being studied:

High-Dose Chemotherapy with Bone Marrow Transplant

High-dose chemotherapy with bone marrow transplant is a method of giving very high doses of chemotherapy and replacing blood-forming cells destroyed by the cancer treatment. Stem cells (immature blood cells) are removed from the bone marrow of the patient or a donor and are frozen and stored. After the chemotherapy is completed, the stored stem cells are thawed and given back to the patient through an infusion. These reinfused stem cells grow into (and restore) the body's blood cells.

Combination Chemotherapy

Combination chemotherapy (the use of more than one chemotherapy drug to fight cancer) is being tested in clinical trials. Patients may want to think about taking part in a clinical trial. For some patients, taking part in a clinical trial may be the best treatment choice. Clinical trials are part of the cancer research process. Clinical trials are done to find out if new cancer treatments are safe and effective or better than the standard treatment.

Follow-Up Tests

Follow-up tests may be needed. Some of the tests that were done to diagnose the cancer or to find out the stage of the cancer may be repeated. Some tests will be repeated in order to see how well the treatment is working. Decisions about whether to continue, change, or stop treatment may be based on the results of these tests. This is sometimes called re-staging.

Some of the tests will continue to be done from time to time after treatment has ended. The results of these tests can show if your condition

has changed or if the cancer has recurred (come back). These tests are sometimes called follow-up tests or check-ups.

Section 16.3

Ovarian Epithelial Cancer

Excerpted from PDQ® Cancer Information Summary. National Cancer Institute; Bethesda, MD. "Ovarian Epithelial Cancer Treatment (PDQ®). Patient Version." Updated 01/2010. Available at: http://cancer.gov. Accessed May 24, 2010.

Ovarian epithelial cancer is a disease in which malignant (cancer) cells form in the tissue covering the ovary. Ovarian epithelial cancer is one type of cancer that affects the ovary. When found in its early stages, ovarian epithelial cancer can often be cured.

Tests that examine the ovaries, pelvic area, blood, and ovarian tissue are used to detect (find) and diagnose ovarian cancer. The prognosis (chance of recovery) and treatment options depend on the following: the stage of the cancer; the type and size of the tumor; the patient's age and general health; and whether the cancer has just been diagnosed or has recurred (come back).

Stages of Ovarian Epithelial Cancer

After ovarian epithelial cancer has been diagnosed, tests are done to find out if cancer cells have spread within the ovaries or to other parts of the body. The process used to find out if cancer has spread within the ovary or to other parts of the body is called staging. The information gathered from the staging process determines the stage of the disease. It is important to know the stage in order to plan treatment.

An operation called a laparotomy is usually done to find out the stage of the disease. A doctor must cut into the abdomen and carefully look at all the organs to see if they contain cancer. The doctor will also perform a biopsy (cut out small pieces of tissue so they can be looked at under a microscope to see whether they contain cancer). Usually the doctor will remove the cancer and organs that contain cancer during the laparotomy.

The following stages are used for ovarian epithelial cancer:

Stage I

In stage I, cancer is found in one or both of the ovaries. Stage I is divided into stage IA, stage IB, and stage IC.

- **Stage IA:** Cancer is found in a single ovary.

- **Stage IB:** Cancer is found in both ovaries.

- **Stage IC:** Cancer is found in one or both ovaries and one of the following is true: cancer is found on the outside surface of one or both ovaries; or the capsule of the tumor has ruptured; or cancer cells are found in the fluid of the peritoneal cavity or in washings of the peritoneum.

Stage II

In stage II, cancer is found in one or both ovaries and has spread into other areas of the pelvis. Stage II is divided into stage IIA, stage IIB, and stage IIC.

- **Stage IIA:** Cancer has spread to the uterus and/or the fallopian tubes.

- **Stage IIB:** Cancer has spread to other tissue within the pelvis.

- **Stage IIC:** Cancer has spread to the uterus and/or fallopian tubes and/or other tissue within the pelvis and cancer cells are found in the fluid of the peritoneal cavity or in washings of the peritoneum.

Stage III

In stage III, cancer is found in one or both ovaries and has spread to other parts of the abdomen. Stage III is divided into stage IIIA, stage IIIB, and stage IIIC.

- **Stage IIIA:** The tumor is found in the pelvis only, but cancer cells have spread to the surface of the peritoneum.

- **Stage IIIB:** Cancer has spread to the peritoneum but is 2 centimeters or smaller in diameter.

- **Stage IIIC:** Cancer has spread to the peritoneum and is larger than 2 centimeters in diameter and/or has spread to lymph nodes in the abdomen.

Cancer that has spread to the surface of the liver is also considered stage III disease.

Stage IV

In stage IV, cancer is found in one or both ovaries and has metastasized (spread) beyond the abdomen to other parts of the body, such as the lungs, liver, lymph nodes, or bones. Cancer that has spread to tissues in the liver is also considered stage IV disease.

Recurrent or Persistent Ovarian Epithelial Cancer

Recurrent ovarian epithelial cancer is cancer that has recurred (come back) after it has been treated. Persistent cancer is cancer that does not go away with treatment.

Treatments for Ovarian Epithelial Cancer

Different types of treatment are available for patients with ovarian epithelial cancer. Some treatments are standard, and some are being tested in clinical trials. Three kinds of standard treatment are used. These include the following:

- **Surgery:** Most patients have surgery to remove as much of the tumor as possible. Different types of surgery may include hysterectomy, total hysterectomy, unilateral salpingo-oophorectomy, bilateral salpingo-oophorectomy, omentectomy (a surgical procedure to remove the omentum, a piece of the tissue lining the abdominal wall), and lymph node biopsy.

- **Radiation therapy:** Radiation therapy is a cancer treatment that uses high-energy x-rays or other types of radiation to kill cancer cells or keep them from growing. Some women receive a treatment called intraperitoneal radiation therapy, in which radioactive liquid is put directly in the abdomen through a catheter.

- **Chemotherapy:** Chemotherapy is a cancer treatment that uses drugs to stop the growth of cancer cells, either by killing the cells or by stopping them from dividing. A type of regional chemotherapy used to treat ovarian cancer is intraperitoneal (IP) chemotherapy. In IP chemotherapy, the anticancer drugs are carried directly into the peritoneal cavity (the space that contains the abdominal organs) through a thin tube. Treatment

with more than one anticancer drug is called combination chemotherapy. The way the chemotherapy is given depends on the type and stage of the cancer being treated.

New types of treatment are being tested in clinical trials.

- **Biologic therapy:** Biologic therapy is a treatment that uses the patient's immune system to fight cancer. Substances made by the body or made in a laboratory are used to boost, direct, or restore the body's natural defenses against cancer. This type of cancer treatment is also called biotherapy or immunotherapy.

- **Targeted therapy:** Targeted therapy is a type of treatment that uses drugs or other substances to identify and attack specific cancer cells without harming normal cells.

Section 16.4

Ovarian Low Malignant Potential Tumors

Excerpted from PDQ® Cancer Information Summary. National Cancer Institute; Bethesda, MD. "Ovarian Low Malignant Potential Tumors Treatment (PDQ®): Patient Version." Updated 10/2009. Available at: http://cancer .gov. Accessed May 24, 2010.

Ovarian low malignant potential tumor is a disease in which abnormal cells form in the tissue covering the ovary. Ovarian low malignant potential tumors have abnormal cells that may become cancer, but usually do not. This disease usually remains in the ovary. When disease is found in one ovary, the other ovary should also be checked carefully for signs of disease.

In most cases, ovarian low malignant potential tumor can be treated successfully. These tumors are usually found early. However, even advanced stage ovarian low malignant potential tumors can be treated successfully. Patients who do not survive usually die from complications of the disease (such as a small bowel obstruction) or the side effects of treatment, but rarely because the tumor has spread.

Stages of Ovarian Low Malignant Potential Tumors

After ovarian low malignant potential tumor has been diagnosed, tests are done to find out if abnormal cells have spread within the ovary or to other parts of the body. The process used to find out whether abnormal cells have spread within the ovary or to other parts of the body is called staging. The following stages are used for ovarian low malignant potential tumor:

- **Stage I:** In stage IA the tumor is found in a single ovary; in stage IB the tumor is found in both ovaries; in stage IC the tumor is found in one or both ovaries and one of the following is true: abnormal cells are found on the outside surface of one or both ovaries; or the capsule (outer covering) of the tumor has ruptured (broken open); or tumor cells are found in the fluid of the peritoneal cavity or in washings of the peritoneum.

- **Stage II:** In stage II, the tumor is found in one or both ovaries and has spread into other areas of the pelvis. In stage IIA the tumor has spread to the uterus and/or the fallopian tubes; in stage IIB the tumor has spread to other tissue within the pelvis; in stage IIC the tumor has spread to the uterus and/or fallopian tubes and/or other tissue within the pelvis and tumor cells are found in the fluid of the peritoneal cavity or in washings of the peritoneum.

- **Stage III:** In stage III, the tumor is found in one or both ovaries and has spread to other parts of the abdomen. In stage IIIA the tumor is found only in the pelvis, but tumor cells have spread to the surface of the peritoneum; in stage IIIB the tumor has spread to the peritoneum but is 2 centimeters or smaller in diameter; in stage IIIC the tumor has spread to the peritoneum and is larger than 2 centimeters in diameter and/or has spread to lymph nodes in the abdomen. The spread of tumor cells to the surface of the liver is also considered stage III disease.

- **Stage IV:** In stage IV, tumor cells are found in one or both ovaries and have metastasized (spread) beyond the abdomen to other parts of the body. The spread of tumor cells to tissues in the liver is also considered stage IV disease. Ovarian low malignant potential tumors almost never reach stage IV.

- **Recurrent ovarian low malignant potential tumors:** Ovarian low malignant potential tumors may recur (come back) after they have been treated. The tumors may come back in the other ovary or in other parts of the body.

Treatment Option Overview

Different types of treatment are available for patients with ovarian low malignant potential tumor. Some treatments are standard (the currently used treatment), and some are being tested in clinical trials. Two types of standard treatment are used:

Surgery

The type of surgery (removing the tumor in an operation) depends on the size and spread of the tumor and the woman's plans for having children. Surgery may include the following:

- **Unilateral salpingo-oophorectomy:** Surgery to remove one ovary and one fallopian tube.

- **Bilateral salpingo-oophorectomy:** Surgery to remove both ovaries and both fallopian tubes.

- **Total hysterectomy and bilateral salpingo-oophorectomy:** Surgery to remove the uterus, cervix, and both ovaries and fallopian tubes.

- **Partial oophorectomy:** Surgery to remove part of one ovary or part of both ovaries.

- **Omentectomy:** Surgery to remove the omentum (a piece of the tissue lining the abdominal wall).

Even if the doctor removes all disease that can be seen at the time of the operation, the patient may be given chemotherapy after surgery to kill any tumor cells that are left. Treatment given after the surgery, to lower the risk that the tumor will come back, is called adjuvant therapy.

Chemotherapy

Chemotherapy is a cancer treatment that uses drugs to stop the growth of cancer cells, either by killing the cells or by stopping them from dividing.

Section 16.5

Oral Contraceptives Reduce Long-Term Risk of Ovarian Cancer

From "Oral Contraceptives Reduce Long-Term Risk of Ovarian Cancer,"
National Cancer Institute (www.cancer.gov), February 20, 2008.

Since they were first licensed nearly 50 years ago, birth control pills containing estrogen have prevented some 200,000 cases of ovarian cancer worldwide, estimate the authors of a study published January 26, 2008, in *The Lancet*. Further, in the absence of having taken oral contraceptives, half of these women would have died of the disease.

The researchers showed that oral contraceptives (OCs) continue to confer protection for years—even decades—after women stop using them. Thus, they surmise, "the number of ovarian cancers prevented [will] rise over the next few decades" to at least 30,000 each year.

These figures emerge from a comprehensive meta-analysis based on prospective and case-control data from 45 epidemiological studies in 21 countries, mostly in Europe and the United States. "These findings set a new standard in prevention for a deadly cancer," wrote the editors of *The Lancet*, "and have important public health implications."

The results showed that women who had ever taken OCs were 27 percent less likely to develop ovarian cancer. The studies included 23,257 women with ovarian cancer, 31 percent of whom had taken OCs; of the 87,303 controls, 37 percent took OCs.

Two trends emerged that were really striking, according to Dr. Beth Karlan, editor-in-chief of the journal *Gynecologic Oncology* and director of the Gilda Radner Cancer Detection Program at Cedars-Sinai Outpatient Cancer Center in Los Angeles. First, the longer OCs were used, the greater the ovarian cancer risk reduction, decreasing about 20 percent for each five years of use.

The second clear trend was the duration of the protective effects, which lasted long after women had stopped using OCs. For each five years of use, risk of developing ovarian cancer was reduced 29 percent in the first 10 years after stopping. The risk reduction was still

significant though smaller (19 percent) for years 10–20, and smaller still (15 percent) 20–29 years after discontinuation.

Another feature of these results is their uniformity. OCs seem to protect against nearly all types of epithelial and nonepithelial tumors, with the possible exception of mucinous ovarian cancer (which accounted for only 12 percent of cases studied in the meta-analysis). *The Lancet* editorial points out that the results show "the benefits of oral contraceptives are independent of the preparation [estrogen dose], and vary little by ethnic origin, parity, family history of breast cancer, body-mass index, and use of hormone replacement therapy."

Representatives from nearly all of these studies—including Drs. Patricia Hartge, James Lacey, Louise Brinton, and Robert Hoover from the Epidemiology and Biostatistics Program in National Cancer Institute's Division of Cancer Epidemiology and Genetics (DCEG)—worked together to ensure the integrity of the analysis, forming the Collaborative Group on Epidemiological Studies of Ovarian Cancer, under the leadership of Dr. Valerie Beral and colleagues at Oxford University's Cancer Research UK Epidemiology Unit.

The absence of proven screening methods for ovarian cancer make these findings all the more welcome. But the issue is not straightforward, because calculating "the net effect on women's health is fraught with uncertainties," wrote Drs. Eduardo L. Franco and Eliane Duarte-Franco of McGill University in Montreal in a comment accompanying the article. They went on to list possible side effects of OCs as increased risk of thromboembolism, heart disease, migraine, liver disease, and several other relatively uncommon conditions.

The analyses were not focused on comparing the benefits and risks of OCs, explains DCEG's Dr. Brinton, but only examined their effect on ovarian cancer risk. In the absence of detailed risk-benefit data, including currently unknown risks, such as cancers in women who have taken OCs and later take long-term hormone replacement therapy, she says, "This meta-analysis does not recommend widespread prescription of OCs as a preventative measure against ovarian cancer."

Dr. Beral commented that while OCs may pose a slight increased risk of breast and cervical cancer, the effect is small and disappears once the drugs are no longer being used, as contrasted with the ongoing protective effect against ovarian cancer.

Dr. Karlan added, "Ovarian cancer remains a disease with a high mortality due [mainly] to our inability to reliably diagnose it at an early stage. Women are concerned about this risk." She noted that it is important for women to be aware that OCs reduce that risk when discussing their contraceptive choices with their health care providers.

Section 16.6

Ovarian Epithelial Tumors Traced to Fallopian Tubes

Excerpted from "Ovarian Epithelial Tumors Traced to Fallopian Tubes,"
National Cancer Institute (www.cancer.gov), April 30, 2008.

Researchers at Dana-Farber Cancer Institute in Boston, Massachusetts, have found that the source of disease in many cases of the most aggressive form of ovarian cancer, serous carcinoma, may not be the ovary at all, but rather the fimbria of the fallopian tube. Dr. Keren Levanon reported these findings at the American Association for Cancer Research annual meeting on April 14, 2008.

"Until now, there was no understanding of the basic pathogenesis or carcinogenesis of [ovarian] serous carcinoma," said Dr. Levanon at the meeting. Noting that the majority of ovarian cancers are diagnosed at an advanced stage, she continued: "We didn't really know what the early cancer lesion or precursor lesion looks like, so we couldn't analyze what went wrong."

Her team, which included collaborators at Brigham and Women's Hospital, searched for these early lesions by identifying cells with a "p53 signature"—mutations in the p53 gene and buildup of p53 protein in cells—in the tissues of women who, due to a high risk for developing ovarian and other cancers, volunteered to have their ovaries and fallopian tubes removed.

The team found a p53 signature most often in the secretory cells lining the finger-like appendages, called fimbria, at the ends of fallopian tubes. Dr. Levanon's team then developed an ex vivo model that they are using to continue studying these cells and the molecular events that lead to cancer. They hope this research will lead to targeted therapies and biomarkers for early detection.

Though they were surprised by their findings, explained Dr. Levanon, they were not surprised that ovarian cancer could begin in the fallopian tubes. "When we look at patients who are diagnosed with later-stage ovarian cancer," she said, "we find that they have these lesions in their fallopian tubes in close to 100 percent of cases." She

also noted that patients who have prophylactic surgery to remove their ovaries sometimes develop tumors in other parts of their abdomen, which could result from shed cancer cells when the fallopian tubes are left intact.

Section 16.7

Removal of Ovaries and Fallopian Tubes Cuts Cancer Risk for BRCA1/2 Carriers

Excerpted from "Removal of Ovaries and Fallopian Tubes Cuts Cancer Risk for BRCA1/2 Carriers." National Cancer Institute (www.cancer.gov), April 24, 2009.

Surgery that removes the ovaries and fallopian tubes, called salpingo-oophorectomy, is one of the most effective ways to decrease a woman's risk of breast and gynecologic cancer if she carries a BRCA1 or BRCA2 gene mutation. However, the true degree of risk reduction has not been precisely defined. A new meta-analysis of 10 independent studies has revealed with greater confidence than ever before that the risk reduction of this surgery can be 80 percent for ovarian or fallopian tube cancer and 50 percent for breast cancer. The full results of the analysis appeared in the January 21, 2009, *Journal of the National Cancer Institute*.

A team of researchers led by Dr. Timothy R. Rebbeck of the University of Pennsylvania looked at overall breast cancer risk, breast cancer risk according to BRCA mutation, and ovarian or fallopian cancer risk. Women who had BRCA1 mutations and women who had BRCA2 mutations benefited equally in terms of breast cancer risk after the surgery, according to their analysis. The authors pointed out, however, that this conflicts with results from their previous prospective cohort study, which indicated that the surgery may have more benefit for BRCA2 mutation carriers.

"[Studies] that used retrospective cohort or case-control approaches did not observe this difference, and therefore, there was no difference in the pooled estimates," they wrote, noting that the issue deserves further investigation. Data were not available for the meta-analysis

to make this BRCA-type distinction for gynecologic cancer risk after the surgery.

In a related editorial, Drs. Mark H. Greene and Phuong L. Mai of National Cancer Institute's Division of Cancer Epidemiology and Genetics commended the study authors, noting that their attempt to "disentangle potential differences between BRCA1 and BRCA2 mutation carriers who, despite having superficial similarities with regard to phenotype, have important biological differences" strengthens the findings of their report. "The risk estimates presented in the study represent the most accurate current measures of potential benefits from risk-reducing salpingo-oophorectomy," said Dr. Greene, "and genetics providers should use them in their daily practice."

Chapter 17

Uterine Cancer

Chapter Contents

Section 17.1

Understanding Cancer of the Uterus

Excerpted from "What You Need to Know about Cancer
of the Uterus," National Cancer Institute (www.cancer.gov), 2002.
Revised by David A. Cooke, MD, FACP, May 2010.

The Uterus

The uterus is part of a woman's reproductive system. It is the hollow, pear-shaped organ where a baby grows. The uterus is in the pelvis between the bladder and the rectum.

The narrow, lower portion of the uterus is the cervix. The broad, middle part of the uterus is the body, or corpus. The dome-shaped top of the uterus is the fundus. The fallopian tubes extend from either side of the top of the uterus to the ovaries.

The wall of the uterus has two layers of tissue. The inner layer, or lining, is the endometrium. The outer layer is muscle tissue called the myometrium.

In women of childbearing age, the lining of the uterus grows and thickens each month to prepare for pregnancy. If a woman does not become pregnant, the thick, bloody lining flows out of the body through the vagina. This flow is called menstruation.

Benign Conditions of the Uterus

Fibroids are common benign tumors that grow in the muscle of the uterus. They occur mainly in women in their forties. Women may have many fibroids at the same time. Fibroids do not develop into cancer. As a woman reaches menopause, fibroids are likely to become smaller, and sometimes they disappear.

Usually, fibroids cause no symptoms and need no treatment. But depending on their size and location, fibroids can cause bleeding, vaginal discharge, and frequent urination. Women with these symptoms should see a doctor. If fibroids cause heavy bleeding, or if they press against nearby organs and cause pain, the doctor may suggest surgery or other treatment.

Endometriosis is another benign condition that affects the uterus. It is most common in women in their thirties and forties, especially in women who have never been pregnant. It occurs when endometrial tissue begins to grow on the outside of the uterus and on nearby organs. This condition may cause painful menstrual periods, abnormal vaginal bleeding, and sometimes loss of fertility (ability to get pregnant), but it does not cause cancer. Women with endometriosis may be treated with hormones or surgery.

Endometrial hyperplasia is an increase in the number of cells in the lining of the uterus. It is not cancer. Sometimes it develops into cancer. Heavy menstrual periods, bleeding between periods, and bleeding after menopause are common symptoms of hyperplasia. It is most common after age 40.

To prevent endometrial hyperplasia from developing into cancer, the doctor may recommend surgery to remove the uterus (hysterectomy) or treatment with hormones (progesterone) and regular followup exams.

Two Types of Uterine Cancer

Malignant tumors are cancer. They are generally more serious and may be life threatening. Cancer cells can invade and damage nearby tissues and organs. Also, cancer cells can break away from a malignant tumor and enter the bloodstream or lymphatic system. That is how cancer cells spread from the original (primary) tumor to form new tumors in other organs. The spread of cancer is called metastasis.

When uterine cancer spreads (metastasizes) outside the uterus, cancer cells are often found in nearby lymph nodes, nerves, or blood vessels. If the cancer has reached the lymph nodes, cancer cells may have spread to other lymph nodes and other organs, such as the lungs, liver, and bones.

When cancer spreads from its original place to another part of the body, the new tumor has the same kind of abnormal cells and the same name as the primary tumor. For example, if cancer of the uterus spreads to the lungs, the cancer cells in the lungs are actually uterine cancer cells. The disease is metastatic uterine cancer, not lung cancer. It is treated as uterine cancer, not lung cancer. Doctors sometimes call the new tumor "distant" disease.

The majority of cancer of the uterus begins in the lining (endometrium). It is called endometrial cancer, and this is what is meant in most cases when someone refers to uterine cancer. For more detailed information on endometrial cancer, see Chapter 14.

A different type of cancer, uterine sarcoma, develops in the muscle (myometrium). This kind of cancer is much rarer than endometrial cancer. For more information about uterine sarcoma, see Section 17.2 later in this chapter.

Diagnosis

If a woman has symptoms that suggest uterine cancer, her doctor may check general signs of health and may order blood and urine tests. The doctor also may perform one or more of the exams or tests described below:

- **Pelvic exam:** A woman has a pelvic exam to check the vagina, uterus, bladder, and rectum. The doctor feels these organs for any lumps or changes in their shape or size. To see the upper part of the vagina and the cervix, the doctor inserts an instrument called a speculum into the vagina.

- **Pap test:** The doctor collects cells from the cervix and upper vagina. A medical laboratory checks for abnormal cells. Although the Pap test can detect cancer of the cervix, cells from inside the uterus usually do not show up on a Pap test. This is why the doctor collects samples of cells from inside the uterus in a procedure called a biopsy.

- **Transvaginal ultrasound:** The doctor inserts an instrument into the vagina. The instrument aims high-frequency sound waves at the uterus. The pattern of the echoes they produce creates a picture. If the endometrium looks too thick, the doctor can do a biopsy.

- **Biopsy:** The doctor removes a sample of tissue from the uterine lining. This usually can be done in the doctor's office. In some cases, however, a woman may need to have a dilation and curettage (D&C). A D&C is usually done as same-day surgery with anesthesia in a hospital. A pathologist examines the tissue to check for cancer cells, hyperplasia, and other conditions. For a short time after the biopsy, some women have cramps and vaginal bleeding.

Section 17.2

Staging and Treating Uterine Sarcoma

Excerpted from PDQ® Cancer Information Summary. National Cancer Institute; Bethesda, MD. "Uterine Sarcoma Treatment (PDQ®): Patient Version." Updated 08/2009. Available at: http://cancer.gov. Accessed May 24, 2010.

Uterine sarcoma is a disease in which malignant (cancer) cells form in the muscles of the uterus or other tissues that support the uterus. Uterine sarcoma is a very rare kind of cancer that forms in the uterine muscles or in tissues that support the uterus. Uterine sarcoma is different from cancer of the endometrium, a disease in which cancer cells start growing inside the lining of the uterus.

Risk factors for uterine sarcoma include the following:

- Past treatment with radiation therapy to the pelvis.

- Treatment with tamoxifen for breast cancer. A patient taking this drug should have a pelvic exam every year and report any vaginal bleeding (other than menstrual bleeding) as soon as possible.

Abnormal bleeding from the vagina and other symptoms may be caused by uterine sarcoma. Other conditions may cause the same symptoms. A doctor should be consulted if any of the following problems occur:

- Bleeding that is not part of menstrual periods

- Bleeding after menopause

- A mass in the vagina

- Pain or a feeling of fullness in the abdomen

- Frequent urination

The prognosis (chance of recovery) and treatment options depend on the following:

- The stage of the cancer

- The type and size of the tumor

- The patient's general health

- Whether the cancer has just been diagnosed or has recurred (come back)

Stages of Uterine Sarcoma

Surgery is used to diagnose, stage, and treat uterine sarcoma. During this surgery, the doctor removes as much of the cancer as possible. The following procedures may be used to diagnose, stage, and treat uterine sarcoma:

- **Laparotomy:** A surgical procedure in which an incision (cut) is made in the wall of the abdomen to check the inside of the abdomen for signs of disease. The size of the incision depends on the reason the laparotomy is being done. Sometimes organs are removed or tissue samples are taken and checked under a microscope for signs of disease.

- **Abdominal and pelvic washings:** A procedure in which a saline solution is placed into the abdominal and pelvic body cavities. After a short time, the fluid is removed and viewed under a microscope to check for cancer cells.

- **Total abdominal hysterectomy:** A surgical procedure to remove the uterus and cervix through a large incision (cut) in the abdomen.

- **Bilateral salpingo-oophorectomy:** Surgery to remove both ovaries and both fallopian tubes.

- **Lymphadenectomy:** A surgical procedure in which lymph nodes are removed and checked under a microscope for signs of cancer. For a regional lymphadenectomy, some of the lymph nodes in the tumor area are removed. For a radical lymphadenectomy, most or all of the lymph nodes in the tumor area are removed. This procedure is also called lymph node dissection.

Stage I

In stage I, cancer is found in the uterus only. Stage I is divided into stage IA, stage IB, and stage IC, based on how far the cancer has spread.

- **Stage IA:** Cancer is in the endometrium only.

- **Stage IB:** Cancer has spread into the inner half of the myometrium (muscle layer of the uterus).

- **Stage IC:** Cancer has spread into the outer half of the myometrium.

Stage II

In stage II, cancer has spread from the uterus to the cervix. Stage II is divided into stage IIA and stage IIB, based on how far the cancer has spread.

- **Stage IIA:** Cancer has spread to the glands where the cervix and uterus meet.

- *Stage IIB:* Cancer has spread into the connective tissue of the cervix.

Stage III

In stage III, cancer has spread beyond the uterus and cervix, but has not spread beyond the pelvis. Stage III is divided into stage IIIA and stage IIIB, based on how far the cancer has spread within the pelvis.

- **Stage IIIA:** Cancer has spread to one or more of the following: the outermost layer of the uterus; and/or tissues just beyond the uterus; and/or the peritoneum.

- **Stage IIIB:** Cancer has spread to lymph nodes in the pelvis and/or near the uterus.

Stage IV

In stage IV, cancer has spread beyond the pelvis. Stage IV is divided into stage IVA and stage IVB, based on how far the cancer has spread.

- **Stage IVA:** Cancer has spread to the lining of the bladder and/or bowel.

- **Stage IVB:** Cancer has spread to other parts of the body beyond the pelvis, including lymph nodes in the abdomen and/or groin.

Recurrent Uterine Sarcoma

Recurrent uterine sarcoma is cancer that has recurred (come back) after it has been treated. The cancer may come back in the uterus or in other parts of the body.

Treatment Option Overview

Different types of treatments are available for patients with uterine sarcoma. Some treatments are standard (the currently used treatment), and some are being tested in clinical trials. Four types of standard treatment are used:

Surgery

Surgery is the most common treatment for uterine sarcoma. Some types are surgery total abdominal hysterectomy, bilateral salpingo-oophorectomy, and lymphadenectomy.

Even if the doctor removes all the cancer that can be seen at the time of the surgery, some patients may be given chemotherapy or radiation therapy after surgery to kill any cancer cells that are left. Treatment given after the surgery, to increase the chances of a cure, is called adjuvant therapy.

Radiation Therapy

Radiation therapy is a cancer treatment that uses high energy x-rays or other types of radiation to kill cancer cells or keep them from growing. There are two types of radiation therapy. External radiation therapy uses a machine outside the body to send radiation toward the cancer. Internal radiation therapy uses a radioactive substance sealed in needles, seeds, wires, or catheters that are placed directly into or near the cancer. The way the radiation therapy is given depends on the type and stage of the cancer being treated.

Chemotherapy

Chemotherapy is a cancer treatment that uses drugs to stop the growth of cancer cells, either by killing the cells or by stopping them from dividing. When chemotherapy is taken by mouth or injected into a vein or muscle, the drugs enter the bloodstream and can reach cancer cells throughout the body (systemic chemotherapy). When chemotherapy is placed directly into the spinal column, an organ, or a body

cavity such as the abdomen, the drugs mainly affect cancer cells in those areas (regional chemotherapy). The way the chemotherapy is given depends on the type and stage of the cancer being treated.

Hormone Therapy

Hormone therapy is a cancer treatment that removes hormones or blocks their action and stops cancer cells from growing. Hormones are substances produced by glands in the body and circulated in the bloodstream. Some hormones can cause certain cancers to grow. If tests show the cancer cells have places where hormones can attach (receptors), drugs, surgery, or radiation therapy are used to reduce the production of hormones or block them from working.

Clinical Trials

New types of treatment are being tested in clinical trials. Some clinical trials only include patients who have not yet received treatment. Other trials test treatments for patients whose cancer has not gotten better. There are also clinical trials that test new ways to stop cancer from recurring (coming back) or reduce the side effects of cancer treatment.

Chapter 18

Vaginal Cancer

Understanding Vaginal Cancer

Vaginal cancer is a disease in which malignant (cancer) cells form in the vagina. The vagina is the canal leading from the cervix (the opening of uterus) to the outside of the body. At birth, a baby passes out of the body through the vagina (also called the birth canal).

Vaginal cancer is not common. When found in early stages, it can often be cured. There are two main types of vaginal cancer:

- **Squamous cell carcinoma:** Cancer that forms in squamous cells, the thin, flat cells lining the vagina. Squamous cell vaginal cancer spreads slowly and usually stays near the vagina, but may spread to the lungs and liver. This is the most common type of vaginal cancer. It is found most often in women aged 60 or older.

- **Adenocarcinoma:** Cancer that begins in glandular (secretory) cells. Glandular cells in the lining of the vagina make and release fluids such as mucus. Adenocarcinoma is more likely than squamous cell cancer to spread to the lungs and lymph nodes. It is found most often in women aged 30 or younger.

Excerpted from PDQ® Cancer Information Summary. National Cancer Institute; Bethesda, MD. "Vaginal Cancer Treatment (PDQ®): Patient Version." Updated 10/2009. Available at: http://cancer.gov. Accessed May 24, 2010.

Risk Factors

Anything that increases your risk of getting a disease is called a risk factor. Risk factors for vaginal cancer include the following:

- Being aged 60 or older.

- Being exposed to DES while in the mother's womb. In the 1950s, the drug DES was given to some pregnant women to prevent miscarriage (premature birth of a fetus that cannot survive). Women who were exposed to DES before birth have an increased risk of developing vaginal cancer. Some of these women develop a rare form of cancer called clear cell adenocarcinoma.

- Having human papilloma virus (HPV) infection.

- Having a history of abnormal cells in the cervix or cervical cancer.

Signs of Vaginal Cancer

Vaginal cancer often does not cause early symptoms and may be found during a routine Pap test. When symptoms occur they may be caused by vaginal cancer or by other conditions. A doctor should be consulted if any of the following problems occur:

- Bleeding or discharge not related to menstrual periods.

- Pain during sexual intercourse.

- Pain in the pelvic area.

- A lump in the vagina.

Diagnosing Vaginal Cancer

The following tests and procedures may be used to diagnose vaginal cancer:

- **Physical exam and history:** An exam of the body to check general signs of health, including checking for signs of disease, such as lumps or anything else that seems unusual. A history of the patient's health habits and past illnesses and treatments will also be taken.

- **Pelvic exam:** An exam of the vagina, cervix, uterus, fallopian tubes, ovaries, and rectum. The doctor or nurse inserts one or two lubricated, gloved fingers of one hand into the vagina and

places the other hand over the lower abdomen to feel the size, shape, and position of the uterus and ovaries. A speculum is also inserted into the vagina and the doctor or nurse looks at the vagina and cervix for signs of disease. A Pap test or Pap smear of the cervix is usually done. The doctor or nurse also inserts a lubricated, gloved finger into the rectum to feel for lumps or abnormal areas.

- **Pap smear:** A procedure to collect cells from the surface of the cervix and vagina. A piece of cotton, a brush, or a small wooden stick is used to gently scrape cells from the cervix and vagina. The cells are viewed under a microscope to find out if they are abnormal. This procedure is also called a Pap test.

- **Biopsy:** The removal of cells or tissues from the vagina and cervix so they can be viewed under a microscope by a pathologist to check for signs of cancer. If a Pap smear shows abnormal cells in the vagina, a biopsy may be done during a colposcopy.

- **Colposcopy:** A procedure in which a colposcope (a lighted, magnifying instrument) is used to check the vagina and cervix for abnormal areas. Tissue samples may be taken using a curette (spoon-shaped instrument) and checked under a microscope for signs of disease.

Certain factors affect prognosis (chance of recovery) and treatment options:

- The stage of the cancer (whether it is in the vagina only or has spread to other areas)
- The size of the tumor
- The grade of tumor cells (how different they are from normal cells)
- Where the cancer is within the vagina
- Whether there are symptoms
- The patient's age and general health
- Whether the cancer has just been diagnosed or has recurred (come back)

Stages of Vaginal Cancer

After vaginal cancer has been diagnosed, tests are done to find out if cancer cells have spread within the vagina or to other parts of

the body. The process used to find out if cancer has spread within the vagina or to other parts of the body is called staging. The information gathered from the staging process determines the stage of the disease. It is important to know the stage in order to plan treatment. The following procedures may be used in the staging process:

- **Biopsy:** A biopsy may be done to find out if cancer has spread to the cervix. A sample of tissue is cut from the cervix and viewed under a microscope. A biopsy that removes only a small amount of tissue is usually done in the doctor's office. A woman may need to go to a hospital for a cone biopsy (removal of a larger, cone-shaped piece of tissue from the cervix and cervical canal). A biopsy of the vulva may also be done to see if cancer has spread there.

- **Chest x-ray:** An x-ray of the organs and bones inside the chest. An x-ray is a type of energy beam that can go through the body and onto film, making a picture of areas inside the body.

- **Cystoscopy:** A procedure to look inside the bladder and urethra to check for abnormal areas. A cystoscope is inserted through the urethra into the bladder. A cystoscope is a thin, tube-like instrument with a light and a lens for viewing. It may also have a tool to remove tissue samples, which are checked under a microscope for signs of cancer.

- **Ureteroscopy:** A procedure to look inside the ureters to check for abnormal areas. A ureteroscope is inserted through the bladder and into the ureters. A ureteroscope is a thin, tube-like instrument with a light and a lens for viewing. It may also have a tool to remove tissue to be checked under a microscope for signs of disease. A ureteroscopy and cystoscopy may be done during the same procedure.

- **Proctoscopy:** A procedure to look inside the rectum to check for abnormal areas. A proctoscope is inserted through the rectum. A proctoscope is a thin, tube-like instrument with a light and a lens for viewing. It may also have a tool to remove tissue to be checked under a microscope for signs of disease.

- **CT scan (CAT scan):** A procedure that makes a series of detailed pictures of areas inside the body, taken from different angles. The pictures are made by a computer linked to an x-ray machine. A dye may be injected into a vein or swallowed to help the organs or tissues show up more clearly. This procedure is

also called computed tomography, computerized tomography, or computerized axial tomography.

- **MRI (magnetic resonance imaging):** A procedure that uses a magnet, radio waves, and a computer to make a series of detailed pictures of areas inside the body. This procedure is also called nuclear magnetic resonance imaging (NMRI).

- **Lymphangiogram:** A procedure used to x-ray the lymph system. A dye is injected into the lymph vessels in the feet. The dye travels upward through the lymph nodes and lymph vessels and x-rays are taken to see if there are any blockages. This test helps find out whether cancer has spread to the lymph nodes.

The following stages are used for vaginal cancer.

Stage 0 (Carcinoma in Situ)

In stage 0, abnormal cells are found in tissue lining the inside of the vagina. These abnormal cells may become cancer and spread into nearby normal tissue. Stage 0 is also called carcinoma in situ.

Stage I

In stage I, cancer has formed and is found in the vagina only.

Stage II

In stage II, cancer has spread from the vagina to the tissue around the vagina.

Stage III

In stage III, cancer has spread from the vagina to the lymph nodes in the pelvis or groin, or to the pelvis, or both.

Stage IV

Stage IV is divided into stage IVA and stage IVB:

- **Stage IVA:** Cancer may have spread to lymph nodes in the pelvis or groin and has spread to one or both of the following areas: the lining of the bladder or rectum; beyond the pelvis.

- **Stage IVB:** Cancer has spread to parts of the body that are not near the vagina, such as the lungs. Cancer may also have spread to the lymph nodes.

Recurrent Vaginal Cancer

Recurrent vaginal cancer is cancer that has recurred (come back) after it has been treated. The cancer may come back in the vagina or in other parts of the body.

Treatment Option Overview

Different types of treatments are available for patients with vaginal cancer. Some treatments are standard (the currently used treatment), and some are being tested in clinical trials. Three types of standard treatment are used for vaginal cancer.

Surgery

Surgery is the most common treatment of vaginal cancer. The following surgical procedures may be used:

- **Laser surgery:** A surgical procedure that uses a laser beam (a narrow beam of intense light) as a knife to make bloodless cuts in tissue or to remove a surface lesion such as a tumor.

- **Wide local excision:** A surgical procedure that takes out the cancer and some of the healthy tissue around it.

- **Vaginectomy:** Surgery to remove all or part of the vagina.

- **Total hysterectomy:** Surgery to remove the uterus, including the cervix. If the uterus and cervix are taken out through the vagina, the operation is called a vaginal hysterectomy. If the uterus and cervix are taken out through a large incision (cut) in the abdomen, the operation is called a total abdominal hysterectomy. If the uterus and cervix are taken out through a small incision in the abdomen using a laparoscope, the operation is called a total laparoscopic hysterectomy.

- **Lymph nodes are removed and checked under a microscope for signs of cancer:** This procedure is also called lymph node dissection. If the cancer is in the upper vagina, the pelvic lymph nodes may be removed. If the cancer is in the lower vagina, lymph nodes in the groin may be removed.

- **Pelvic exenteration:** Surgery to remove the lower colon, rectum, and bladder. In women, the cervix, vagina, ovaries, and nearby lymph nodes are also removed. Artificial openings (stoma) are made for urine and stool to flow from the body into a collection bag.

- **Skin grafting may follow surgery, to repair or reconstruct the vagina:** Skin grafting is a surgical procedure in which skin is moved from one part of the body to another. A piece of healthy skin is taken from a part of the body that is usually hidden, such as the buttock or thigh, and used to repair or rebuild the area treated with surgery.

Even if the doctor removes all the cancer that can be seen at the time of the surgery, some patients may be given radiation therapy after surgery to kill any cancer cells that are left. Treatment given after the surgery, to lower the risk that the cancer will come back, is called adjuvant therapy.

Radiation Therapy

Radiation therapy is a cancer treatment that uses high-energy x-rays or other types of radiation to kill cancer cells or keep them from growing. There are two types of radiation therapy. External radiation therapy uses a machine outside the body to send radiation toward the cancer. Internal radiation therapy uses a radioactive substance sealed in needles, seeds, wires, or catheters that are placed directly into or near the cancer. The way the radiation therapy is given depends on the type and stage of the cancer being treated.

Chemotherapy

Chemotherapy is a cancer treatment that uses drugs to stop the growth of cancer cells, either by killing the cells or by stopping them from dividing. When chemotherapy is taken by mouth or injected into a vein or muscle, the drugs enter the bloodstream and can affect cancer cells throughout the body (systemic chemotherapy). When chemotherapy is placed directly into the spinal column, an organ, or a body cavity such as the abdomen, the drugs mainly affect cancer cells in those areas (regional chemotherapy). The way the chemotherapy is given depends on the type and stage of the cancer being treated.

Topical chemotherapy for squamous cell vaginal cancer may be applied to the vagina in a cream or lotion.

Clinical Trials

For some patients, taking part in a clinical trial may be the best treatment choice. Clinical trials are part of the cancer research process.

Clinical trials are done to find out if new cancer treatments are safe and effective or better than the standard treatment.

Many of today's standard treatments for cancer are based on earlier clinical trials. Patients who take part in a clinical trial may receive the standard treatment or be among the first to receive a new treatment.

Patients who take part in clinical trials also help improve the way cancer will be treated in the future. Even when clinical trials do not lead to effective new treatments, they often answer important questions and help move research forward.

Some clinical trials only include patients who have not yet received treatment. Other trials test treatments for patients whose cancer has not gotten better. There are also clinical trials that test new ways to stop cancer from recurring (coming back) or reduce the side effects of cancer treatment.

Clinical trials are taking place in many parts of the country.

Radiosensitizers

Radiosensitizers are being tested in clinical trials. Radiosensitizers are drugs that make tumor cells more sensitive to radiation therapy. Combining radiation therapy with radiosensitizers may kill more tumor cells.

Follow-Up Tests

Some of the tests that were done to diagnose the cancer or to find out the stage of the cancer may be repeated. Some tests will be repeated in order to see how well the treatment is working. Decisions about whether to continue, change, or stop treatment may be based on the results of these tests. This is sometimes called re-staging.

Some of the tests will continue to be done from time to time after treatment has ended. The results of these tests can show if your condition has changed or if the cancer has recurred (come back). These tests are sometimes called follow-up tests or check-ups.

Chapter 19

Vulvar Cancer

Vulvar cancer is a rare disease in which malignant (cancer) cells form in the tissues of the vulva. The vulva includes the inner and outer lips of the vagina, the clitoris (sensitive tissue between the lips), and the opening of the vagina and its glands. Vulvar cancer most often affects the outer vaginal lips. Less often, cancer affects the inner vaginal lips or the clitoris.

Vulvar cancer usually develops slowly over a period of years. Abnormal cells can grow on the surface of the vulvar skin for a long time. This precancerous condition is called vulvar intraepithelial neoplasia (VIN) or dysplasia. Because it is possible for VIN or dysplasia to develop into vulvar cancer, treatment of this condition is very important.

Risk Factors and Signs

Risk factors include the following:

- Having human papillomavirus (HPV) infection.

- Older age.

Vulvar cancer often does not cause early symptoms. When symptoms occur, they may be caused by vulvar cancer or by other conditions. A doctor should be consulted if any of the following problems occur:

PDQ® Cancer Information Summary. National Cancer Institute; Bethesda, MD. "Vulvar Cancer Treatment PDQ®): Patient Version. Updated 08/2009." Available at: http://cancer.gov. Accessed May 24, 2010.

- A lump in the vulva.

- Itching that does not go away in the vulvar area.

- Bleeding not related to menstruation (periods).

- Tenderness in the vulvar area.

Diagnosing Vulvar Cancer

The following tests and procedures may be used to diagnose vulvar cancer:

- **Physical exam and history:** An exam of the body to check general signs of health, including checking the vulva for signs of disease, such as lumps or anything else that seems unusual. A history of the patient's health habits and past illnesses and treatments will also be taken.

- **Biopsy:** The removal of cells or tissues from the vulva so they can be viewed under a microscope by a pathologist to check for signs of cancer.

The prognosis (chance of recovery) and treatment options depend on the stage of the cancer, the patient's age and general health, and whether the cancer has just been diagnosed or has recurred (come back).

Stages of Vulvar Cancer

After vulvar cancer has been diagnosed, tests are done to find out if cancer cells have spread within the vulva or to other parts of the body.

The process used to find out if cancer has spread within the vulva or to other parts of the body is called staging. The information gathered from the staging process determines the stage of the disease. It is important to know the stage in order to plan treatment. The following tests and procedures may be used in the staging process:

- **Pelvic exam:** An exam of the vagina, cervix, uterus, fallopian tubes, ovaries, and rectum. The doctor or nurse inserts one or two lubricated, gloved fingers of one hand into the vagina and places the other hand over the lower abdomen to feel the size, shape, and position of the uterus and ovaries. A speculum is also inserted into the vagina and the doctor or nurse looks at the vagina and cervix for signs of disease. A Pap test or Pap smear of the cervix is usually done. The doctor or nurse also inserts a

lubricated, gloved finger into the rectum to feel for lumps or abnormal areas.

- **Cystoscopy:** A procedure to look inside the bladder and urethra to check for abnormal areas. A cystoscope (a thin, lighted tube) is inserted through the urethra into the bladder. Tissue samples may be taken for biopsy.

- **Proctoscopy:** A procedure to look inside the rectum and anus to check for abnormal areas. A proctoscope (a thin, lighted tube) is inserted into the anus and rectum. Tissue samples may be taken for biopsy.

- **X-rays:** An x-ray is a type of energy beam that can go through the body and onto film, making a picture of areas inside the body. To stage vulvar cancer, x-rays may be taken of the organs and bones inside the chest, and the pelvic bones.

- **Intravenous pyelogram (IVP):** A series of x-rays of the kidneys, ureters, and bladder to find out if cancer has spread to these organs. A contrast dye is injected into a vein. As the contrast dye moves through the kidneys, ureters and bladder, x-rays are taken to see if there are any blockages. This procedure is also called intravenous urography.

- **CT scan (CAT scan):** A procedure that makes a series of detailed pictures of areas inside the body, taken from different angles. The pictures are made by a computer linked to an x-ray machine. A dye may be injected into a vein or swallowed to help the organs or tissues show up more clearly. This procedure is also called computed tomography, computerized tomography, or computerized axial tomography.

- **MRI (magnetic resonance imaging):** A procedure that uses a magnet, radio waves, and a computer to make a series of detailed pictures of areas inside the body. This procedure is also called nuclear magnetic resonance imaging (NMRI).

The following stages are used for vulvar cancer:

Stage 0 (Carcinoma in Situ)

In stage 0, abnormal cells are found on the surface of the vulvar skin. These abnormal cells may become cancer and spread into nearby normal tissue. Stage 0 is also called carcinoma in situ.

Stage I

In stage I, cancer has formed and is found in the vulva only or in the vulva and perineum (area between the rectum and the vagina). The tumor is 2 centimeters or smaller and has spread to tissue under the skin. Stage I vulvar cancer is further divided into stage IA and stage IB.

- **Stage IA:** The tumor has spread 1 millimeter or less into the tissue of the vulva.

- **Stage IB:** The tumor has spread more than 1 millimeter into the tissue of the vulva.

Stage II

In stage II, cancer is found in the vulva or the vulva and perineum (space between the rectum and the vagina), and the tumor is larger than 2 centimeters.

Stage III

In stage III vulvar cancer, the cancer is of any size and either is found only in the vulva or the vulva and perineum and has spread to tissue under the skin and to nearby lymph nodes on one side of the groin; or has spread to nearby tissues such as the lower part of the urethra and/or vagina or anus, and may have spread to nearby lymph nodes on one side of the groin.

Stage IV

Stage IV is divided into stage IVA and stage IVB, based on where the cancer has spread.

- **Stage IVA:** Cancer has spread to nearby lymph nodes on both sides of the groin, or has spread beyond nearby tissues to the upper part of the urethra, bladder, or rectum, or has attached to the pelvic bone and may have spread to lymph nodes.

- **Stage IVB:** Cancer has spread to distant parts of the body.

Recurrent Vulvar Cancer

Recurrent vulvar cancer is cancer that has recurred (come back) after it has been treated. The cancer may come back in the vulva or in other parts of the body.

Treatment Option Overview

Different types of treatments are available for patients with vulvar cancer. Some treatments are standard (the currently used treatment), and some are being tested in clinical trials. Four types of standard treatment are used for vulvar cancer:

Laser Therapy

Laser therapy is a cancer treatment that uses a laser beam (a narrow beam of intense light) to kill cancer cells.

Surgery

Surgery is the most common treatment for cancer of the vulva. The goal of surgery is to remove all the cancer without any loss of the woman's sexual function. One of the following types of surgery may be done:

- **Wide local excision:** A surgical procedure to remove the cancer and some of the normal tissue around the cancer.

- **Radical local excision:** A surgical procedure to remove the cancer and a large amount of normal tissue around it. Nearby lymph nodes in the groin may also be removed.

- **Vulvectomy:** A surgical procedure to remove part or all of the vulva:

  - **Skinning vulvectomy:** The top layer of vulvar skin where the cancer is found is removed. Skin grafts from other parts of the body may be needed to cover the area.

  - **Simple vulvectomy:** The entire vulva is removed.

  - **Modified radical vulvectomy:** The part of the vulva that contains cancer and some of the normal tissue around it are removed.

  - **Radical vulvectomy:** The entire vulva, including the clitoris, and nearby tissue are removed. Nearby lymph nodes may also be removed.

- **Pelvic exenteration:** A surgical procedure to remove the lower colon, rectum, and bladder. The cervix, vagina, ovaries, and nearby lymph nodes are also removed. Artificial openings (stoma) are made for urine and stool to flow from the body into a collection bag.

Even if the doctor removes all the cancer that can be seen at the time of the surgery, some patients may have chemotherapy or radiation therapy after surgery to kill any cancer cells that are left. Treatment given after the surgery, to lower the risk that the cancer will come back, is called adjuvant therapy.

Radiation therapy

Radiation therapy is a cancer treatment that uses high-energy x-rays or other types of radiation to kill cancer cells. There are two types of radiation therapy. External radiation therapy uses a machine outside the body to send radiation toward the cancer. Internal radiation therapy uses a radioactive substance sealed in needles, seeds, wires, or catheters that are placed directly into or near the cancer. The way the radiation therapy is given depends on the type and stage of the cancer being treated.

Chemotherapy

Chemotherapy is a cancer treatment that uses drugs to stop the growth of cancer cells, either by killing the cells or by stopping the cells from dividing. The way the chemotherapy is given depends on the type and stage of the cancer being treated. Topical chemotherapy for vulvar cancer may be applied to the skin in a cream or lotion.

Clinical Trials

New types of treatment are being tested in clinical trials. For some patients, taking part in a clinical trial may be the best treatment choice. Clinical trials are part of the cancer research process. Clinical trials are done to find out if new cancer treatments are safe and effective or better than the standard treatment.

Some clinical trials only include patients who have not yet received treatment. Other trials test treatments for patients whose cancer has not gotten better. There are also clinical trials that test new ways to stop cancer from recurring (coming back) or reduce the side effects of cancer treatment.

Follow-Up Tests

Some of the tests that were done to diagnose the cancer or to find out the stage of the cancer may be repeated. Some tests will be repeated in order to see how well the treatment is working. Decisions

about whether to continue, change, or stop treatment may be based on the results of these tests. This is sometimes called re-staging.

Some of the tests will continue to be done from time to time after treatment has ended. The results of these tests can show if your condition has changed or if the cancer has recurred (come back). These tests are sometimes called follow-up tests or check-ups.

Part Four

Other Cancers of Special Concern to Women

Chapter 20

Anal Cancer

Anal cancer is a disease in which malignant (cancer) cells form in the tissues of the anus. The anus is the end of the large intestine, below the rectum, through which stool (solid waste) leaves the body. The anus is formed partly from the outer, skin layers of the body and partly from the intestine. Two ring-like muscles, called sphincter muscles, open and close the anal opening to let stool pass out of the body. The anal canal, the part of the anus between the rectum and the anal opening, is about 1½ inches long.

The skin around the outside of the anus is called the perianal area. Tumors in this area are skin tumors, not anal cancer.

Risk Factors

Risk factors for anal cancer include the following:

- Being over 50 years old

- Being infected with human papillomavirus (HPV)

- Having many sexual partners

- Having receptive anal intercourse (anal sex)

- Frequent anal redness, swelling, and soreness

Excerpted from PDQ® Cancer Information Summary. National Cancer Institute; Bethesda, MD. "Anal Cancer Treatment (PDQ®): Patient Version." Updated 06/2008. Available at: http://cancer.gov. Accessed July 23, 2009.

- Having anal fistulas (abnormal openings)

- Smoking cigarettes

Possible signs of anal cancer include bleeding from the anus or rectum or a lump near the anus.

These and other symptoms may be caused by anal cancer. Other conditions may cause the same symptoms. A doctor should be consulted if any of the following problems occur:

- Bleeding from the anus or rectum

- Pain or pressure in the area around the anus

- Itching or discharge from the anus

- A lump near the anus

- A change in bowel habits

Diagnosing Anal Cancer

Tests that examine the rectum and anus are used to detect (find) and diagnose anal cancer.

- **Physical exam and history:** An exam of the body to check general signs of health, including checking for signs of disease, such as lumps or anything else that seems unusual. A history of the patient's health habits and past illnesses and treatments will also be taken.

- **Digital rectal examination (DRE):** An exam of the anus and rectum. The doctor or nurse inserts a lubricated, gloved finger into the lower part of the rectum to feel for lumps or anything else that seems unusual.

- **Anoscopy:** An exam of the anus and lower rectum using a short, lighted tube called an anoscope.

- **Proctoscopy:** An exam of the rectum using a short, lighted tube called a proctoscope.

- **Endo-anal or endorectal ultrasound:** A procedure in which an ultrasound transducer (probe) is inserted into the anus or rectum and used to bounce high-energy sound waves (ultrasound) off internal tissues or organs and make echoes. The echoes form a picture of body tissues called a sonogram.

- **Biopsy:** The removal of cells or tissues so they can be viewed under a microscope by a pathologist to check for signs of cancer.

If an abnormal area is seen during the anoscopy, a biopsy may be done at that time.

The prognosis (chance of recovery) depends on the size of the tumor, where the tumor is in the anus, and whether the cancer has spread to the lymph nodes. The treatment options depend on the stage of the cancer, where the tumor is in the anus, whether the patient has human immunodeficiency virus (HIV), and whether cancer remains after initial treatment or has recurred.

Stages of Anal Cancer

After anal cancer has been diagnosed, tests are done to find out if cancer cells have spread within the anus or to other parts of the body.

The process used to find out if cancer has spread within the anus or to other parts of the body is called staging. The information gathered from the staging process determines the stage of the disease. It is important to know the stage in order to plan treatment. The following tests may be used in the staging process:

- **CT scan (CAT scan):** A procedure that makes a series of detailed pictures of areas inside the body, taken from different angles. The pictures are made by a computer linked to an x-ray machine. A dye may be injected into a vein or swallowed to help the organs or tissues show up more clearly. This procedure is also called computed tomography, computerized tomography, or computerized axial tomography. For anal cancer, a CT scan of the pelvis and abdomen may be done.

- **Chest x-ray:** An x-ray of the organs and bones inside the chest. An x-ray is a type of energy beam that can go through the body and onto film, making a picture of areas inside the body.

- **Endo-anal or endorectal ultrasound:** A procedure in which an ultrasound transducer (probe) is inserted into the anus or rectum and used to bounce high-energy sound waves (ultrasound) off internal tissues or organs and make echoes. The echoes form a picture of body tissues called a sonogram.

There are three ways that cancer spreads in the body:

- **Through tissue:** Cancer invades the surrounding normal tissue.

- **Through the lymph system:** Cancer invades the lymph system and travels through the lymph vessels to other places in the body.

- **Through the blood:** Cancer invades the veins and capillaries and travels through the blood to other places in the body.

When cancer cells break away from the primary (original) tumor and travel through the lymph or blood to other places in the body, another (secondary) tumor may form. This process is called metastasis. The secondary (metastatic) tumor is the same type of cancer as the primary tumor.

The following stages are used for anal cancer:

- **Stage 0 (carcinoma in situ):** In stage 0, abnormal cells are found in the innermost lining of the anus. These abnormal cells may become cancer and spread into nearby normal tissue. Stage 0 is also called carcinoma in situ.

- **Stage I:** In stage I, cancer has formed and the tumor is two centimeters or smaller.

- **Stage II:** In stage II, the tumor is larger than two centimeters.

- **Stage IIIA:** In stage IIIA, the tumor may be any size and has spread to either lymph nodes near the rectum; or nearby organs, such as the vagina, urethra, and bladder.

- **Stage IIIB:** In stage IIIB, the tumor may be any size and has spread to nearby organs and to lymph nodes near the rectum; or to lymph nodes on one side of the pelvis and/or groin, and may have spread to nearby organs; or to lymph nodes near the rectum and in the groin, and/or to lymph nodes on both sides of the pelvis and/or groin, and may have spread to nearby organs.

- **Stage IV:** In stage IV, the tumor may be any size and cancer may have spread to lymph nodes or nearby organs and has spread to distant parts of the body.

- **Recurrent anal cancer:** Recurrent anal cancer is cancer that has recurred (come back) after it has been treated. The cancer may come back in the anus or in other parts of the body.

Treatment Option Overview

Different types of treatments are available for patients with anal cancer. Some treatments are standard (the currently used treatment), and some are being tested in clinical trials. Three types of standard treatment are used:

Radiation Therapy

Radiation therapy is a cancer treatment that uses high-energy x-rays or other types of radiation to kill cancer cells. There are two types of radiation therapy. External radiation therapy uses a machine outside the body to send radiation toward the cancer. Internal radiation therapy uses a radioactive substance sealed in needles, seeds, wires, or catheters that are placed directly into or near the cancer. The way the radiation therapy is given depends on the type and stage of the cancer being treated.

Chemotherapy

Chemotherapy is a cancer treatment that uses drugs to stop the growth of cancer cells, either by killing the cells or by stopping the cells from dividing. When chemotherapy is taken by mouth or injected into a vein or muscle, the drugs enter the bloodstream and can reach cancer cells throughout the body (systemic chemotherapy). When chemotherapy is placed directly into the spinal column, an organ, or a body cavity such as the abdomen, the drugs mainly affect cancer cells in those areas (regional chemotherapy). The way the chemotherapy is given depends on the type and stage of the cancer being treated.

Surgery

- **Local resection:** A surgical procedure in which the tumor is cut from the anus along with some of the healthy tissue around it. Local resection may be used if the cancer is small and has not spread. This procedure may save the sphincter muscles so the patient can still control bowel movements. Tumors that develop in the lower part of the anus can often be removed with local resection.

- **Abdominoperineal resection:** A surgical procedure in which the anus, the rectum, and part of the sigmoid colon are removed through an incision made in the abdomen. The doctor sews the end of the intestine to an opening, called a stoma, made in the surface of the abdomen so body waste can be collected in a disposable bag outside of the body. This is called a colostomy. Lymph nodes that contain cancer may also be removed during this operation.

- **Anal cancer surgery with colostomy:** The anus, rectum, and part of the colon are removed, a stoma is created, and a colostomy bag is attached to the stoma.

Cancer therapy can further damage the already weakened immune systems of patients who have the human immunodeficiency virus (HIV). For this reason, patients who have anal cancer and HIV are usually treated with lower doses of anticancer drugs and radiation than patients who do not have HIV.

Clinical Trials

For some patients, taking part in a clinical trial may be the best treatment choice. Clinical trials are part of the cancer research process. Clinical trials are done to find out if new cancer treatments are safe and effective or better than the standard treatment.

Patients can enter clinical trials before, during, or after starting their cancer treatment. Some clinical trials only include patients who have not yet received treatment. Other trials test treatments for patients whose cancer has not gotten better. There are also clinical trials that test new ways to stop cancer from recurring (coming back) or reduce the side effects of cancer treatment.

Radiosensitizers

Radiosensitizers are being tested in clinical trials. Radiosensitizers are drugs that make tumor cells more sensitive to radiation therapy. Combining radiation therapy with radiosensitizers may kill more tumor cells.

Follow-Up Tests

Some of the tests that were done to diagnose the cancer or to find out the stage of the cancer may be repeated. Some tests will be repeated in order to see how well the treatment is working. Decisions about whether to continue, change, or stop treatment may be based on the results of these tests. This is sometimes called re-staging.

Some of the tests will continue to be done from time to time after treatment has ended. The results of these tests can show if your condition has changed or if the cancer has recurred (come back). These tests are sometimes called follow-up tests or check-ups.

Chapter 21

Colorectal Cancer

Chapter Contents

Section 21.1

Cancers of the Colon and Rectum

Excerpted from "What You Need to Know about Cancer of the Colon and Rectum," National Cancer Institute (www.cancer.gov), May 26, 2006.

The Colon and Rectum

The colon and rectum are parts of the digestive system. They form a long, muscular tube called the large intestine (also called the large bowel). The colon is the first four to five feet of the large intestine, and the rectum is the last several inches.

Partly digested food enters the colon from the small intestine. The colon removes water and nutrients from the food and turns the rest into waste (stool). The waste passes from the colon into the rectum and then out of the body through the anus.

No one knows the exact causes of colorectal cancer. Doctors often cannot explain why one person develops this disease and another does not. However, it is clear that colorectal cancer is not contagious. No one can catch this disease from another person.

Research has shown that people with certain risk factors are more likely than others to develop colorectal cancer. A risk factor is something that may increase the chance of developing a disease. Studies have found the following risk factors for colorectal cancer:

- **Age over 50:** Colorectal cancer is more likely to occur as people get older. More than 90 percent of people with this disease are diagnosed after age 50. The average age at diagnosis is 72.

- **Colorectal polyps:** Polyps are growths on the inner wall of the colon or rectum. They are common in people over age 50. Most polyps are benign (not cancer), but some polyps (adenomas) can become cancer. Finding and removing polyps may reduce the risk of colorectal cancer.

- **Family history of colorectal cancer:** Close relatives (parents, brothers, sisters, or children) of a person with a history of colorectal cancer are somewhat more likely to develop this disease

themselves, especially if the relative had the cancer at a young age. If many close relatives have a history of colorectal cancer, the risk is even greater.

- **Genetic alterations:** Changes in certain genes increase the risk of colorectal cancer. Hereditary nonpolyposis colon cancer (HNPCC) is the most common type of inherited (genetic) colorectal cancer. It accounts for about two percent of all colorectal cancer cases. It is caused by changes in an HNPCC gene. Most people with an altered HNPCC gene develop colon cancer, and the average age at diagnosis of colon cancer is 44. Familial adenomatous polyposis (FAP) is a rare, inherited condition in which hundreds of polyps form in the colon and rectum. It is caused by a change in a specific gene called APC. Unless FAP is treated, it usually leads to colorectal cancer by age 40. FAP accounts for less than one percent of all colorectal cancer cases. Family members of people who have HNPCC or FAP can have genetic testing to check for specific genetic changes. For those who have changes in their genes, health care providers may suggest ways to try to reduce the risk of colorectal cancer, or to improve the detection of this disease. For adults with FAP, the doctor may recommend an operation to remove all or part of the colon and rectum.

- **Personal history of cancer:** A person who has already had colorectal cancer may develop colorectal cancer a second time. Also, women with a history of cancer of the ovary, uterus (endometrium), or breast are at a somewhat higher risk of developing colorectal cancer.

- **Ulcerative colitis or Crohn disease:** A person who has had a condition that causes inflammation of the colon (such as ulcerative colitis or Crohn disease) for many years is at increased risk of developing colorectal cancer.

- **Diet:** Studies suggest that diets high in fat (especially animal fat) and low in calcium, folate, and fiber may increase the risk of colorectal cancer. Also, some studies suggest that people who eat a diet very low in fruits and vegetables may have a higher risk of colorectal cancer. However, results from diet studies do not always agree, and more research is needed to better understand how diet affects the risk of colorectal cancer.

- **Cigarette smoking:** A person who smokes cigarettes may be at increased risk of developing polyps and colorectal cancer.

Because people who have colorectal cancer may develop colorectal cancer a second time, it is important to have checkups. If you have colorectal cancer, you also may be concerned that your family members may develop the disease. People who think they may be at risk should talk to their doctor. The doctor may be able to suggest ways to reduce the risk and can plan an appropriate schedule for checkups.

Screening for Colorectal Cancers

Screening tests help your doctor find polyps or cancer before you have symptoms. Finding and removing polyps may prevent colorectal cancer. Also, treatment for colorectal cancer is more likely to be effective when the disease is found early.

To find polyps or early colorectal cancer, people in their 50s and older should be screened. People who are at higher-than-average risk of colorectal cancer should talk with their doctor about whether to have screening tests before age 50, what tests to have, the benefits and risks of each test, and how often to schedule appointments.

The following screening tests can be used to detect polyps, cancer, or other abnormal areas. Your doctor can explain more about each test:

- **Fecal occult blood test (FOBT):** Sometimes cancers or polyps bleed, and the FOBT can detect tiny amounts of blood in the stool. If this test detects blood, other tests are needed to find the source of the blood. Benign conditions (such as hemorrhoids) also can cause blood in the stool.

- **Sigmoidoscopy:** Your doctor checks inside your rectum and the lower part of the colon with a lighted tube called a sigmoidoscope. If polyps are found, the doctor removes them. The procedure to remove polyps is called a polypectomy.

- **Colonoscopy:** Your doctor examines inside the rectum and entire colon using a long, lighted tube called a colonoscope. Your doctor removes polyps that may be found.

- **Double-contrast barium enema:** You are given an enema with a barium solution, and air is pumped into your rectum. Several x-ray pictures are taken of your colon and rectum. The barium and air help your colon and rectum show up on the pictures. Polyps or tumors may show up.

- **Digital rectal exam:** A rectal exam is often part of a routine physical examination. Your doctor inserts a lubricated, gloved finger into your rectum to feel for abnormal areas.

- **Virtual colonoscopy:** This method, which uses virtual reality technology to permit a minimally invasive evaluation of the colon and rectum, is under study.

Symptoms

A common symptom of colorectal cancer is a change in bowel habits. Symptoms include the following:

- Having diarrhea or constipation
- Feeling that your bowel does not empty completely
- Finding blood (either bright red or very dark) in your stool
- Finding your stools are narrower than usual
- Frequently having gas pains or cramps, or feeling full or bloated
- Losing weight with no known reason
- Feeling very tired all the time
- Having nausea or vomiting

Most often, these symptoms are not due to cancer. Other health problems can cause the same symptoms. Anyone with these symptoms should see a doctor to be diagnosed and treated as early as possible.

Usually, early cancer does not cause pain. It is important not to wait to feel pain before seeing a doctor.

Diagnosis

If you have screening test results that suggest cancer or you have symptoms, your doctor must find out whether they are due to cancer or some other cause. Your doctor asks about your personal and family medical history and gives you a physical exam.

If tests show an abnormal area (such as a polyp), a biopsy to check for cancer cells may be necessary. Often, the abnormal tissue can be removed during colonoscopy or sigmoidoscopy. A pathologist checks the tissue for cancer cells using a microscope.

Section 21.2

Staging and Treating Cancer of the Colon

Excerpted from PDQ® Cancer Information Summary. National Cancer Institute; Bethesda, MD. "Colon Cancer Treatment (PDQ®): Patient Version." Updated 10/2009. Available at: http://cancer.gov. Accessed May 25, 2010.

Stages of Colon Cancer

After colon cancer has been diagnosed, tests are done to find out if cancer cells have spread within the colon or to other parts of the body.

The process used to find out if cancer has spread within the colon or to other parts of the body is called staging. The information gathered from the staging process determines the stage of the disease. It is important to know the stage in order to plan treatment. The following tests and procedures may be used in the staging process:

- **CT scan (CAT scan):** A procedure that makes a series of detailed pictures of areas inside the body, taken from different angles. The pictures are made by a computer linked to an x-ray machine. A dye may be injected into a vein or swallowed to help the organs or tissues show up more clearly. This procedure is also called computed tomography, computerized tomography, or computerized axial tomography.

- **Lymph node biopsy:** The removal of all or part of a lymph node. A pathologist views the tissue under a microscope to look for cancer cells.

- **Complete blood count (CBC):** A procedure in which a sample of blood is drawn and checked for the following:

  - The number of red blood cells, white blood cells, and platelets.

  - The amount of hemoglobin (the protein that carries oxygen) in the red blood cells.

  - The portion of the blood sample made up of red blood cells.

- **Carcinoembryonic antigen (CEA) assay:** A test that measures the level of CEA in the blood. CEA is released into the bloodstream from both cancer cells and normal cells. When found in higher than normal amounts, it can be a sign of colon cancer or other conditions.

- **MRI (magnetic resonance imaging):** A procedure that uses a magnet, radio waves, and a computer to make a series of detailed pictures of areas inside the colon. A substance called gadolinium is injected into the patient through a vein. The gadolinium collects around the cancer cells so they show up brighter in the picture. This procedure is also called nuclear magnetic resonance imaging (NMRI).

- **Chest x-ray:** An x-ray of the organs and bones inside the chest. An x-ray is a type of energy beam that can go through the body and onto film, making a picture of areas inside the body.

- **Surgery:** A procedure to remove the tumor and see how far it has spread through the colon.

The following stages are used for colon cancer:

Stage 0 (Carcinoma in Situ)

In stage 0, abnormal cells are found in the innermost lining of the colon. These abnormal cells may become cancer and spread into nearby normal tissue. Stage 0 is also called carcinoma in situ.

Stage I

In stage I, cancer has formed and spread beyond the innermost tissue layer of the colon wall to the middle layers. Stage I colon cancer is sometimes called Dukes A colon cancer.

Stage II

Stage II colon cancer is divided into stage IIA and stage IIB.

- **Stage IIA:** Cancer has spread beyond the middle tissue layers of the colon wall or has spread to nearby tissues around the colon or rectum.

- **Stage IIB:** Cancer has spread beyond the colon wall into nearby organs and/or through the peritoneum.

Stage II colon cancer is sometimes called Dukes B colon cancer.

Stage III

Stage III colon cancer is divided into stage IIIA, stage IIIB, and stage IIIC.

- **Stage IIIA:** Cancer has spread from the innermost tissue layer of the colon wall to the middle layers and has spread to as many as three lymph nodes.

- **Stage IIIB:** Cancer has spread to as many as three nearby lymph nodes and has spread:

  - beyond the middle tissue layers of the colon wall; or

  - to nearby tissues around the colon or rectum; or

  - beyond the colon wall into nearby organs and/or through the peritoneum.

- **Stage IIIC:** Cancer has spread to 4 or more nearby lymph nodes and has spread:

  - to or beyond the middle tissue layers of the colon wall; or

  - to nearby tissues around the colon or rectum; or

- to nearby organs and/or through the peritoneum.

Stage III colon cancer is sometimes called Dukes C colon cancer.

Stage IV

In stage IV, cancer may have spread to nearby lymph nodes and has spread to other parts of the body, such as the liver or lungs. Stage IV colon cancer is sometimes called Dukes D colon cancer.

Recurrent Colon Cancer

Recurrent colon cancer is cancer that has recurred (come back) after it has been treated. The cancer may come back in the colon or in other parts of the body, such as the liver, lungs, or both.

Treatment Option Overview

Different types of treatment are available for patients with colon cancer. Some treatments are standard (the currently used treatment), and some are being tested in clinical trials. Three types of standard treatment are used:

Surgery

Surgery (removing the cancer in an operation) is the most common treatment for all stages of colon cancer. A doctor may remove the cancer using one of the following types of surgery:

- **Local excision:** If the cancer is found at a very early stage, the doctor may remove it without cutting through the abdominal wall. Instead, the doctor may put a tube through the rectum into the colon and cut the cancer out. This is called a local excision. If the cancer is found in a polyp (a small bulging piece of tissue), the operation is called a polypectomy.

- **Resection:** If the cancer is larger, the doctor will perform a partial colectomy (removing the cancer and a small amount of healthy tissue around it). The doctor may then perform an anastomosis (sewing the healthy parts of the colon together). The doctor will also usually remove lymph nodes near the colon and examine them under a microscope to see whether they contain cancer.

- **Resection and colostomy:** If the doctor is not able to sew the two ends of the colon back together, a stoma (an opening) is made on the outside of the body for waste to pass through. This procedure is called a colostomy. A bag is placed around the stoma to collect the waste. Sometimes the colostomy is needed only until the lower colon has healed, and then it can be reversed. If the doctor needs to remove the entire lower colon, however, the colostomy may be permanent.

- **Radiofrequency ablation:** The use of a special probe with tiny electrodes that kill cancer cells. Sometimes the probe is inserted directly through the skin and only local anesthesia is needed. In other cases, the probe is inserted through an incision in the abdomen. This is done in the hospital with general anesthesia.

- **Cryosurgery:** A treatment that uses an instrument to freeze and destroy abnormal tissue, such as carcinoma in situ. This type of treatment is also called cryotherapy.

Even if the doctor removes all the cancer that can be seen at the time of the operation, some patients may be given chemotherapy or radiation therapy after surgery to kill any cancer cells that are left. Treatment given after the surgery, to lower the risk that the cancer will come back, is called adjuvant therapy.

Chemotherapy

Chemotherapy is a cancer treatment that uses drugs to stop the growth of cancer cells, either by killing the cells or by stopping them from dividing. The way the chemotherapy is given depends on the type and stage of the cancer being treated.

Chemoembolization of the hepatic artery may be used to treat cancer that has spread to the liver. This involves blocking the hepatic artery (the main artery that supplies blood to the liver) and injecting anticancer drugs between the blockage and the liver. The liver's arteries then deliver the drugs throughout the liver. Only a small amount of the drug reaches other parts of the body. The blockage may be temporary or permanent, depending on what is used to block the artery. The liver continues to receive some blood from the hepatic portal vein, which carries blood from the stomach and intestine.

Radiation Therapy

Radiation therapy is a cancer treatment that uses high-energy x-rays or other types of radiation to kill cancer cells or keep them from growing. There are two types of radiation therapy. External radiation therapy uses a machine outside the body to send radiation toward the cancer. Internal radiation therapy uses a radioactive substance sealed in needles, seeds, wires, or catheters that are placed directly into or near the cancer. The way the radiation therapy is given depends on the type and stage of the cancer being treated.

Clinical Trials

For some patients, taking part in a clinical trial may be the best treatment choice. Clinical trials are part of the cancer research process. Clinical trials are done to find out if new cancer treatments are safe and effective or better than the standard treatment.

Patients can enter clinical trials before, during, or after starting their cancer treatment. Some clinical trials only include patients who have not yet received treatment. Other trials test treatments for patients whose cancer has not gotten better. There are also clinical trials that test new ways to stop cancer from recurring (coming back) or reduce the side effects of cancer treatment.

Targeted Therapy

Targeted therapy is a treatment that is being studied in clinical trials. It is a type of treatment that uses drugs or other substances

to identify and attack specific cancer cells without harming normal cells. Monoclonal antibody therapy is a type of targeted therapy being studied in the treatment of colon cancer.

Monoclonal antibody therapy uses antibodies made in the laboratory from a single type of immune system cell. These antibodies can identify substances on cancer cells or normal substances that may help cancer cells grow. The antibodies attach to the substances and kill the cancer cells, block their growth, or keep them from spreading. Monoclonal antibodies are given by infusion. They may be used alone or to carry drugs, toxins, or radioactive material directly to cancer cells.

Follow-Up Tests

Some of the tests that were done to diagnose the cancer or to find out the stage of the cancer may be repeated. Some tests will be repeated in order to see how well the treatment is working. Decisions about whether to continue, change, or stop treatment may be based on the results of these tests. This is sometimes called re-staging.

Some of the tests will continue to be done from time to time after treatment has ended. The results of these tests can show if your condition has changed or if the cancer has recurred (come back). These tests are sometimes called follow-up tests or check-ups.

For colon cancer, a blood test to measure carcinoembryonic antigen (CEA; a substance in the blood that may be increased when colon cancer is present) may be done along with other tests to see if the cancer has come back.

Section 21.3

Staging and Treating Cancer of the Rectum

Excerpted from PDQ® Cancer Information Summary. National Cancer Institute; Bethesda, MD. "Rectal Cancer Treatment (PDQ®): Patient Version." Updated 10/2009. Available at: http://cancer.gov. Accessed May 25, 2010.

Stages of Rectal Cancer

After rectal cancer has been diagnosed, tests are done to find out if cancer cells have spread within the rectum or to other parts of the body.

The process used to find out whether cancer has spread within the rectum or to other parts of the body is called staging. The information gathered from the staging process determines the stage of the disease. It is important to know the stage in order to plan treatment. The following tests and procedures may be used in the staging process:

- **Chest x-ray:** An x-ray of the organs and bones inside the chest.*

- **CT scan (CAT scan):** A procedure that makes a series of detailed pictures of areas inside the body, taken from different angles.*

- **MRI (magnetic resonance imaging):** A procedure that uses a magnet, radio waves, and a computer to make a series of detailed pictures of areas inside the body.*

- **Endoscopic ultrasound (EUS):** A procedure in which an endoscope or rigid probe is inserted into the body through the rectum. The endoscope or probe has a light and a lens for viewing. A device at the end is used to bounce high-energy sound waves (ultrasound) off internal tissues or organs and make echoes. The echoes form a picture of body tissues called a sonogram. This procedure is also called endosonography.

- **PET scan (positron emission tomography scan):** A procedure to find malignant tumor cells in the body. A small amount of radioactive glucose (sugar) is injected into a vein. The PET scanner rotates around the body and makes a picture of where glucose is being used in the body. Malignant tumor cells show

up brighter in the picture because they are more active and take up more glucose than normal cells do.

- **Carcinoembryonic antigen (CEA) assay:** A test that measures the level of CEA in the blood. CEA is released into the bloodstream from both cancer cells and normal cells.*

Tests marked with an asterisk (*) are also used in staging cancer of the colon; they are described in greater detail in the previous section. The following stages are used for rectal cancer:

- **Stage 0 (carcinoma in situ):** In stage 0, abnormal cells are found in the innermost lining of the rectum. These abnormal cells may become cancer and spread into nearby normal tissue. Stage 0 is also called carcinoma in situ.

- **Stage I:** In stage I, cancer has formed and spread beyond the innermost lining of the rectum to the second and third layers and involves the inside wall of the rectum, but it has not spread to the outer wall of the rectum or outside the rectum. Stage I rectal cancer is sometimes called Dukes A rectal cancer.

- **Stage II:** In stage II, cancer has spread outside the rectum to nearby tissue, but it has not gone into the lymph nodes (small, bean-shaped structures found throughout the body that filter substances in a fluid called lymph and help fight infection and disease). Stage II rectal cancer is sometimes called Dukes B rectal cancer.

- **Stage III:** In stage III, cancer has spread to nearby lymph nodes, but it has not spread to other parts of the body. Stage III rectal cancer is sometimes called Dukes C rectal cancer.

- **Stage IV:** In stage IV, cancer has spread to other parts of the body, such as the liver, lungs, or ovaries. Stage IV rectal cancer is sometimes called Dukes D rectal cancer.

- **Recurrent rectal cancer:** Recurrent rectal cancer is cancer that has recurred (come back) after it has been treated. The cancer may come back in the rectum or in other parts of the body, such as the colon, pelvis, liver, or lungs.

Treatment Option Overview

Different types of treatment are available for patients with rectal cancer. Some treatments are standard (the currently used treatment),

and some are being tested in clinical trials. Three types of standard treatment are used:

Surgery

Surgery is the most common treatment for all stages of rectal cancer. The cancer is removed using one of the following types of surgery:

- **Polypectomy:** If the cancer is found in a polyp (a small piece of bulging tissue), the polyp is often removed during a colonoscopy.

- **Local excision:** If the cancer is found on the inside surface of the rectum and has not spread into the wall of the rectum, the cancer and a small amount of surrounding healthy tissue is removed.

- **Resection:** If the cancer has spread into the wall of the rectum, the section of the rectum with cancer and nearby healthy tissue is removed. Sometimes the tissue between the rectum and the abdominal wall is also removed. The lymph nodes near the rectum are removed and checked under a microscope for signs of cancer.

- **Pelvic exenteration:** If the cancer has spread to other organs near the rectum, the lower colon, rectum, and bladder are removed. In women, the cervix, vagina, ovaries, and nearby lymph nodes may be removed. In men, the prostate may be removed. Artificial openings (stoma) are made for urine and stool to flow from the body to a collection bag.

After the cancer is removed, the surgeon will either do an anastomosis (sew the healthy parts of the rectum together, sew the remaining rectum to the colon, or sew the colon to the anus); or make a stoma (an opening) from the rectum to the outside of the body for waste to pass through. This procedure is done if the cancer is too close to the anus and is called a colostomy. A bag is placed around the stoma to collect the waste. Sometimes the colostomy is needed only until the rectum has healed, and then it can be reversed. If the entire rectum is removed, however, the colostomy may be permanent.

Radiation therapy or chemotherapy may be given before surgery to shrink the tumor, make it easier to remove the cancer, and lessen problems with bowel control after surgery. Treatment given before surgery is called neoadjuvant therapy. Even if all the cancer that can be seen at the time of the operation is removed, some patients may

be given radiation therapy or chemotherapy after surgery to kill any cancer cells that are left. Treatment given after the surgery, to lower the risk that the cancer will come back, is called adjuvant therapy.

Other Treatments

The other two types of standard treatment for rectal cancer are radiation therapy and chemotherapy. Targeted therapy is a treatment that is currently being studied in clinical trials. In addition to these, follow-up tests that repeat the initial staging tests may need to be done, and a blood test to measure amounts of carcinoembryonic antigen may be done to see if the cancer has returned. These treatments and tests are also used for colon cancer, and they are described more completely in the previous section.

Chapter 22

Gallbladder and Bile Duct Cancer

Gallbladder Cancer

Gallbladder cancer is a rare disease in which malignant (cancer) cells are found in the tissues of the gallbladder. The gallbladder is a pear-shaped organ that lies just under the liver in the upper abdomen. The gallbladder stores bile, a fluid made by the liver to digest fat. When food is being broken down in the stomach and intestines, bile is released from the gallbladder through a tube called the common bile duct, which connects the gallbladder and liver to the first part of the small intestine.

The wall of the gallbladder has three main layers of tissue:

- Mucosal (innermost) layer

- Muscularis (middle, muscle) layer

- Serosal (outer) layer

Between these layers is supporting connective tissue. Primary gallbladder cancer starts in the innermost layer and spreads through the outer layers as it grows. Anything that increases your chance of getting a

Excerpted from PDQ® Cancer Information Summary. National Cancer Institute; Bethesda, MD. "Gallbladder Cancer Treatment (PDQ®): Patient Version." Updated 06/2008. Available at: http://cancer.gov. Accessed July 23, 2009; and PDQ® Cancer Information Summary. National Cancer Institute; Bethesda, MD. "Extrahepatic Bile Duct Cancer Treatment (PDQ®): Patient Version." Updated 07/2008. Available at: http://cancer.gov. Accessed July 23, 2009.

disease is called a risk factor. Risk factors for gallbladder cancer include being female and being Native American.

Possible signs of gallbladder cancer include jaundice (yellowing of the skin and whites of the eyes), pain above the stomach, fever, nausea and vomiting, bloating, and lumps in the abdomen. These and other symptoms may be caused by gallbladder cancer. Other conditions may cause the same symptoms. A doctor should be consulted if any of the following problems occur:

Diagnosing Gallbladder Cancer

Gallbladder cancer is difficult to detect and diagnose early for the following reasons:

- There aren't any noticeable signs or symptoms in the early stages of gallbladder cancer.

- The symptoms of gallbladder cancer, when present, are like the symptoms of many other illnesses.

- The gallbladder is hidden behind the liver.

- Gallbladder cancer is sometimes found when the gallbladder is removed for other reasons. Patients with gallstones rarely develop gallbladder cancer.

Procedures that create pictures of the gallbladder and the area around it help diagnose gallbladder cancer and show how far the cancer has spread. The process used to find out if cancer cells have spread within and around the gallbladder is called staging.

In order to plan treatment, it is important to know if the gallbladder cancer can be removed by surgery. Tests and procedures to detect, diagnose, and stage gallbladder cancer are usually done at the same time.

The prognosis (chance of recovery) and treatment options depend on the following:

- The stage of the cancer (whether the cancer has spread from the gallbladder to other places in the body)

- Whether the cancer can be completely removed by surgery

- The type of gallbladder cancer (how the cancer cell looks under a microscope)

- Whether the cancer has just been diagnosed or has recurred (come back)

Treatment may also depend on the age and general health of the patient and whether the cancer is causing symptoms.

Gallbladder cancer can be cured only if it is found before it has spread, when it can be removed by surgery. If the cancer has spread, palliative treatment can improve the patient's quality of life by controlling the symptoms and complications of this disease. Taking part in one of the clinical trials being done to improve treatment should be considered.

Stages of Gallbladder Cancer

The following stages are used for gallbladder cancer:

- **Stage 0 (carcinoma in situ):** In stage 0, abnormal cells are found in the innermost (mucosal) layer of the gallbladder. These abnormal cells may become cancer and spread into nearby normal tissue. Stage 0 is also called carcinoma in situ.

- **Stage I:** In stage I, cancer has formed. Stage I is divided into stage IA and stage IB.

  - **Stage IA:** Cancer has spread beyond the innermost (mucosal) layer to the connective tissue or to the muscle (muscularis) layer.

  - **Stage IB:** Cancer has spread beyond the muscle layer to the connective tissue around the muscle.

- **Stage II:** Stage II is divided into stage IIA and stage IIB.

  - **Stage IIA:** Cancer has spread beyond the visceral peritoneum (tissue that covers the gallbladder) and/or to the liver and/or one nearby organ (such as the stomach, small intestine, colon, pancreas, or bile ducts outside the liver).

  - **Stage IIB:** Cancer has spread beyond the innermost layer to the connective tissue and to nearby lymph nodes; or to the muscle layer and nearby lymph nodes; or beyond the muscle layer to the connective tissue around the muscle and to nearby lymph nodes; or through the visceral peritoneum (tissue that covers the gallbladder) and/or to the liver and/or to one nearby organ (such as the stomach, small intestine, colon, pancreas, or bile ducts outside the liver), and to nearby lymph nodes.

- **Stage III:** In stage III, cancer has spread to a main blood vessel in the liver or to nearby organs and may have spread to nearby lymph nodes.

- **Stage IV:** In stage IV, cancer has spread to nearby lymph nodes and/or to organs far away from the gallbladder.

- **Recurrent gallbladder cancer:** Recurrent gallbladder cancer is cancer that has recurred (come back) after it has been treated. The cancer may come back in the gallbladder or in other parts of the body.

For gallbladder cancer, stages are also grouped according to how the cancer may be treated. There are two treatment groups:

- **Localized (Stage I):** Cancer is found in the wall of the gallbladder and can be completely removed by surgery.

- **Unresectable (Stage II, Stage III, and Stage IV):** Cancer has spread through the wall of the gallbladder to surrounding tissues or organs or throughout the abdominal cavity. Except in patients whose cancer has spread only to lymph nodes, the cancer is unresectable (cannot be completely removed by surgery).

Standard Treatment for Gallbladder Cancer

Different types of treatments are available for patients with gallbladder cancer. Some treatments are standard (the currently used treatment), and some are being tested in clinical trials. Three types of standard treatment are used:

Surgery: Gallbladder cancer may be treated with a cholecystectomy, surgery to remove the gallbladder and some of the tissues around it. Nearby lymph nodes may be removed. A laparoscope is sometimes used to guide gallbladder surgery. The laparoscope is attached to a video camera and inserted through an incision (port) in the abdomen. Surgical instruments are inserted through other ports to perform the surgery. Because there is a risk that gallbladder cancer cells may spread to these ports, tissue surrounding the port sites may also be removed.

If the cancer has spread and cannot be removed, the following types of palliative surgery may relieve symptoms:

- **Surgical biliary bypass:** If the tumor is blocking the small intestine and bile is building up in the gallbladder, a biliary bypass may be done. During this operation, the gallbladder or bile duct will be cut and sewn to the small intestine to create a new pathway around the blocked area.

- **Endoscopic stent placement:** If the tumor is blocking the bile duct, surgery may be done to put in a stent (a thin, flexible tube) to drain bile that has built up in the area. The stent may be placed through a catheter that drains to the outside of the body or the stent may go around the blocked area and drain the bile into the small intestine.

- **Percutaneous transhepatic biliary drainage:** A procedure done to drain bile when there is a blockage and endoscopic stent placement is not possible. An x-ray of the liver and bile ducts is done to locate the blockage. Images made by ultrasound are used to guide placement of a stent, which is left in the liver to drain bile into the small intestine or a collection bag outside the body. This procedure may be done to relieve jaundice before surgery.

Radiation therapy: Radiation therapy is a cancer treatment that uses high-energy x-rays or other types of radiation to kill cancer cells. There are two types of radiation therapy. External radiation therapy uses a machine outside the body to send radiation toward the cancer. Internal radiation therapy uses a radioactive substance sealed in needles, seeds, wires, or catheters that are placed directly into or near the cancer. The way the radiation therapy is given depends on the type and stage of the cancer being treated.

Chemotherapy: Chemotherapy is a cancer treatment that uses drugs to stop the growth of cancer cells, either by killing the cells or by stopping the cells from dividing. When chemotherapy is taken by mouth or injected into a vein or muscle, the drugs enter the bloodstream and can reach cancer cells throughout the body (systemic chemotherapy). When chemotherapy is placed directly into the spinal column, an organ, or a body cavity such as the abdomen, the drugs mainly affect cancer cells in those areas (regional chemotherapy). The way the chemotherapy is given depends on the type and stage of the cancer being treated.

Clinical Trials

A treatment clinical trial is a research study meant to help improve current treatments or obtain information on new treatments for patients with cancer. When clinical trials show that a new treatment is better than the standard treatment, the new treatment may become the standard treatment. Patients may want to think about taking part in a clinical trial. Some clinical trials are open only to patients who have not started treatment.

Radiosensitizers: Radiosensitizers are being tested in clinical trials. Radiosensitizers are drugs that make tumor cells more sensitive to radiation therapy. Combining radiation therapy with radiosensitizers may kill more tumor cells.

Extrahepatic Bile Duct Cancer

Extrahepatic bile duct cancer is a rare disease in which malignant (cancer) cells form in the part of bile duct that is outside the liver.

A network of bile ducts (tubes) connects the liver and the gallbladder to the small intestine. This network begins in the liver where many small ducts collect bile, a fluid made by the liver to break down fats during digestion. The small ducts come together to form the right and left hepatic bile ducts, which lead out of the liver. The two ducts join outside the liver to become the common hepatic duct. The part of the common hepatic duct that is outside the liver is called the extrahepatic bile duct. The extrahepatic bile duct is joined by a duct from the gallbladder (which stores bile) to form the common bile duct. Bile is released from the gallbladder through the common bile duct into the small intestine when food is being digested.

Anything that increases your risk of getting a disease is called a risk factor. Having a risk factor does not mean that you will get cancer; not

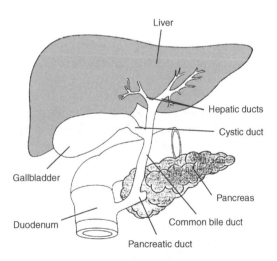

Figure 22.1. *The liver, gallbladder, and surrounding organs (Source: From "Gallstones," National Digestive Diseases Information Clearinghouse, July 2007).*

having risk factors doesn't mean that you will not get cancer. People who think they may be at risk should discuss this with their doctor. Risk factors include primary sclerosing cholangitis, chronic ulcerative colitis, choledochal cysts, and infection with a Chinese liver fluke parasite.

Possible signs of extrahepatic bile duct cancer include jaundice and pain. These and other symptoms may be caused by extrahepatic bile duct cancer or by other conditions. A doctor should be consulted if any of the following problems occur: jaundice (yellowing of the skin or whites of the eyes), pain in the abdomen, fever, or itchy skin.

The prognosis (chance of recovery) and treatment options depend on the stage of the cancer (whether it affects only the bile duct or has spread to other places in the body), whether the tumor can be completely removed by surgery, whether the tumor is in the upper or lower part of the duct, and whether the cancer has just been diagnosed or has recurred (come back).

Treatment options may also depend on the symptoms caused by the tumor. Extrahepatic bile duct cancer is usually found after it has spread and can rarely be removed completely by surgery. Palliative therapy may relieve symptoms and improve the patient's quality of life.

Stages of Extrahepatic Bile Duct Cancer

After extrahepatic bile duct cancer has been diagnosed, tests are done to find out if cancer cells have spread within the bile duct or to other parts of the body.

The process used to find out if cancer has spread within the extrahepatic bile duct or to other parts of the body is called staging. The information gathered from the staging process determines the stage of the disease. It is important to know the stage in order to plan treatment.

Extrahepatic bile duct cancer is usually staged following a laparotomy. A surgical incision is made in the wall of the abdomen to check the inside of the abdomen for signs of disease and to remove tissue and fluid for examination under a microscope. The results of the diagnostic imaging tests, laparotomy, and biopsy are viewed together to determine the stage of the cancer. Sometimes, a laparoscopy will be done before the laparotomy to see if the cancer has spread. If the cancer has spread and cannot be removed by surgery, the surgeon may decide not to do a laparotomy.

The following stages are used for extrahepatic bile duct cancer:

- **Stage 0 (carcinoma in situ):** In stage 0, abnormal cells are found in the innermost layer of tissue lining the extrahepatic

bile duct. These abnormal cells may become cancer and spread into nearby normal tissue. Stage 0 is also called carcinoma in situ.

- **Stage I:** In stage I, cancer has formed. Stage I is divided into stage IA and stage IB.

  - **Stage IA:** Cancer is found in the bile duct only.

  - **Stage IB:** Cancer has spread through the wall of the bile duct.

- **Stage II**: Stage II is divided into stage IIA and stage IIB.

  - **Stage IIA:** Cancer has spread to the liver, gallbladder, pancreas, and/or to either the right or left branch of the hepatic artery or to the right or left branch of the portal vein.

  - **Stage IIB:** Cancer has spread to nearby lymph nodes and: is found in the bile duct; or has spread through the wall of the bile duct; or has spread to the liver, gallbladder, pancreas, and/or the right or left branches of the hepatic artery or portal vein.

- **Stage III:** In stage III, cancer has spread: to the main portal vein or to both right and left branches of the portal vein; or to the hepatic artery; or to other nearby organs or tissues, such as the colon, stomach, small intestine, or abdominal wall. Cancer may have spread to nearby lymph nodes also.

- **Stage IV:** In stage IV, cancer has spread to lymph nodes and/or organs far away from the extrahepatic bile duct.

- **Recurrent extrahepatic bile duct cancer:** Recurrent extrahepatic bile duct cancer is cancer that has recurred (come back) after it has been treated. The cancer may come back in the bile duct or in other parts of the body.

Extrahepatic bile duct cancer can also be grouped according to how the cancer may be treated. There are two treatment groups:

- **Localized (and resectable):** The cancer is in an area where it can be removed completely by surgery.

- **Unresectable:** The cancer cannot be removed completely by surgery. The cancer may have spread to nearby blood vessels, the liver, the common bile duct, nearby lymph nodes, or other parts of the abdominal cavity.

Treatments for Extrahepatic Bile Duct Cancer

Different types of treatment are available for patients with extrahepatic bile duct cancer. Some treatments are standard (the currently used treatment), and some are being tested in clinical trials. Two types of standard treatment are used: surgery and radiation therapy.

The following types of surgery are used to treat extrahepatic bile duct cancer:

- **Removal of the bile duct:** If the tumor is small and only in the bile duct, the entire bile duct may be removed. A new duct is made by connecting the duct openings in the liver to the intestine. Lymph nodes are removed and viewed under a microscope to see if they contain cancer.

- **Partial hepatectomy:** Removal of the part of the liver where cancer is found. The part removed may be a wedge of tissue, an entire lobe, or a larger part of the liver, along with some normal tissue around it.

- **Whipple procedure:** A surgical procedure in which the head of the pancreas, the gallbladder, part of the stomach, part of the small intestine, and the bile duct are removed. Enough of the pancreas is left to make digestive juices and insulin.

- **Surgical biliary bypass:** If the tumor cannot be removed but is blocking the small intestine and causing bile to build up in the gallbladder, a biliary bypass may be done. During this operation, the gallbladder or bile duct will be cut and sewn to the small intestine to create a new pathway around the blocked area. This procedure helps to relieve jaundice caused by the build-up of bile.

- **Stent placement:** If the tumor is blocking the bile duct, a stent (a thin tube) may be placed in the duct to drain bile that has built up in the area. The stent may drain to the outside of the body or it may go around the blocked area and drain the bile into the small intestine. The doctor may place the stent during surgery or PTC, or with an endoscope.

Radiation therapy is a cancer treatment that uses high-energy x-rays or other types of radiation to kill cancer cells or keep them from growing. There are two types of radiation therapy. External radiation therapy uses a machine outside the body to send radiation toward the cancer. Internal radiation therapy uses a radioactive substance sealed in needles, seeds, wires, or catheters that are placed directly into or

271

near the cancer. The way the radiation therapy is given depends on the type and stage of the cancer being treated.

Clinical Trials

A treatment clinical trial is a research study meant to help improve current treatments or obtain information on new treatments for patients with cancer. When clinical trials show that a new treatment is better than the standard treatment, the new treatment may become the standard treatment. Patients may want to think about taking part in a clinical trial. Some clinical trials are open only to patients who have not started treatment. The following types of treatment are being tested in clinical trials for extrahepatic bile duct cancer:

- **Hyperthermia therapy:** A treatment in which body tissue is exposed to high temperatures to damage and kill cancer cells or to make cancer cells more sensitive to the effects of radiation therapy and certain anticancer drugs.

- **Radiosensitizers:** Drugs that make tumor cells more sensitive to radiation therapy. Combining radiation therapy with radiosensitizers may kill more tumor cells.

- **Chemotherapy:** Chemotherapy is a cancer treatment that uses drugs to stop the growth of cancer cells, either by killing the cells or by stopping them from dividing.

- **Biologic therapy:** Biologic therapy is a treatment that uses the patient's immune system to fight cancer. Substances made by the body or made in a laboratory are used to boost, direct, or restore the body's natural defenses against cancer. This type of cancer treatment is also called biotherapy or immunotherapy.

Follow-Up Tests

Some of the tests that were done to diagnose either gallbladder cancer or extrahepatic bile duct cancer or to find out the stage of the cancer may be repeated. Some tests will be repeated in order to see how well the treatment is working. Decisions about whether to continue, change, or stop treatment may be based on the results of these tests. This is sometimes called re-staging.

Some of the tests will continue to be done from time to time after treatment has ended. The results of these tests can show if your condition has changed or if the cancer has recurred (come back). These tests are sometimes called follow-up tests or check-ups.

Chapter 23

Lung Cancer

Chapter Contents

Section 23.1

What You Need to Know about Lung Cancer

Excerpted from "What You Need to Know about Lung Cancer,"
National Cancer Institute (www.cancer.gov), July 26, 2007.

The Lungs

Your lungs are a pair of large organs in your chest. They are part of your respiratory system. Air enters your body through your nose or mouth. It passes through your windpipe (trachea) and through each bronchus and goes into your lungs.

When you breathe in, your lungs expand with air. This is how your body gets oxygen. When you breathe out, air goes out of your lungs. This is how your body gets rid of carbon dioxide.

Your right lung has three parts (lobes). Your left lung is smaller and has two lobes. A thin tissue (the pleura) covers the lungs and lines the inside of the chest. Between the two layers of the pleura is a very small amount of fluid (pleural fluid). Normally, this fluid does not build up.

Lung Cancer Risk Factors

Doctors cannot always explain why one person develops lung cancer and another does not. However, we do know that a person with certain risk factors may be more likely than others to develop lung cancer. A risk factor is something that may increase the chance of developing a disease. Studies have found the following risk factors for lung cancer:

- **Tobacco smoke:** Tobacco smoke causes most cases of lung cancer. It's by far the most important risk factor for lung cancer. Harmful substances in smoke damage lung cells. That's why smoking cigarettes, pipes, or cigars can cause lung cancer and why secondhand smoke can cause lung cancer in nonsmokers. The more a person is exposed to smoke, the greater the risk of lung cancer.

- **Radon:** Radon is a radioactive gas that you cannot see, smell, or taste. It forms in soil and rocks. People who work in mines may be

exposed to radon. In some parts of the country, radon is found in houses. Radon damages lung cells, and people exposed to radon are at increased risk of lung cancer. The risk of lung cancer from radon is even higher for smokers.

- **Asbestos and other substances:** People who have certain jobs (such as those who work in the construction and chemical industries) have an increased risk of lung cancer. Exposure to asbestos, arsenic, chromium, nickel, soot, tar, and other substances can cause lung cancer. The risk is highest for those with years of exposure. The risk of lung cancer from these substances is even higher for smokers.

- **Air pollution:** Air pollution may slightly increase the risk of lung cancer. The risk from air pollution is higher for smokers.

- **Family history of lung cancer:** People with a father, mother, brother, or sister who had lung cancer may be at slightly increased risk of the disease, even if they don't smoke.

- **Personal history of lung cancer:** People who have had lung cancer are at increased risk of developing a second lung tumor.

- **Age over 65:** Most people are older than 65 years when diagnosed with lung cancer.

Researchers have studied other possible risk factors. For example, having certain lung diseases (such as tuberculosis or bronchitis) for many years may increase the risk of lung cancer. It's not yet clear whether having certain lung diseases is a risk factor for lung cancer.

People who think they may be at risk for developing lung cancer should talk to their doctor. The doctor may be able to suggest ways to reduce their risk and can plan an appropriate schedule for checkups. For people who have been treated for lung cancer, it's important to have checkups after treatment. The lung tumor may come back after treatment, or another lung tumor may develop.

How to Quit Smoking

Quitting is important for anyone who smokes tobacco—even people who have smoked for many years. For people who already have cancer, quitting may reduce the chance of getting another cancer. Quitting also can help cancer treatments work better. There are many ways to get help:

- Ask your doctor about medicine or nicotine replacement therapy, such as a patch, gum, lozenge, nasal spray, or inhaler. Your doctor can suggest a number of treatments that help people quit.

- Ask your doctor to help you find local programs or trained professionals who help people stop using tobacco.

- Call staff at the National Cancer Institute (NCI)'s Smoking Quitline (877-44U-QUIT) or instant message them through Live-Help (www.cancer.gov/livehelp). They can tell you about ways to quit smoking, groups that help smokers who want to quit, NCI publications about quitting smoking, and how to take part in a study of methods to help smokers quit.

- Go online to Smokefree.gov (http://www.smokefree.gov, a federal government website. It offers a guide to quitting smoking and a list of other resources.

Screening for Lung Cancer

Although screening tests to help doctors find and treat cancer early have been shown to be very helpful in some cancers such as breast cancer, there is no generally accepted screening test for lung cancer. Several methods of detecting lung cancer have been studied as possible screening tests. The methods under study include tests of sputum (mucus brought up from the lungs by coughing), chest x-rays, or spiral (helical) CT scans. However, screening tests have risks. For example, an abnormal x-ray result could lead to other procedures (such as surgery to check for cancer cells), but a person with an abnormal test result might not have lung cancer. Studies so far have not shown that screening tests lower the number of deaths from lung cancer.

Symptoms of Lung Cancer

Early lung cancer often does not cause symptoms. But as the cancer grows, common symptoms may include the following:

- A cough that gets worse or does not go away

- Breathing trouble, such as shortness of breath

- Constant chest pain

- Coughing up blood

- A hoarse voice

- Frequent lung infections, such as pneumonia
- Feeling very tired all the time
- Weight loss with no known cause

Most often these symptoms are not due to cancer. Other health problems can cause some of these symptoms. Anyone with such symptoms should see a doctor to be diagnosed and treated as early as possible.

Diagnosing Lung Cancer

If you have a symptom that suggests lung cancer, your doctor must find out whether it's from cancer or something else. Your doctor may ask about your personal and family medical history. Your doctor may order blood tests, and you may have one or more of the following tests:

- **Physical exam:** Your doctor checks for general signs of health, listens to your breathing, and checks for fluid in the lungs. Your doctor may feel for swollen lymph nodes and a swollen liver.

- **Chest x-ray:** X-ray pictures of your chest may show tumors or abnormal fluid.

- **CT scan:** Doctors often use CT scans to take pictures of tissue inside the chest. An x-ray machine linked to a computer takes several pictures. For a spiral CT scan, the CT scanner rotates around you as you lie on a table. The table passes through the center of the scanner. The pictures may show a tumor, abnormal fluid, or swollen lymph nodes.

Finding Lung Cancer Cells

The only sure way to know if lung cancer is present is for a pathologist to check samples of cells or tissue. The pathologist studies the sample under a microscope and performs other tests. There are many ways to collect samples. Your doctor may order one or more of the following tests to collect samples:

- **Sputum cytology:** Thick fluid (sputum) is coughed up from the lungs. The lab checks samples of sputum for cancer cells.

- **Thoracentesis:** The doctor uses a long needle to remove fluid (pleural fluid) from the chest. The lab checks the fluid for cancer cells.

277

- **Bronchoscopy:** The doctor inserts a thin, lighted tube (a bronchoscope) through the nose or mouth into the lung. This allows an exam of the lungs and the air passages that lead to them. The doctor may take a sample of cells with a needle, brush, or other tool. The doctor also may wash the area with water to collect cells in the water.

- **Fine-needle aspiration:** The doctor uses a thin needle to remove tissue or fluid from the lung or lymph node. Sometimes the doctor uses a CT scan or other imaging method to guide the needle to a lung tumor or lymph node.

- **Thoracoscopy:** The surgeon makes several small incisions in your chest and back. The surgeon looks at the lungs and nearby tissues with a thin, lighted tube. If an abnormal area is seen, a biopsy to check for cancer cells may be needed.

- **Thoracotomy:** The surgeon opens the chest with a long incision. Lymph nodes and other tissue may be removed.

- **Mediastinoscopy:** The surgeon makes an incision at the top of the breastbone. A thin, lighted tube is used to see inside the chest. The surgeon may take tissue and lymph node samples.

Types of Lung Cancer

The pathologist checks the sputum, pleural fluid, tissue, or other samples for cancer cells. If cancer is found, the pathologist reports the type. The types of lung cancer are treated differently. The most common types are named for how the lung cancer cells look under a microscope:

- **Small cell lung cancer:** About 13 percent of lung cancers are small cell lung cancers. This type tends to spread quickly.

- **Non-small cell lung cancer:** Most lung cancers (about 87 percent) are non-small cell lung cancers. This type spreads more slowly than small cell lung cancer.

Section 23.2

Staging and Treating Small Cell Lung Cancer

PDQ® Cancer Information Summary. National Cancer Institute; Bethesda, MD. "Small Cell Lung Cancer Treatment (PDQ®): Patient Version." Updated 08/2009. Available at: http://cancer.gov. Accessed May 31, 2010.

Stages of Small Cell Lung Cancer

After small cell lung cancer has been diagnosed, tests are done to find out if cancer cells have spread within the chest or to other parts of the body.

The process used to find out if cancer has spread within the chest or to other parts of the body is called staging. The information gathered from the staging process determines the stage of the disease. It is important to know the stage in order to plan treatment. Some of the tests used to diagnose small cell lung cancer are also used to stage the disease. Other tests and procedures that may be used in the staging process include the following:

- **Laboratory tests:** Medical procedures that test samples of tissue, blood, urine, or other substances in the body. These tests help to diagnose disease, plan and check treatment, or monitor the disease over time.

- **Bone marrow aspiration and biopsy:** The removal of bone marrow, blood, and a small piece of bone by inserting a hollow needle into the hipbone or breastbone. A pathologist views the bone marrow, blood, and bone under a microscope to look for signs of cancer.

- **MRI (magnetic resonance imaging) of the brain:** A procedure that uses a magnet, radio waves, and a computer to make a series of detailed pictures of areas inside the body. This procedure is also called nuclear magnetic resonance imaging (NMRI).

- **Endoscopic ultrasound (EUS):** A procedure in which an endoscope is inserted into the body. An endoscope is a thin, tube-like

instrument with a light and a lens for viewing. A probe at the end of the endoscope is used to bounce high-energy sound waves (ultrasound) off internal tissues or organs and make echoes. The echoes form a picture of body tissues called a sonogram. This procedure is also called endosonography. EUS may be used to guide fine-needle aspiration (FNA) biopsy of the lung, lymph nodes, or other areas.

- **Lymph node biopsy:** The removal of all or part of a lymph node. A pathologist views the tissue under a microscope to look for cancer cells.

- **Radionuclide bone scan:** A procedure to check if there are rapidly dividing cells, such as cancer cells, in the bone. A very small amount of radioactive material is injected into a vein and travels through the bloodstream. The radioactive material collects in the bones and is detected by a scanner.

When cancer cells break away from the primary (original) tumor and travel through the lymph or blood to other places in the body, another (secondary) tumor may form. This process is called metastasis. The secondary (metastatic) tumor is the same type of cancer as the primary tumor.

The following stages are used for small cell lung cancer:

- **Limited-stage small cell lung cancer:** In limited-stage, cancer is found in one lung, the tissues between the lungs, and nearby lymph nodes only.

- **Extensive-stage small cell lung cancer:** In extensive-stage, cancer has spread outside of the lung in which it began or to other parts of the body.

- **Recurrent small cell lung cancer:** Recurrent small cell lung cancer is cancer that has recurred (come back) after it has been treated. The cancer may come back in the chest, central nervous system, or in other parts of the body.

Treatment Option Overview

Different types of treatment are available for patients with small cell lung cancer. Some treatments are standard (the currently used treatment), and some are being tested in clinical trials. Five types of standard treatment are used:

Surgery

Surgery may be used if the cancer is found in one lung and in nearby lymph nodes only. Because this type of lung cancer is usually found in both lungs, surgery alone is not often used. Occasionally, surgery may be used to help determine the patient's exact type of lung cancer. During surgery, the doctor will also remove lymph nodes to see if they contain cancer.

Even if the doctor removes all the cancer that can be seen at the time of the operation, some patients may be given chemotherapy or radiation therapy after surgery to kill any cancer cells that are left. Treatment given after the surgery, to lower the risk that the cancer will come back, is called adjuvant therapy.

Chemotherapy

Chemotherapy is a cancer treatment that uses drugs to stop the growth of cancer cells, either by killing the cells or by stopping them from dividing. When chemotherapy is taken by mouth or injected into a vein or muscle, the drugs enter the bloodstream and can reach cancer cells throughout the body (systemic chemotherapy). When chemotherapy is placed directly into the spinal column, an organ, or a body cavity such as the abdomen, the drugs mainly affect cancer cells in those areas (regional chemotherapy). The way the chemotherapy is given depends on the type and stage of the cancer being treated.

Radiation Therapy

Radiation therapy is a cancer treatment that uses high-energy x-rays or other types of radiation to kill cancer cells or keep them from growing. There are two types of radiation therapy. External radiation therapy uses a machine outside the body to send radiation toward the cancer. Internal radiation therapy uses a radioactive substance sealed in needles, seeds, wires, or catheters that are placed directly into or near the cancer. Prophylactic cranial irradiation (radiation therapy to the brain to reduce the risk that cancer will spread to the brain) may also be given. The way the radiation therapy is given depends on the type and stage of the cancer being treated.

Laser Therapy

Laser therapy is a cancer treatment that uses a laser beam (a narrow beam of intense light) to kill cancer cells.

Endoscopic Stent Placement

An endoscope is a thin, tube-like instrument used to look at tissues inside the body. An endoscope has a light and a lens for viewing and may be used to place a stent in a body structure to keep the structure open. Endoscopic stent placement can be used to open an airway blocked by abnormal tissue.

Clinical Trials

New types of treatment are being tested in clinical trials. A treatment clinical trial is a research study meant to help improve current treatments or obtain information on new treatments for patients with cancer. When clinical trials show that a new treatment is better than the standard treatment, the new treatment may become the standard treatment. Patients may want to think about taking part in a clinical trial. Some clinical trials are open only to patients who have not started treatment.

You can check for U.S. clinical trials that are now accepting patients with small cell lung cancer from NCI's PDQ Cancer Clinical Trials Registry, available online through the NCI website at www.cancer.gov.

Follow-Up Tests

Some of the tests that were done to diagnose the cancer or to find out the stage of the cancer may be repeated. Some tests will be repeated in order to see how well the treatment is working. Decisions about whether to continue, change, or stop treatment may be based on the results of these tests. This is sometimes called re-staging.

Some of the tests will continue to be done from time to time after treatment has ended. The results of these tests can show if your condition has changed or if the cancer has recurred (come back). These tests are sometimes called follow-up tests or check-ups.

Section 23.3

Staging and Treating Non-Small Cell Lung Cancer

PDQ® Cancer Information Summary. National Cancer Institute; Bethesda, MD. "Non-Small Cell Lung Cancer Treatment (PDQ®): Patient Version." Updated 01/2010. Available at: http://cancer.gov. Accessed May 31, 2010.

Stages of Non-Small Cell Lung Cancer

Some of the tests used to diagnose non-small cell lung cancer are also used to stage the disease. Other tests and procedures are the same as those described in the section above on staging small cell lung cancer. Another test that may be used is called a mediastinoscopy.

Mediastinoscopy is a surgical procedure to look at the organs, tissues, and lymph nodes between the lungs for abnormal areas. An incision is made at the top of the breastbone and a mediastinoscope is inserted into the chest. A mediastinoscope is a thin, tube-like instrument with a light and a lens for viewing. It may also have a tool to remove tissue or lymph node samples, which are checked under a microscope for signs of cancer.

An anterior mediastinotomy is a little different. It is a surgical procedure to look at the organs and tissues between the lungs and between the breastbone and heart for abnormal areas. An incision is made next to the breastbone. This is also called the Chamberlain procedure.

The following stages are used for non-small cell lung cancer:

Occult (Hidden) Stage

In the occult (hidden) stage, cancer cells are found in sputum (mucus coughed up from the lungs), but no tumor can be found in the lung by imaging or bronchoscopy, or the primary tumor is too small to be checked.

Stage 0 (Carcinoma in Situ)

In stage 0, abnormal cells are found in the innermost lining of the lung. These abnormal cells may become cancer and spread into nearby normal tissue. Stage 0 is also called carcinoma in situ.

Stage I

In stage I, cancer has formed. Stage I is divided into stages IA and IB:

- **Stage IA:** The tumor is in the lung only and is three centimeters or smaller.

- **Stage IB:** One or more of the following is true:

  - The tumor is larger than three centimeters.

  - Cancer has spread to the main bronchus of the lung, and is at least two centimeters from the carina (where the trachea joins the bronchi).

  - Cancer has spread to the innermost layer of the membrane that covers the lungs.

  - The tumor partly blocks the bronchus or bronchioles and part of the lung has collapsed or developed pneumonitis (inflammation of the lung).

Stage II

Stage II is divided into stages IIA and IIB:

- **Stage IIA:** The tumor is 3 centimeters or smaller and cancer has spread to nearby lymph nodes on the same side of the chest as the tumor.

- **Stage IIB:** Cancer has spread to nearby lymph nodes on the same side of the chest as the tumor and one or more of the following is true:

  - Cancer has spread to nearby lymph nodes on the same side of the chest as the tumor and one or more of the following is true: the tumor is larger than three centimeters; cancer has spread to the main bronchus of the lung and is two centimeters or more from the carina (where the trachea joins the bronchi); cancer has spread to the innermost layer of the membrane that covers the lungs; the tumor partly blocks the bronchus or bronchioles and part of the lung has collapsed or developed pneumonitis (inflammation of the lung).

  or

  - Cancer has not spread to lymph nodes and one or more of the following is true: the tumor may be any size and cancer has spread to the chest wall, or the diaphragm, or the pleura between the lungs, or membranes surrounding the heart; cancer has spread to the main bronchus of the lung and is no more

than two centimeters from the carina (where the trachea meets the bronchi), but has not spread to the trachea; cancer blocks the bronchus or bronchioles and the whole lung has collapsed or developed pneumonitis (inflammation of the lung).

Stage IIIA

In stage IIIA, cancer has spread to lymph nodes on the same side of the chest as the tumor. Also the tumor may be any size. Cancer may have spread to the main bronchus, the chest wall, the diaphragm, the pleura around the lungs, or the membrane around the heart, but has not spread to the trachea. Part or all of the lung may have collapsed or developed pneumonitis (inflammation of the lung).

Stage IIIB

In stage IIIB, the tumor may be any size and has spread to lymph nodes above the collarbone or in the opposite side of the chest from the tumor; and/or to any of the following:

- Heart
- Major blood vessels that lead to or from the heart
- Chest wall
- Diaphragm
- Trachea
- Esophagus
- Sternum (chest bone) or backbone
- More than one place in the same lobe of the lung
- The fluid of the pleural cavity surrounding the lung

Stage IV

In stage IV, cancer may have spread to lymph nodes and has spread to another lobe of the lungs or to other parts of the body, such as the brain, liver, adrenal glands, kidneys, or bone.

Recurrent Non-Small Cell Lung Cancer

Recurrent non-small cell lung cancer is cancer that has recurred (come back) after it has been treated. The cancer may come back in the brain, lung, or other parts of the body.

Treatment Option Overview

Different types of treatments are available for patients with non-small cell lung cancer. Some treatments are standard (the currently used treatment), and some are being tested in clinical trials. Nine types of standard treatment are used:

Surgery

Four types of surgery are used:

- **Wedge resection:** Surgery to remove a tumor and some of the normal tissue around it. When a slightly larger amount of tissue is taken, it is called a segmental resection.

- **Lobectomy:** Surgery to remove a whole lobe (section) of the lung.

- **Pneumonectomy:** Surgery to remove one whole lung.

- **Sleeve resection:** Surgery to remove part of the bronchus.

Even if the doctor removes all the cancer that can be seen at the time of the surgery, some patients may be given chemotherapy or radiation therapy after surgery to kill any cancer cells that are left. Treatment given after the surgery, to lower the risk that the cancer will come back, is called adjuvant therapy.

Radiation Therapy

Radiation therapy is a cancer treatment that uses high-energy x-rays or other types of radiation to kill cancer cells or keep them from growing. Radiosurgery is a method of delivering radiation directly to the tumor with little damage to healthy tissue. It does not involve surgery and may be used to treat certain tumors in patients who cannot have surgery. The way the radiation therapy is given depends on the type and stage of the cancer being treated.

Chemotherapy

Chemotherapy is a cancer treatment that uses drugs to stop the growth of cancer cells, either by killing the cells or by stopping them from dividing. When chemotherapy is taken by mouth or injected into a vein or muscle, the drugs enter the bloodstream and can reach cancer cells throughout the body (systemic chemotherapy). When chemotherapy is placed directly into the spinal column, an organ, or a body cavity such as the abdomen, the drugs mainly affect cancer cells in

those areas (regional chemotherapy). The way the chemotherapy is given depends on the type and stage of the cancer being treated.

Targeted Therapy

Targeted therapy is a type of treatment that uses drugs or other substances to identify and attack specific cancer cells without harming normal cells. Monoclonal antibodies and tyrosine kinase inhibitors are two types of targeted therapy being used in the treatment of non-small cell lung cancer.

Monoclonal antibody therapy is a cancer treatment that uses antibodies made in the laboratory from a single type of immune system cell. These antibodies can identify substances on cancer cells or normal substances that may help cancer cells grow. The antibodies attach to the substances and kill the cancer cells, block their growth, or keep them from spreading. Monoclonal antibodies are given by infusion. They may be used alone or to carry drugs, toxins, or radioactive material directly to cancer cells.

Tyrosine kinase inhibitors are targeted therapy drugs that block signals needed for tumors to grow. Tyrosine kinase inhibitors may be used with other anticancer drugs as adjuvant therapy.

Laser Therapy

Laser therapy is a cancer treatment that uses a laser beam (a narrow beam of intense light) to kill cancer cells.

Photodynamic Therapy (PDT)

Photodynamic therapy (PDT) is a cancer treatment that uses a drug and a certain type of laser light to kill cancer cells. A drug that is not active until it is exposed to light is injected into a vein. The drug collects more in cancer cells than in normal cells. Fiberoptic tubes are then used to carry the laser light to the cancer cells, where the drug becomes active and kills the cells. Photodynamic therapy causes little damage to healthy tissue. It is used mainly to treat tumors on or just under the skin or in the lining of internal organs.

Cryosurgery

Cryosurgery is a treatment that uses an instrument to freeze and destroy abnormal tissue, such as carcinoma in situ. This type of treatment is also called cryotherapy.

Electrocautery

Electrocautery is a treatment that uses a probe or needle heated by an electric current to destroy abnormal tissue.

Watchful Waiting

Watchful waiting is closely monitoring a patient's condition without giving any treatment until symptoms appear or change. This may be done in certain rare cases of non-small cell lung cancer.

Clinical Trials

A treatment clinical trial is a research study meant to help improve current treatments or obtain information on new treatments for patients with cancer. When clinical trials show that a new treatment is better than the standard treatment, the new treatment may become the standard treatment. Patients may want to think about taking part in a clinical trial. Some clinical trials are open only to patients who have not started treatment.

Chemoprevention is being studied in clinical trials. It is the use of drugs, vitamins, or other substances to reduce the risk of developing cancer or to reduce the risk cancer will recur (come back).

New combinations of treatments are also being studied in clinical trials. Clinical trials are taking place in many parts of the country. Visit www.cancer.gov to find information about current treatment clinical trials.

Follow-Up Tests

Some of the tests that were done to diagnose the cancer or to find out the stage of the cancer may be repeated. Some tests will be repeated in order to see how well the treatment is working. Decisions about whether to continue, change, or stop treatment may be based on the results of these tests. This is sometimes called re-staging.

Some of the tests will continue to be done from time to time after treatment has ended. The results of these tests can show if your condition has changed or if the cancer has recurred (come back). These tests are sometimes called follow-up tests or check-ups.

Chapter 24

Pancreatic Cancer

Chapter Contents

Section 24.1

What You Need to Know
about Cancer of the Pancreas

Excerpted from, "What You Need to Know about Cancer of the Pancreas," National Cancer Institute, 2002; accessed July 23, 2009.

The Pancreas

The pancreas is a gland located deep in the abdomen between the stomach and the spine (backbone). The liver, intestine, and other organs surround the pancreas.

The pancreas is about six inches long and is shaped like a flat pear. The widest part of the pancreas is the head, the middle section is the body, and the thinnest part is the tail.

The pancreas makes insulin and other hormones. These hormones enter the bloodstream and travel throughout the body. They help the body use or store the energy that comes from food. For example, insulin helps control the amount of sugar in the blood.

The pancreas also makes pancreatic juices. These juices contain enzymes that help digest food. The pancreas releases the juices into a system of ducts leading to the common bile duct. The common bile duct empties into the duodenum, the first section of the small intestine.

Most pancreatic cancers begin in the ducts that carry pancreatic juices. Cancer of the pancreas may be called pancreatic cancer or carcinoma of the pancreas.

A rare type of pancreatic cancer begins in the cells that make insulin and other hormones. Cancer that begins in these cells is called islet cell cancer. This chapter does not deal with this rare disease. The National Cancer Institute (NCI)'s Cancer Information Service (800-4-CANCER or www.cancer.gov) can provide information about islet cell cancer.

When cancer of the pancreas spreads (metastasizes) outside the pancreas, cancer cells are often found in nearby lymph nodes. If the cancer has reached these nodes, it means that cancer cells may have spread to other lymph nodes or other tissues, such as the liver or lungs.

Sometimes cancer of the pancreas spreads to the peritoneum, the tissue that lines the abdomen.

When cancer spreads from its original place to another part of the body, the new tumor has the same kind of abnormal cells and the same name as the primary tumor. For example, if cancer of the pancreas spreads to the liver, the cancer cells in the liver are pancreatic cancer cells. The disease is metastatic pancreatic cancer, not liver cancer. It is treated as pancreatic cancer, not liver cancer.

Risk Factors

No one knows the exact causes of pancreatic cancer. Doctors can seldom explain why one person gets pancreatic cancer and another does not. However, it is clear that this disease is not contagious. No one can "catch" cancer from another person. Research has shown that people with certain risk factors are more likely than others to develop pancreatic cancer. A risk factor is anything that increases a person's chance of developing a disease. Studies have found the following risk factors for pancreatic cancer:

- **Age:** The likelihood of developing pancreatic cancer increases with age. Most pancreatic cancers occur in people over the age of 60.

- **Smoking:** Cigarette smokers are two or three times more likely than nonsmokers to develop pancreatic cancer.

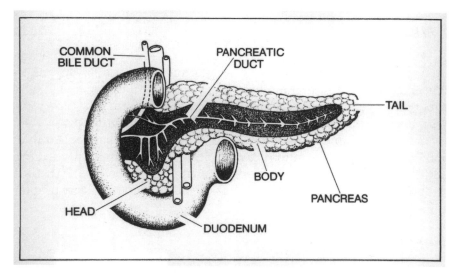

Figure 24.1. Detail of the pancreas (Source: National Cancer Institute, AV-0000-4104).

- **Diabetes:** Pancreatic cancer occurs more often in people who have diabetes than in people who do not.

- **Being male:** More men than women are diagnosed with pancreatic cancer.

- **Being African American:** African Americans are more likely than Asians, Hispanics, or whites to get pancreatic cancer.

- **Family history:** The risk for developing pancreatic cancer triples if a person's mother, father, sister, or brother had the disease. Also, a family history of colon or ovarian cancer increases the risk of pancreatic cancer.

- **Chronic pancreatitis:** Chronic pancreatitis is a painful condition of the pancreas. Some evidence suggests that chronic pancreatitis may increase the risk of pancreatic cancer.

- **Other factors:** Other studies suggest that exposure to certain chemicals in the workplace or a diet high in fat may increase the chance of getting pancreatic cancer.

Most people with known risk factors do not get pancreatic cancer. On the other hand, many who do get the disease have none of these factors. People who think they may be at risk for pancreatic cancer should discuss this concern with their doctor. The doctor may suggest ways to reduce the risk and can plan an appropriate schedule for checkups.

Symptoms

Pancreatic cancer is sometimes called a "silent disease" because early pancreatic cancer often does not cause symptoms. But, as the cancer grows, symptoms may include pain in the upper abdomen or upper back, yellow skin and eyes, and dark urine from jaundice, weakness, loss of appetite, nausea and vomiting. and weight loss.

These symptoms are not sure signs of pancreatic cancer. An infection or other problem could also cause these symptoms. Only a doctor can diagnose the cause of a person's symptoms. Anyone with these symptoms should see a doctor so that the doctor can treat any problem as early as possible.

Diagnosis

If a patient has symptoms that suggest pancreatic cancer, the doctor asks about the patient's medical history. The doctor may perform a number of procedures, including one or more of the following:

- **Physical exam:** The doctor examines the skin and eyes for signs of jaundice. The doctor then feels the abdomen to check for changes in the area near the pancreas, liver, and gallbladder. The doctor also checks for ascites, an abnormal buildup of fluid in the abdomen.

- **Lab tests:** The doctor may take blood, urine, and stool samples to check for bilirubin and other substances. Bilirubin is a substance that passes from the liver to the gallbladder to the intestine. If the common bile duct is blocked by a tumor, the bilirubin cannot pass through normally. Blockage may cause the level of bilirubin in the blood, stool, or urine to become very high. High bilirubin levels can result from cancer or from noncancerous conditions.

- **CT scan (Computed tomography):** An x-ray machine linked to a computer takes a series of detailed pictures. The x-ray machine is shaped like a donut with a large hole. The patient lies on a bed that passes through the hole. As the bed moves slowly through the hole, the machine takes many x-rays. The computer puts the x-rays together to create pictures of the pancreas and other organs and blood vessels in the abdomen.

- **Ultrasonography:** The ultrasound device uses sound waves that cannot be heard by humans. The sound waves produce a pattern of echoes as they bounce off internal organs. The echoes create a picture of the pancreas and other organs inside the abdomen. The echoes from tumors are different from echoes made by healthy tissues. The ultrasound procedure may use an external or internal device, or both types:

  - **Transabdominal ultrasound:** To make images of the pancreas, the doctor places the ultrasound device on the abdomen and slowly moves it around.

  - **EUS (Endoscopic ultrasound):** The doctor passes a thin, lighted tube (endoscope) through the patient's mouth and stomach, down into the first part of the small intestine. At the tip of the endoscope is an ultrasound device. The doctor slowly withdraws the endoscope from the intestine toward the stomach to make images of the pancreas and surrounding organs and tissues.

- **ERCP (endoscopic retrograde cholangiopancreatography):** The doctor passes an endoscope through the patient's mouth and stomach, down into the first part of the small intestine. The doctor slips a smaller tube (catheter) through the endoscope into the bile ducts and pancreatic ducts. After injecting dye through the catheter

into the ducts, the doctor takes x-ray pictures. The x-rays can show whether the ducts are narrowed or blocked by a tumor or other condition.

- **PTC (percutaneous transhepatic cholangiography):** A dye is injected through a thin needle inserted through the skin into the liver. Unless there is a blockage, the dye should move freely through the bile ducts. The dye makes the bile ducts show up on x-ray pictures. From the pictures, the doctor can tell whether there is a blockage from a tumor or other condition.

- **Biopsy:** In some cases, the doctor may remove tissue. A pathologist then uses a microscope to look for cancer cells in the tissue. The doctor may obtain tissue in several ways. One way is by inserting a needle into the pancreas to remove cells. This is called fine-needle aspiration. The doctor uses x-ray or ultrasound to guide the needle. Sometimes the doctor obtains a sample of tissue during EUS or ERCP. Another way is to open the abdomen during an operation.

Section 24.2

Staging and Treating Pancreatic Cancer

Excerpted from PDQ® Cancer Information Summary. National Cancer Institute; Bethesda, MD. "Pancreatic Cancer Treatment (PDQ®): Patient Version." Updated 05/2009. Available at: http://cancer.gov. Accessed July 23, 2009.

Stages of Pancreatic Cancer

Tests and procedures to stage pancreatic cancer are usually done at the same time as diagnosis. The following stages are used for pancreatic cancer:

Stage 0 (Carcinoma in Situ)

In stage 0, abnormal cells are found in the lining of the pancreas. These abnormal cells may become cancer and spread into nearby normal tissue. Stage 0 is also called carcinoma in situ.

Stage I

In stage I, cancer has formed and is found in the pancreas only. Stage I is divided into stage IA and stage IB, based on the size of the tumor.

- **Stage IA:** The tumor is 2 centimeters or smaller.
- **Stage IB:** The tumor is larger than 2 centimeters.

Stage II

In stage II, cancer may have spread to nearby tissue and organs, and may have spread to lymph nodes near the pancreas. Stage II is divided into stage IIA and stage IIB, based on where the cancer has spread.

- **Stage IIA:** Cancer has spread to nearby tissue and organs but has not spread to nearby lymph nodes.
- **Stage IIB:** Cancer has spread to nearby lymph nodes and may have spread to nearby tissue and organs.

Stage III

In stage III, cancer has spread to the major blood vessels near the pancreas and may have spread to nearby lymph nodes.

Stage IV

In stage IV, cancer may be of any size and has spread to distant organs, such as the liver, lung, and peritoneal cavity. It may have also spread to organs and tissues near the pancreas or to lymph nodes.

Recurrent Pancreatic Cancer

Recurrent pancreatic cancer is cancer that has recurred (come back) after it has been treated. The cancer may come back in the pancreas or in other parts of the body.

Treatment

Different types of treatment are available for patients with pancreatic cancer. Some treatments are standard (the currently used treatment), and some are being tested in clinical trials. Three types of standard treatment are used:

Surgery

One of the following types of surgery may be used to take out the tumor:

- **Whipple procedure:** A surgical procedure in which the head of the pancreas, the gallbladder, part of the stomach, part of the small intestine, and the bile duct are removed. Enough of the pancreas is left to produce digestive juices and insulin.

- **Total pancreatectomy:** This operation removes the whole pancreas, part of the stomach, part of the small intestine, the common bile duct, the gallbladder, the spleen, and nearby lymph nodes.

- **Distal pancreatectomy:** The body and the tail of the pancreas and usually the spleen are removed.

If the cancer has spread and cannot be removed, the following types of palliative surgery may be done to relieve symptoms:

- **Surgical biliary bypass:** If cancer is blocking the small intestine and bile is building up in the gallbladder, a biliary bypass may be done. During this operation, the doctor will cut the gallbladder or bile duct and sew it to the small intestine to create a new pathway around the blocked area.

- **Endoscopic stent placement:** If the tumor is blocking the bile duct, surgery may be done to put in a stent (a thin tube) to drain bile that has built up in the area. The doctor may place the stent through a catheter that drains to the outside of the body or the stent may go around the blocked area and drain the bile into the small intestine.

- **Gastric bypass:** If the tumor is blocking the flow of food from the stomach, the stomach may be sewn directly to the small intestine so the patient can continue to eat normally.

Radiation Therapy

Radiation therapy is a cancer treatment that uses high-energy x-rays or other types of radiation to kill cancer cells or keep them from growing. There are two types of radiation therapy. External radiation therapy uses a machine outside the body to send radiation toward the cancer. Internal radiation therapy uses a radioactive substance sealed in needles, seeds, wires, or catheters that are placed directly into or near the cancer. The way the radiation therapy is given depends on the type and stage of the cancer being treated.

Chemotherapy

Chemotherapy is a cancer treatment that uses drugs to stop the growth of cancer cells, either by killing the cells or by stopping them from dividing. When chemotherapy is taken by mouth or injected into a vein or muscle, the drugs enter the bloodstream and can reach cancer cells throughout the body (systemic chemotherapy). When chemotherapy is placed directly into the spinal column, an organ, or a body cavity such as the abdomen, the drugs mainly affect cancer cells in those areas (regional chemotherapy). The way the chemotherapy is given depends on the type and stage of the cancer being treated.

Pain and Nutrition

Pain can occur when the tumor presses on nerves or other organs near the pancreas. When pain medicine is not enough, there are treatments that act on nerves in the abdomen to relieve the pain. The doctor may inject medicine into the area around affected nerves or may cut the nerves to block the feeling of pain. Radiation therapy with or without chemotherapy can also help relieve pain by shrinking the tumor.

Surgery to remove the pancreas may interfere with the production of pancreatic enzymes that help to digest food. As a result, patients may have problems digesting food and absorbing nutrients into the body. To prevent malnutrition, the doctor may prescribe medicines that replace these enzymes.

Clinical Trials

A treatment clinical trial is a research study meant to help improve current treatments or obtain information on new treatments for patients with cancer. When clinical trials show that a new treatment is better than the standard treatment, the new treatment may become the standard treatment. Patients may want to think about taking part in a clinical trial. Some clinical trials are open only to patients who have not started treatment. For more information on clinical trials, visit the NCI website at www.cancer.gov.

Biologic Therapy

Biologic therapy is being studied in clinical trials. It is a treatment that uses the patient's immune system to fight cancer. Substances made by the body or made in a laboratory are used to boost, direct, or

restore the body's natural defenses against cancer. This type of cancer treatment is also called biotherapy or immunotherapy.

Follow-Up Tests

Some of the tests that were done to diagnose the cancer or to find out the stage of the cancer may be repeated. Some tests will be repeated in order to see how well the treatment is working. Decisions about whether to continue, change, or stop treatment may be based on the results of these tests. This is sometimes called re-staging.

Some of the tests will continue to be done from time to time after treatment has ended. The results of these tests can show if your condition has changed or if the cancer has recurred (come back). These tests are sometimes called follow-up tests or check-ups.

Chapter 25

Skin Cancer

Chapter Contents

Section 25.1

Facts about Skin Cancer

From "Skin Cancer Facts," (to view the entire document, including references, visit http://www.skincancer.org/skin-cancer-facts/), © 2009 Skin Cancer Foundation (www.skincancer.org). Reprinted with permission.

General

- Skin cancer is the most common form of cancer in the United States. More than one million skin cancers are diagnosed annually.

- Each year there are more new cases of skin cancer than the combined incidence of cancers of the breast, prostate, lung and colon.

- One in five Americans will develop skin cancer in the course of a lifetime.

- Basal cell carcinoma (BCC) is the most common form of skin cancer; about one million of the cases diagnosed annually are basal cell carcinomas. Basal cell carcinomas are rarely fatal, but can be highly disfiguring.

- Squamous cell carcinoma (SCC) is the second most common form of skin cancer. More than 250,000 cases are diagnosed each year, resulting in approximately 2,500 deaths.

- Basal cell carcinoma and squamous cell carcinoma are the two major forms of non-melanoma skin cancer. Between 40 and 50 percent of Americans who live to age 65 will have either skin cancer at least once.

- In 2004, the total direct cost associated with the treatment for non-melanoma skin cancers was more than $1 billion.

- About 90 percent of non-melanoma skin cancers are associated with exposure to ultraviolet (UV) radiation from the sun.

- Up to 90 percent of the visible changes commonly attributed to aging are caused by the sun.

- Contrary to popular belief, 80 percent of a person's lifetime sun exposure is not acquired before age 18; only about 23 percent of lifetime exposure occurs by age 18.

Melanoma

- The incidence of many common cancers is falling, but the incidence of melanoma continues to rise significantly, at a rate faster than that of any of the seven most common cancers.

- Approximately 68,720 melanomas will be diagnosed this year, with nearly 8,650 resulting in death.

- Melanoma accounts for about three percent of skin cancer cases, but it causes more than 75 percent of skin cancer deaths.

- Melanoma mortality increased by about 33 percent from 1975–90, but has remained relatively stable since 1990.

- Survival with melanoma increased from 49 percent between 1950 and 1954 to 92 percent between 1996 and 2003.

- More than 20 Americans die each day from skin cancer, primarily melanoma. One person dies of melanoma almost every hour (every 62 minutes).

- The survival rate for patients whose melanoma is detected early, before the tumor has penetrated the epidermis, is about 99 percent. The survival rate falls to 15 percent for those with advanced disease.

- Melanoma is the fifth most common cancer for males and sixth most common for females.

Table 25.1. Lifetime UV Exposure in the United States

Ages	Average Accumulated Exposure*
1–18	22.73%
19–40	46.53%
41–59	73.7%
60–78	100*

*Based on a 78 year lifespan

- Women aged 39 and under have a higher probability of developing melanoma than any other cancer except breast cancer.

- Melanoma is the second most common form of cancer for young adults 15–29 years old.

- About 65 percent of melanoma cases can be attributed to ultraviolet (UV) radiation from the sun.

- One in 55 people will be diagnosed with melanoma during their lifetime.

- One blistering sunburn in childhood or adolescence more than doubles a person's chances of developing melanoma later in life.

- A person's risk for melanoma doubles if he or she has had five or more sunburns at any age.

Men and Women

- The majority of people diagnosed with melanoma are white men over age 50.

- Five percent of all cancers in men are melanomas; four percent of all cancers in women are melanomas.

- Contrary to popular belief, recent studies show that people receive a fairly consistent dose of ultraviolet radiation over their entire lifetime. Adults over age 40, especially men, have the highest annual exposure to UV.

- Between 1980 and 2004, the annual incidence of melanoma among young women increased by 50 percent, from 9.4 cases to 13.9 cases per 100,000 women.

- The number of women under age 40 diagnosed with basal cell carcinoma has more than doubled in the last 30 years; the squamous cell carcinoma rate for women has also increased significantly.

- Until age 39, women are almost twice as likely to develop melanoma as men. Starting at age 40, melanoma incidence in men exceeds incidence in women, and this trend becomes more pronounced with each decade.

- One in 39 men and one in 58 women will develop melanoma in their lifetime.

- Melanoma is one of only three cancers with an increasing mortality rate for men.

Indoor Tanning

- Ultraviolet radiation (UVR) is a proven human carcinogen, according to the U.S. Department of Health and Human Services.

- Frequent tanners using new high-pressure sunlamps may receive as much as 12 times the annual UVA dose compared to the dose they receive from sun exposure.

- Nearly 30 million people tan indoors in the U.S. every year; 2.3 million of them are teens.

- On an average day, more than one million Americans use tanning salons.

- Seventy one percent of tanning salon patrons are girls and women aged 16–29.

- First exposure to tanning beds in youth increases melanoma risk by 75 percent.

- People who use tanning beds are 2.5 times more likely to develop squamous cell carcinoma and 1.5 times more likely to develop basal cell carcinoma.

- The indoor tanning industry has an annual estimated revenue of $5 billion.

Pediatrics

- Melanoma accounts for up to three percent of all pediatric cancers.

- Between 1973 and 2001, melanoma incidence in those under 20 rose 2.9 percent.

- Melanoma is seven times more common between the ages of 10 and 20 than it is between 0 and 10 years.

- Diagnoses—and treatment—are delayed in 40 percent of childhood melanoma cases.

- Ninety percent of pediatric melanoma cases occur in girls aged 10–19.

Ethnicity

- Asian American and African American melanoma patients have a greater tendency than Caucasians to present with advanced disease at time of diagnosis.

- The average annual melanoma rate among Caucasians is about 22 cases per 100,000 people. In comparison, African Americans have an incidence of one case per 100,000 people. However, the overall melanoma survival rate for African Americans is only 77 percent, versus 91 percent for Caucasians.

- While melanoma is uncommon in African Americans, Latinos, and Asians, it is frequently fatal for these populations.

- Melanomas in African Americans, Asians, Filipinos, Indonesians, and native Hawaiians most often occur on non-exposed skin with less pigment, with up to 60–75 percent of tumors arising on the palms, soles, mucous membranes and nail regions.

- Basal cell carcinoma (BCC) is the most common cancer in Caucasians, Hispanics, Chinese, and Japanese, and other Asian populations.

- Squamous cell carcinoma (SCC) is the most common skin cancer among African Americans and Asian Indians.

- Among non-Caucasians, melanoma is a higher risk for children than adults: 6.5 percent of pediatric melanomas occur in non-Caucasians.

These facts and statistics have been reviewed by David Polsky, MD, Assistant Professor of Dermatology and Pathology, New York University Medical Center and Steven Q. Wang, MD, Director of Dermatologic Surgery and Dermatology, Memorial Sloan-Kettering Cancer Center, Basking Ridge, New Jersey.

Section 25.2

Can Skin Cancer Be Prevented?

PDQ® Cancer Information Summary. National Cancer Institute; Bethesda, MD. "Skin Cancer Prevention (PDQ®): Patient Version." Updated 06/2009. Available at: http://cancer.gov. Accessed August 11, 2009.

Cancer Prevention

Cancer prevention is action taken to lower the chance of getting cancer. By preventing cancer, the number of new cases of cancer in a group or population is lowered. Hopefully, this will lower the number of deaths caused by cancer.

To prevent new cancers from starting, scientists look at risk factors and protective factors. Anything that increases your chance of developing cancer is called a cancer risk factor; anything that decreases your chance of developing cancer is called a cancer protective factor.

Some risk factors for cancer can be avoided, but many cannot. For example, both smoking and inheriting certain genes are risk factors for some types of cancer, but only smoking can be avoided. Regular exercise and a healthy diet may be protective factors for some types of cancer. Avoiding risk factors and increasing protective factors may lower your risk but it does not mean that you will not get cancer.

Different ways to prevent cancer are being studied, including changing lifestyle or eating habits, avoiding things known to cause cancer, and taking medicines to treat a precancerous condition or to keep cancer from starting.

Skin Cancer

Skin cancer is a disease in which malignant (cancer) cells form in the tissues of the skin. The skin is the body's largest organ. It protects against heat, sunlight, injury, and infection. Skin also helps control body temperature and stores water, fat, and vitamin D. The skin has several layers, but the two main layers are the epidermis (upper or outer layer) and the dermis (lower or inner layer).

The epidermis is made up of three kinds of cells. Squamous cells are the thin, flat cells that make up most of the epidermis. Basal cells are the round cells under the squamous cells. Melanocytes are found throughout the lower part of the epidermis. They make melanin, the pigment that gives skin its natural color. When skin is exposed to the sun, melanocytes make more pigment, causing the skin to tan, or darken. The dermis contains blood and lymph vessels, hair follicles, and glands.

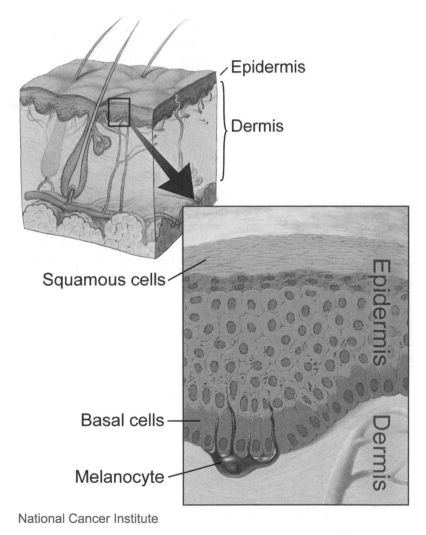

National Cancer Institute

Figure 25.1. *The layers of the skin and types of cells (Source: Don Bliss, National Cancer Institute, 2005).*

There are several types of skin cancer. The most common types of skin cancer are squamous cell carcinoma, which forms in the squamous cells and basal cell carcinoma, which forms in the basal cells. Squamous cell carcinoma and basal cell carcinoma are also called nonmelanoma skin cancers. Melanoma, which forms in the melanocytes, is a less common type of skin cancer.

Studies suggest that being exposed to ultraviolet (UV) radiation and the sensitivity of a person's skin to UV radiation are risk factors for skin cancer. UV radiation is the name for the invisible rays that are part of the energy that comes from the sun. Sunlamps and tanning booths also give off UV radiation.

Risk factors for nonmelanoma and melanoma cancers are not the same:

- **Nonmelanoma skin cancer:** The total amount of time the skin is exposed to UV radiation may affect the risk of nonmelanoma skin cancer. Spending more time in the sun may increase the risk. People may have an increased risk of nonmelanoma skin cancer if their skin burns easily in the sun.

- **Melanoma skin cancer:** Being exposed to strong UV radiation for short periods (as with sunburns), especially in childhood and teen years, may increase the risk of melanoma. People may have an increased risk of melanoma from UV radiation if they burn easily in the sun or have freckles or a lot of moles.

It is not known if nonmelanoma skin cancer risk is decreased by staying out of the sun, using sunscreens, or wearing long sleeve shirts, long pants, sun hats, and sunglasses when outdoors.

Sunscreen may help decrease the amount of UV radiation to the skin. One study found that wearing sunscreen can help prevent actinic keratoses, scaly patches of skin that may become squamous cell carcinoma. However, the use of sunscreen has not been proven to lower the risk of melanoma skin cancer.

Although protecting the skin and eyes from the sun has not been proven to lower the chance of getting skin cancer, skin experts suggest the following:

- Use sunscreen that protects against UV radiation.

- Do not stay out in the sun for long periods of time, especially when the sun is at its strongest.

- Wear long sleeve shirts, long pants, sun hats, and sunglasses, when outdoors.

Section 25.3

Diagnosing and Treating Melanoma

Excerpted from "What You Need to Know about Melanoma,"
National Cancer Institute (www.cancer.gov), March 31, 2003;
accessed August 11, 2009.

Diagnosing Melanoma

If the doctor suspects that a spot on the skin is melanoma, the patient will need to have a biopsy. A biopsy is the only way to make a definite diagnosis. In this procedure, the doctor tries to remove all of the suspicious-looking growth. This is an excisional biopsy. If the growth is too large to be removed entirely, the doctor removes a sample of the tissue. The doctor will never "shave off" or cauterize a growth that might be melanoma.

A biopsy can usually be done in the doctor's office using local anesthesia. A pathologist then examines the tissue under a microscope to check for cancer cells. Sometimes it is helpful for more than one pathologist to check the tissue for cancer cells.

Staging

If the diagnosis is melanoma, the doctor needs to learn the extent, or stage, of the disease before planning treatment. Staging is a careful attempt to learn how thick the tumor is, how deeply the melanoma has invaded the skin, and whether melanoma cells have spread to nearby lymph nodes or other parts of the body. The doctor may remove nearby lymph nodes to check for cancer cells. (Such surgery may be considered part of the treatment because removing cancerous lymph nodes may help control the disease.) The doctor also does a careful physical exam and, if the tumor is thick, may order chest x-rays, blood tests, and scans of the liver, bones, and brain.

The following stages are used for melanoma:

- **Stage 0:** In stage 0, the melanoma cells are found only in the outer layer of skin cells and have not invaded deeper tissues.

- **Stage I:** Melanoma in stage I is thin: The tumor is no more than one millimeter (1/25 inch) thick. The outer layer (epidermis) of skin may appear scraped. (This is called an ulceration). Or, the tumor is between onc and two millimeters (1/12 inch) thick. There is no ulceration. The melanoma cells have not spread to nearby lymph nodes.

- **Stage II:** The tumor is at least one millimeter thick: The tumor is between one and two millimeters thick. There is ulceration. Or, the thickness of the tumor is more than two millimeters. There may be ulceration. The melanoma cells have not spread to nearby lymph nodes.

- **Stage III:** The melanoma cells have spread to nearby tissues: The melanoma cells have spread to one or more nearby lymph nodes. Or, the melanoma cells have spread to tissues just outside the original tumor but not to any lymph nodes.

- **Stage IV:** The melanoma cells have spread to other organs, to lymph nodes, or to skin areas far away from the original tumor.

- **Recurrent:** Recurrent disease means that the cancer has come back (recurred) after it has been treated. It may have come back in the original site or in another part of the body.

Treatment

The doctor can describe treatment choices and discuss the results expected with each treatment option. The doctor and patient can work together to develop a treatment plan that fits the patient's needs. Treatment for melanoma depends on the extent of the disease, the patient's age and general health, and other factors.

People with melanoma are often treated by a team of specialists. The team may include a dermatologist, surgeon, medical oncologist, radiation oncologist, and plastic surgeon.

Getting a Second Opinion

Before starting treatment, the patient might want a second opinion about the diagnosis and the treatment plan. Some insurance companies require a second opinion; others may cover a second opinion if the patient or doctor requests it. There are a number of ways to find a doctor for a second opinion:

- The patient's doctor may refer the patient to one or more specialists. At cancer centers, several specialists often work together as a team.

- The Cancer Information Service, at 800-4-CANCER, can tell callers about nearby treatment centers.

- A local or state medical society, a nearby hospital, or a medical school can usually provide the names of specialists.

- The American Board of Medical Specialties (ABMS) has a list of doctors who have met certain education and training requirements and have passed specialty examinations. The Official ABMS Directory of Board Certified Medical Specialists lists doctors' names along with their specialty and their educational background. The directory is available in most public libraries. Also, ABMS offers this information on the internet at http://www.abms.org/. (Click on "Who's Certified.")

Methods of Treatment

People with melanoma may have surgery, chemotherapy, biological therapy, or radiation therapy. Patients may have a combination of treatments. In addition, at any stage of disease, people with melanoma may have treatment to control pain and other symptoms of the cancer, to relieve the side effects of therapy, and to ease emotional and practical problems. This kind of treatment is called symptom management, supportive care, or palliative care.

Surgery

Surgery is the usual treatment for melanoma. The surgeon removes the tumor and some normal tissue around it. This procedure reduces the chance that cancer cells will be left in the area. The width and depth of surrounding skin that needs to be removed depends on the thickness of the melanoma and how deeply it has invaded the skin.

The doctor may be able to completely remove a very thin melanoma during the biopsy. Further surgery may not be necessary.

If the melanoma was not completely removed during the biopsy, the doctor takes out the remaining tumor. In most cases, additional surgery is performed to remove normal-looking tissue around the tumor (called the margin) to make sure all melanoma cells are removed. This is often necessary, even for thin melanomas. If the melanoma is thick, the doctor may need to remove a larger margin of tissue.

If a large area of tissue is removed, the surgeon may do a skin graft. For this procedure, the doctor uses skin from another part of the body to replace the skin that was removed.

310

Lymph nodes near the tumor may be removed because cancer can spread through the lymphatic system. If the pathologist finds cancer cells in the lymph nodes, it may mean that the disease has also spread to other parts of the body. Two procedures are used to remove the lymph nodes:

- **Sentinel lymph node biopsy:** The sentinel lymph node biopsy is done after the biopsy of the melanoma but before the wider excision of the tumor. A radioactive substance is injected near the melanoma. The surgeon follows the movement of the substance on a computer screen. The first lymph node(s) to take up the substance is called the sentinel lymph node(s). (The imaging study is called lymphoscintigraphy. The procedure to identify the sentinel node(s) is called sentinel lymph node mapping.) The surgeon removes the sentinel node(s) to check for cancer cells. If a sentinel node contains cancer cells, the surgeon removes the rest of the lymph nodes in the area. However, if a sentinel node does not contain cancer cells, no additional lymph nodes are removed.

- **Lymph node dissection:** The surgeon removes all the lymph nodes in the area of the melanoma.

Therapy may be given after surgery to kill cancer cells that remain in the body. This treatment is called adjuvant therapy. The patient may receive biological therapy.

Surgery is generally not effective in controlling melanoma that has spread to other parts of the body. In such cases, doctors may use other methods of treatment, such as chemotherapy, biological therapy, radiation therapy, or a combination of these methods.

Chemotherapy

Chemotherapy, the use of drugs to kill cancer cells, is sometimes used to treat melanoma. The drugs are usually given in cycles: a treatment period followed by a recovery period, then another treatment period, and so on. Usually a patient has chemotherapy as an outpatient (at the hospital, at the doctor's office, or at home). However, depending on which drugs are given and the patient's general health, a short hospital stay may be needed.

People with melanoma may receive chemotherapy by mouth or injection. Either way, the drugs enter the bloodstream and travel throughout the body. Chemotherapy may also be given by isolated limb perfusion (also called isolated arterial perfusion). For melanoma on an arm or leg, chemotherapy drugs are put directly into the bloodstream

of that limb. The flow of blood to and from the limb is stopped for a while. This allows most of the drug to reach the tumor directly. Most of the chemotherapy remains in that limb. The drugs may be heated before injection. This type of chemotherapy is called hyperthermic perfusion.

Biological Therapy

Biological therapy (also called immunotherapy) is a form of treatment that uses the body's immune system, either directly or indirectly, to fight cancer or to reduce side effects caused by some cancer treatments. Biological therapy for melanoma uses substances called cytokines. The body normally produces cytokines in small amounts in response to infections and other diseases. Using modern laboratory techniques, scientists can produce cytokines in large amounts. In some cases, biological therapy given after surgery can help prevent melanoma from recurring. For patients with metastatic melanoma or a high risk of recurrence, interferon alpha and interleukin-2 (also called IL-2 or aldesleukin) may be recommended after surgery.

Radiation Therapy

Radiation therapy (also called radiotherapy) uses high-energy rays to kill cancer cells. A large machine directs radiation at the body. The patient usually has treatment at a hospital or clinic, five days a week for several weeks. Radiation therapy may be used to help control melanoma that has spread to the brain, bones, and other parts of the body. It may shrink the tumor and relieve symptoms.

Section 25.4

Diagnosing and Treating Non-Melanoma Skin Cancers

Excerpted from "What You Need to Know about Skin Cancer,"
National Cancer Institute (www.cancer.gov), July 30, 2009; accessed
August 11, 2009.

Diagnosing Skin Cancer

If you have a change on the skin, the doctor must find out whether it is due to cancer or to some other cause. Your doctor removes all or part of the area that does not look normal. The sample goes to a lab. A pathologist checks the sample under a microscope. This is a biopsy. A biopsy is the only sure way to diagnose skin cancer.

You may have the biopsy in a doctor's office or as an outpatient in a clinic or hospital. Where it is done depends on the size and place of the abnormal area on your skin. You probably will have local anesthesia.

There are four common types of skin biopsies:

- **Punch biopsy:** The doctor uses a sharp, hollow tool to remove a circle of tissue from the abnormal area.

- **Incisional biopsy:** The doctor uses a scalpel to remove part of the growth.

- **Excisional biopsy:** The doctor uses a scalpel to remove the entire growth and some tissue around it.

- **Shave biopsy:** The doctor uses a thin, sharp blade to shave off the abnormal growth.

Staging Skin Cancer

If the biopsy shows that you have cancer, your doctor needs to know the extent (stage) of the disease. In very few cases, the doctor may check your lymph nodes to stage the cancer. The stage is based on the size of the growth, how deeply it has grown beneath the top layer of skin, and whether it has spread to nearby lymph nodes or to other parts of the body. These are the stages of skin cancer:

- **Stage 0:** The cancer involves only the top layer of skin. It is carcinoma in situ.

- **Stage I:** The growth is two centimeters wide (three-quarters of an inch) or smaller.

- **Stage II:** The growth is larger than two centimeters wide (three-quarters of an inch).

- **Stage III:** The cancer has spread below the skin to cartilage, muscle, bone, or to nearby lymph nodes. It has not spread to other places in the body.

- **Stage IV:** The cancer has spread to other places in the body.

Treatment

Treatment for skin cancer depends on the type and stage of the disease, the size and place of the growth, and your general health and medical history. In most cases, the aim of treatment is to remove or destroy the cancer completely. Sometimes all of the cancer is removed during the biopsy. In such cases, no more treatment is needed. If you do need more treatment, your doctor will describe your options.

Surgery is the usual treatment for people with skin cancer. In some cases, the doctor may suggest topical chemotherapy, photodynamic therapy, or radiation therapy.

Because skin cancer treatment may damage healthy cells and tissues, unwanted side effects sometimes occur. Side effects depend mainly on the type and extent of the treatment. Side effects may not be the same for each person.

Before treatment starts, your doctor will tell you about possible side effects and suggest ways to help you manage them.

Surgery

Surgery to treat skin cancer may be done in one of several ways. The method your doctor uses depends on the size and place of the growth and other factors.

Excisional skin surgery is a common treatment to remove skin cancer. After numbing the area, the surgeon removes the growth with a scalpel. The surgeon also removes a border of skin around the growth. This skin is the margin. The margin is examined under a microscope to be certain that all the cancer cells have been removed. The size of the margin depends on the size of the growth.

Mohs surgery (also called Mohs micrographic surgery) is often used for skin cancer. The area of the growth is numbed. A specially trained surgeon shaves away thin layers of the growth. Each layer is immediately examined under a microscope. The surgeon continues to shave away tissue until no cancer cells can be seen under the microscope. In this way, the surgeon can remove all the cancer and only a small bit of healthy tissue.

Electrodesiccation and curettage is often used to remove small basal cell skin cancers. The doctor numbs the area to be treated. The cancer is removed with a sharp tool shaped like a spoon. This tool is a curette. An electric current is sent into the treated area to control bleeding and kill any cancer cells that may be left. Electrodesiccation and curettage is usually a fast and simple procedure.

Cryosurgery is often used for people who are not able to have other types of surgery. It uses extreme cold to treat early stage or very thin skin cancer. Liquid nitrogen creates the cold. The doctor applies liquid nitrogen directly to the skin growth. This treatment may cause swelling. It also may damage nerves, which can cause a loss of feeling in the damaged area.

Laser surgery uses a narrow beam of light to remove or destroy cancer cells. It is most often used for growths that are on the outer layer of skin only.

Grafts are sometimes needed to close an opening in the skin left by surgery. The surgeon first numbs and then removes a patch of healthy skin from another part of the body, such as the upper thigh. The patch is then used to cover the area where skin cancer was removed. If you have a skin graft, you may have to take special care of the area until it heals.

The time it takes to heal after surgery is different for each person. You may be uncomfortable for the first few days. However, medicine can usually control the pain. Before surgery, you should discuss the plan for pain relief with your doctor or nurse. After surgery, your doctor can adjust the plan if you need more pain relief.

Surgery nearly always leaves some type of scar. The size and color of the scar depend on the size of the cancer, the type of surgery, and how your skin heals.

For any type of surgery, including skin grafts or reconstructive surgery, it is important to follow your doctor's advice on bathing, shaving, exercise, or other activities.

Topical Chemotherapy

Chemotherapy uses anticancer drugs to kill skin cancer cells. When a drug is put directly on the skin, the treatment is topical chemotherapy.

It is most often used when the skin cancer is too large for surgery. It is also used when the doctor keeps finding new cancers.

Most often, the drug comes in a cream or lotion. It is usually applied to the skin one or two times a day for several weeks. A drug called fluorouracil (5-FU) is used to treat basal cell and squamous cell cancers that are in the top layer of the skin only. A drug called imiquimod also is used to treat basal cell cancer only in the top layer of skin.

These drugs may cause your skin to turn red or swell. It also may itch, hurt, ooze, or develop a rash. It may be sore or sensitive to the sun. These skin changes usually go away after treatment is over. Topical chemotherapy usually does not leave a scar. If healthy skin becomes too red or raw when the skin cancer is treated, your doctor may stop treatment.

Photodynamic Therapy

Photodynamic therapy (PDT) uses a chemical along with a special light source, such as a laser light, to kill cancer cells. The chemical is a photosensitizing agent. A cream is applied to the skin or the chemical is injected. It stays in cancer cells longer than in normal cells. Several hours or days later, the special light is focused on the growth. The chemical becomes active and destroys nearby cancer cells.

PDT is used to treat cancer on or very near the surface of the skin.

The side effects of PDT are usually not serious. PDT may cause burning or stinging pain. It also may cause burns, swelling, or redness. It may scar healthy tissue near the growth. If you have PDT, you will need to avoid direct sunlight and bright indoor light for at least six weeks after treatment.

Radiation Therapy

Radiation therapy (also called radiotherapy) uses high-energy rays to kill cancer cells. The rays come from a large machine outside the body. They affect cells only in the treated area. This treatment is given at a hospital or clinic in one dose or many doses over several weeks.

Radiation is not a common treatment for skin cancer. But it may be used for skin cancer in areas where surgery could be difficult or leave a bad scar. You may have this treatment if you have a growth on your eyelid, ear, or nose. It also may be used if the cancer comes back after surgery to remove it.

Side effects depend mainly on the dose of radiation and the part of your body that is treated. During treatment your skin in the treated

area may become red, dry, and tender. Your doctor can suggest ways to relieve the side effects of radiation therapy.

Follow-Up Care

Follow-up care after treatment for skin cancer is important. Your doctor will monitor your recovery and check for new skin cancer. New skin cancers are more common than having a treated skin cancer spread. Regular checkups help ensure that any changes in your health are noted and treated if needed. Between scheduled visits, you should check your skin regularly. You will find a guide for checking your skin below. You should contact the doctor if you notice anything unusual. It also is important to follow your doctor's advice about how to reduce your risk of developing skin cancer again.

Chapter 26

Thyroid Cancer

Chapter Contents

Section 26.1

What You Need to Know about Thyroid Cancer

Excerpting from "What You Need to Know about Thyroid Cancer,"
National Cancer Institute (www.cancer.gov), 2007.

The Thyroid

Your thyroid is a gland at the front of your neck beneath your voice
box (larynx). A healthy thyroid is a little larger than a quarter. It usually cannot be felt through the skin. The thyroid has two parts (lobes).
A thin piece of tissue (the isthmus) separates the lobes. The thyroid
makes hormones:

- **Thyroid hormone:** Thyroid hormone is made by thyroid follicular cells. It affects heart rate, blood pressure, body temperature,
  and weight.

- **Calcitonin:** Calcitonin is made by C cells in the thyroid. It plays
  a small role in keeping a healthy level of calcium in the body.

Four or more tiny parathyroid glands are behind the thyroid. They
are on its surface. They make parathyroid hormone, which plays a big
role in helping the body maintain a healthy level of calcium.

There are several types of thyroid cancer:

- **Papillary thyroid cancer:** In the United States, this type
  makes up about 80 percent of all thyroid cancers. It begins in
  follicular cells and grows slowly. If diagnosed early, most people
  with papillary thyroid cancer can be cured.

- **Follicular thyroid cancer:** This type makes up about 15 percent of all thyroid cancers. It begins in follicular cells and grows
  slowly. If diagnosed early, most people with follicular thyroid
  cancer can be treated successfully.

- **Medullary thyroid cancer:** This type makes up about three
  percent of all thyroid cancers. It begins in the C cells of the thyroid. Cancer that starts in the C cells can make abnormally high
  levels of calcitonin. Medullary thyroid cancer tends to grow

320

slowly. It can be easier to control if it's found and treated before it spreads to other parts of the body.

- **Anaplastic thyroid cancer:** This type makes up about two percent of all thyroid cancers. It begins in the follicular cells of the thyroid. The cancer cells tend to grow and spread very quickly. Anaplastic thyroid cancer is very hard to control.

Risk Factors

Doctors often cannot explain why one person develops thyroid cancer and another does not. However, it is clear that no one can catch thyroid cancer from another person. Research has shown that people with certain risk factors are more likely than others to develop thyroid cancer. A risk factor is something that may increase the chance of developing a disease.

Studies have found the following risk factors for thyroid cancer:

Radiation

People exposed to high levels of radiation are much more likely than others to develop papillary or follicular thyroid cancer. One important source of radiation exposure is treatment with x-rays. Between the

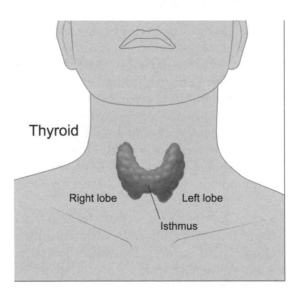

Figure 26.1. The thyroid gland (Source: Don Bliss, National Cancer Institute, 2001).

1920s and the 1950s, doctors used high-dose x-rays to treat children who had enlarged tonsils, acne, and other problems affecting the head and neck. Later, scientists found that some people who had received this kind of treatment developed thyroid cancer. (Routine diagnostic x-rays—such as dental x-rays or chest x-rays—use very low doses of radiation. Their benefits usually outweigh their risks. However, repeated exposure could be harmful, so it's a good idea to talk with your dentist and doctor about the need for each x-ray and to ask about the use of shields to protect other parts of the body.)

Another source of radiation is radioactive fallout. This includes fallout from atomic weapons testing (such as the testing in the United States and elsewhere in the world, mainly in the 1950s and 1960s), nuclear power plant accidents (such as the Chornobyl [also called Chernobyl] accident in 1986), and releases from atomic weapons production plants (such as the Hanford facility in Washington state in the late 1940s). Such radioactive fallout contains radioactive iodine (I-131) and other radioactive elements. People who were exposed to one or more sources of I-131, especially if they were children at the time of their exposure, may have an increased risk of thyroid diseases. For example, children exposed to radioactive iodine from the Chornobyl accident have an increased risk of thyroid cancer.

Family and Personal History

A family history of medullary thyroid cancer increases risks. Medullary thyroid cancer sometimes runs in families. A change in a gene called RET can be passed from parent to child. Nearly everyone with the changed RET gene develops medullary thyroid cancer. The disease occurs alone as familial medullary thyroid cancer or with other cancers as multiple endocrine neoplasia (MEN) syndrome.

A blood test can detect the changed RET gene. If it's found in a person with medullary thyroid cancer, the doctor may suggest that family members be tested. For those who have the changed gene, the doctor may recommend frequent lab tests or surgery to remove the thyroid before cancer develops.

A family history of goiters or colon growths is also associated with increased risk. A small number of people with a family history of having goiters (swollen thyroids) with multiple thyroid nodules are at risk for developing papillary thyroid cancer. Also, a small number of people with a family history of having multiple growths on the inside of the colon or rectum (familial polyposis) are at risk for developing papillary thyroid cancer.

People with a goiter or benign thyroid nodules have an increased risk of thyroid cancer.

Other Risks

- **Being female:** In the United States, women are almost three times more likely than men to develop thyroid cancer.

- **Age over 45:** Most people with thyroid cancer are more than 45 years old. Most people with anaplastic thyroid cancer are more than 60 years old.

- **Iodine:** Iodine is a substance found in shellfish and iodized salt. Scientists are studying iodine as a possible risk factor for thyroid cancer. Too little iodine in the diet may increase the risk of follicular thyroid cancer. However, other studies show that too much iodine in the diet may increase the risk of papillary thyroid cancer. More studies are needed to know whether iodine is a risk factor.

Having one or more risk factors does not mean that a person will get thyroid cancer. Most people who have risk factors never develop cancer.

Symptoms

Early thyroid cancer often does not have symptoms. But as the cancer grows, symptoms may include a lump in the front of the neck, hoarseness or voice changes, swollen lymph nodes in the neck, trouble swallowing or breathing, and pain in the throat or neck that does not go away.

Most often, these symptoms are not due to cancer. An infection, a benign goiter, or another health problem is usually the cause of these symptoms. Anyone with symptoms that do not go away in a couple of weeks should see a doctor to be diagnosed and treated as early as possible.

Diagnosis

If you have symptoms that suggest thyroid cancer, your doctor will help you find out whether they are from cancer or some other cause. Your doctor will ask you about your personal and family medical history. You may have one or more of the following tests:

- **Physical exam:** Your doctor feels your thyroid for lumps (nodules). Your doctor also checks your neck and nearby lymph nodes for growths or swelling.

- **Blood tests:** Your doctor may check for abnormal levels of thyroid-stimulating hormone (TSH) in the blood. Too much or too little TSH means the thyroid is not working well. If your doctor thinks you may have medullary thyroid cancer, you may be checked for a high level of calcitonin and have other blood tests.

- **Ultrasound:** An ultrasound device uses sound waves that people cannot hear. The device aims sound waves at the thyroid, and a computer creates a picture of the waves that bounce off the thyroid. The picture can show thyroid nodules that are too small to be felt. The doctor uses the picture to learn the size and shape of each nodule and whether the nodules are solid or filled with fluid. Nodules that are filled with fluid are usually not cancer. Nodules that are solid may be cancer.

- **Thyroid scan:** Your doctor may order a scan of your thyroid. You swallow a small amount of a radioactive substance, and it travels through the bloodstream. Thyroid cells that absorb the radioactive substance can be seen on a scan. Nodules that take up more of the substance than the thyroid tissue around them are called "hot" nodules. Hot nodules are usually not cancer. Nodules that take up less substance than the thyroid tissue around them are called "cold" nodules. Cold nodules may be cancer.

- **Biopsy:** A biopsy is the only sure way to diagnose thyroid cancer. A pathologist checks a sample of tissue for cancer cells with a microscope.

Your doctor may take tissue for a biopsy in one of two ways:

- **Fine-needle aspiration:** Most people have this type of biopsy. Your doctor removes a sample of tissue from a thyroid nodule with a thin needle. An ultrasound device can help your doctor see where to place the needle.

- **Surgical biopsy:** If a diagnosis cannot be made from fine-needle aspiration, a surgeon removes the whole nodule during an operation. If the doctor suspects follicular thyroid cancer, surgical biopsy may be needed for diagnosis.

Section 26.2

Staging and Treating Thyroid Cancer

Excerpted PDQ® Cancer Information Summary. National Cancer Institute; Bethesda, MD. "Thyroid Cancer Treatment (PDQ®): Patient Version." Updated 09/2009. Available at: http://cancer.gov. Accessed May 31, 2010.

Stages of Thyroid Cancer

After thyroid cancer has been diagnosed, tests are done to find out if cancer cells have spread within the thyroid or to other parts of the body.

The process used to find out if cancer has spread within the thyroid or to other parts of the body is called staging. The information gathered from the staging process determines the stage of the disease. It is important to know the stage in order to plan treatment. The following tests and procedures may be used in the staging process:

- **CT scan (CAT scan):** A procedure that makes a series of detailed pictures of areas inside the body, taken from different angles. The pictures are made by a computer linked to an x-ray machine. A dye may be injected into a vein or swallowed to help the organs or tissues show up more clearly. This procedure is also called computed tomography, computerized tomography, or computerized axial tomography.

- **MRI (magnetic resonance imaging):** A procedure that uses a magnet, radio waves, and a computer to make a series of detailed pictures of areas inside the body. This procedure is also called nuclear magnetic resonance imaging (NMRI).

- **Ultrasound exam:** A procedure in which high-energy sound waves (ultrasound) are bounced off internal tissues or organs and make echoes. The echoes form a picture of body tissues called a sonogram. The picture can be printed to be looked at later.

- **Radioactive iodine scan (RAI scan):** A procedure to find areas in the body where thyroid cancer cells may be dividing

quickly. Radioactive iodine (RAI) is used because only thyroid cells take up iodine. A very small amount of RAI is swallowed, travels through the blood, and collects in thyroid tissue and thyroid cancer cells anywhere in the body. Abnormal thyroid cells take up less iodine than normal thyroid cells. Areas that do not absorb the iodine normally (cold spots) show up lighter in the picture made by the scan. Cold spots can be either benign (not cancer) or malignant, so more tests are needed to find out if they are cancer. A scan of the whole body may be done to find out the stage of the cancer.

- **Lymph node biopsy:** The removal of all or part of a lymph node. A pathologist views the tissue under a microscope to look for cancer cells.

- **Bone scan:** A procedure to check if there are rapidly dividing cells, such as cancer cells, in the bone. A very small amount of radioactive material is injected into a vein and travels through the bloodstream. The radioactive material collects in the bones and is detected by a scanner.

- **Chest x-ray:** An x-ray of the organs and bones inside the chest. An x-ray is a type of energy beam that can go through the body and onto film, making a picture of areas inside the body.

Papillary and Follicular Thyroid Cancer

The following stages are used for papillary and follicular thyroid cancer in patients younger than 45 years:

- **Stage I:** In stage I papillary and follicular thyroid cancer, the tumor is any size, may be in the thyroid, or may have spread to nearby tissues and lymph nodes. Cancer has not spread to other parts of the body.

- **Stage II:** In stage II papillary and follicular thyroid cancer, cancer has spread from the thyroid to other parts of the body, such as the lungs or bone.

The following stages are used for papillary and follicular thyroid cancer in patients 45 years and older:

- **Stage I:** In stage I papillary and follicular thyroid cancer, cancer is found only in the thyroid and the tumor is two centimeters or smaller.

- **Stage II:** In stage II papillary and follicular thyroid cancer, cancer is only in the thyroid and the tumor is larger than two centimeters but not larger than four centimeters.

- **Stage III:** In stage III papillary and follicular thyroid cancer, either of the following is found: the tumor is larger than four centimeters or the tumor is any size and cancer has spread to tissues just outside the thyroid, but not to lymph nodes; or the tumor is any size and cancer may have spread to tissues just outside the thyroid and has spread to lymph nodes near the trachea or the larynx (voice box).

- **Stage IV:** Stage IV papillary and follicular thyroid cancer is divided into stages IVA, IVB, and IVC.

  - **Stage IVA:** In stage IVA, either of the following is found: the tumor is any size and cancer has spread outside the thyroid to tissues under the skin, the trachea, the esophagus, the larynx (voice box), and/or the recurrent laryngeal nerve (a nerve with two branches that go to the larynx); cancer may have spread to lymph nodes; or the tumor is any size and cancer may have spread to tissues just outside the thyroid. Cancer has spread to lymph nodes on one or both sides of the neck or between the lungs.

  - **Stage IVB:** In stage IVB, cancer has spread to tissue in front of the spinal column or has surrounded the carotid artery or the blood vessels in the area between the lungs.

  - **Stage IVC:** In stage IVC, cancer has spread to other parts of the body, such as the lungs and bones.

Medullary Thyroid Cancer

The following stages are used for medullary thyroid cancer:

- **Stage 0:** Stage 0 medullary thyroid cancer is found only with a special screening test. No tumor can be found in the thyroid.

- **Stage I:** Stage I medullary thyroid cancer is found only in the thyroid and is two centimeters or smaller.

- **Stage II:** Stage II medullary thyroid cancer is only in the thyroid and is larger than two centimeters but not larger than four centimeters.

- **Stage III:** In stage III medullary thyroid cancer: the tumor is larger than 4 centimeters or cancer has spread to tissues just outside the thyroid, but not to lymph nodes; or the tumor is any size and cancer may have spread to tissues just outside the thyroid and has spread to lymph nodes near the trachea or the larynx (voice box).

- **Stage IV:** Stage IV medullary thyroid cancer is divided into stages IVA, IVB, and IVC.

  - **Stage IVA:** In stage IVA, it may be possible to remove the tumor by surgery; either of the following is found: cancer has spread out of the thyroid to tissues under the skin, the trachea, the esophagus, the larynx (voice box), and/or the recurrent laryngeal nerve (a nerve with two branches that go to the larynx); cancer may have spread to lymph nodes; or cancer may have spread to tissues just outside the thyroid and has spread to lymph nodes on one or both sides of the neck or between the lungs.

  - **Stage IVB:** In stage IVB, the tumor cannot be removed by surgery; cancer has spread to tissue in front of the spinal column or has surrounded the carotid artery or the blood vessels in the area between the lungs. Cancer may have spread to lymph nodes.

  - **Stage IVC:** In stage IVC, cancer has spread to other parts of the body, such as the lungs and bones.

Anaplastic Thyroid Cancer

Anaplastic thyroid cancer is considered stage IV thyroid cancer. Anaplastic thyroid cancer grows quickly and has usually spread within the neck when it is found. Stage IV anaplastic thyroid cancer is divided into stages IVA, IVB, and IVC.

- **Stage IVA:** In stage IVA, cancer is found in the thyroid and may have spread to lymph nodes. The cancer can be removed by surgery.

- **Stage IVB:** In stage IVB, cancer has spread outside the thyroid and may have spread to lymph nodes. The cancer cannot be removed by surgery.

- **Stage IVC:** In stage IVC, cancer has spread to other parts of the body, such as the lungs and bones.

Recurrent Thyroid Cancer

Recurrent thyroid cancer is cancer that has recurred (come back) after it has been treated. Thyroid cancer may come back in the thyroid or in other parts of the body.

Treatment

Different types of treatment are available for patients with thyroid cancer. Some treatments are standard (the currently used treatment), and some are being tested in clinical trials. Four types of standard treatment are used:

Surgery

Surgery is the most common treatment of thyroid cancer. One of the following procedures may be used:

- **Lobectomy:** Removal of the lobe in which thyroid cancer is found. Biopsies of lymph nodes in the area may be done to see if they contain cancer.

- **Near-total thyroidectomy:** Removal of all but a very small part of the thyroid.

- **Total thyroidectomy:** Removal of the whole thyroid.

- **Lymphadenectomy:** Removal of lymph nodes in the neck that contain cancer.

Radiation Therapy and Radioactive Iodine Therapy

Radiation therapy is a cancer treatment that uses high-energy x-rays or other types of radiation to kill cancer cells or keep them from growing. There are two types of radiation therapy. External radiation therapy uses a machine outside the body to send radiation toward the cancer. Internal radiation therapy uses a radioactive substance sealed in needles, seeds, wires, or catheters that are placed directly into or near the cancer. The way the radiation therapy is given depends on the type and stage of the cancer being treated.

Radiation therapy may be given after surgery to kill any thyroid cancer cells that were not removed. Follicular and papillary thyroid cancers are sometimes treated with radioactive iodine (RAI) therapy. Higher doses than the amounts used to diagnose thyroid cancer are used. RAI is taken by mouth and collects in any remaining thyroid

tissue, including thyroid cancer cells that have spread to other places in the body. Since only thyroid tissue takes up iodine, the RAI destroys thyroid tissue and thyroid cancer cells without harming other tissue. Before a full treatment dose of RAI is given, a small test-dose is given to see if the tumor takes up the iodine.

Chemotherapy

Chemotherapy is a cancer treatment that uses drugs to stop the growth of cancer cells, either by killing the cells or by stopping them from dividing. When chemotherapy is taken by mouth or injected into a vein or muscle, the drugs enter the bloodstream and can reach cancer cells throughout the body (systemic chemotherapy). When chemotherapy is placed directly into the spinal column, an organ, or a body cavity such as the abdomen, the drugs mainly affect cancer cells in those areas (regional chemotherapy). The way the chemotherapy is given depends on the type and stage of the cancer being treated.

Thyroid Hormone Therapy

Hormone therapy is a cancer treatment that removes hormones or blocks their action and stops cancer cells from growing. Hormones are substances made by glands in the body and circulated in the bloodstream. In the treatment of thyroid cancer, drugs may be given to prevent the body from making thyroid-stimulating hormone (TSH), a hormone that can increase the chance that thyroid cancer will grow or recur.

Also, because thyroid cancer treatment kills thyroid cells, the thyroid is not able to make enough thyroid hormone. Patients are given thyroid hormone replacement pills.

Clinical Trials

A treatment clinical trial is a research study meant to help improve current treatments or obtain information on new treatments for patients with cancer. When clinical trials show that a new treatment is better than the standard treatment, the new treatment may become the standard treatment. Patients may want to think about taking part in a clinical trial. Some clinical trials are open only to patients who have not started treatment.

Targeted therapy is being tested in clinical trials. Targeted therapy is a type of treatment that uses drugs or other substances to identify and attack specific cancer cells without harming normal cells.

Tyrosine kinase inhibitor therapy is a type of targeted therapy being studied in the treatment of thyroid cancer. Tyrosine kinase inhibitors block signals needed for tumors to grow.

Follow-Up Tests

Some of the tests that were done to diagnose the cancer or to find out the stage of the cancer may be repeated. Some tests will be repeated in order to see how well the treatment is working. Decisions about whether to continue, change, or stop treatment may be based on the results of these tests. This is sometimes called re-staging.

Some of the tests will continue to be done from time to time after treatment has ended. The results of these tests can show if your condition has changed or if the cancer has recurred (come back). These tests are sometimes called follow-up tests or check-ups.

Part Five

Diagnosing and Treating Cancer

Chapter 27

You and Your Healthcare Team

Chapter Contents

Section 27.1

How to Find a Doctor or Treatment Facility If You Have Cancer

Excerpted from "How To Find a Doctor or Treatment Facility If You Have Cancer," National Cancer Institute (www.cancer.gov), 2009.

Physician Training and Credentials

When choosing a doctor for your cancer care, you may find it helpful to know some of the terms used to describe a doctor's training and credentials. Most physicians who treat people with cancer are medical doctors (they have an M.D. degree) or osteopathic doctors (they have a D.O. degree). The basic training for both types of physicians includes four years of premedical education at a college or university, four years of medical school to earn an M.D. or D.O. degree, and postgraduate medical education through internships and residences. This training usually lasts three to seven years. Physicians must pass an exam to become licensed (legally permitted) to practice medicine in their state. Each state or territory has its own procedures and general standards for licensing physicians.

Specialists are physicians who have completed their residency training in a specific area, such as internal medicine. Independent specialty boards certify physicians after they have fulfilled certain requirements. These requirements include meeting specific education and training criteria, being licensed to practice medicine, and passing an examination given by the specialty board. Doctors who have met all of the requirements are given the status of "Diplomate" and are board-certified as specialists. Doctors who are board-eligible have obtained the required education and training, but have not completed the specialty board examination.

After being trained and certified as a specialist, a physician may choose to become a subspecialist. A subspecialist has at least one additional year of full-time education in a particular area of a specialty. This training is designed to increase the physician's expertise in a specific field. Specialists can be board-certified in their subspecialty as well.

The following are some specialties and subspecialties that pertain to cancer treatment:

- Medical oncology is a subspecialty of internal medicine. Doctors who specialize in internal medicine treat a wide range of medical problems. Medical oncologists treat cancer and manage the patient's course of treatment. A medical oncologist may also consult with other physicians about the patient's care or refer the patient to other specialists.

- Hematology is a subspecialty of internal medicine. Hematologists focus on diseases of the blood and related tissues, including the bone marrow, spleen, and lymph nodes.

- Radiation oncology is a subspecialty of radiology. Radiology is the use of x-rays and other forms of radiation to diagnose and treat disease. Radiation oncologists specialize in the use of radiation to treat cancer.

- Surgery is a specialty that pertains to the treatment of disease by surgical operation. General surgeons perform operations on almost any area of the body. Physicians can also choose to specialize in a certain type of surgery; for example, thoracic surgeons are specialists who perform operations specifically in the chest area, including the lungs and the esophagus.

The American Board of Medical Specialties® (ABMS) is a not-for-profit organization that assists medical specialty boards with the development and use of standards for evaluation and certification of physicians. Information about other specialties that treat cancer is available from the ABMS website, which can be accessed at http://www.abms.org/ on the internet.

Almost all board-certified specialists are members of their medical specialty society. Physicians can attain Fellowship status in a specialty society, such as the American College of Surgeons (ACS), if they demonstrate outstanding achievement in their profession. Criteria for Fellowship status may include the number of years of membership in the specialty society, years practicing in the specialty, and professional recognition by peers.

Finding a Doctor

One way to find a doctor who specializes in cancer care is to ask for a referral from your primary care physician. You may know a specialist

yourself, or through the experience of a family member, coworker, or friend.

The following resources may also be able to provide you with names of doctors who specialize in treating specific diseases or conditions. However, these resources may not have information about the quality of care that the doctors provide. Your local hospital or its patient referral service may be able to provide you with a list of specialists who practice at that hospital.

- The ABMS has a list of doctors who have met certain education and training requirements and have passed specialty examinations. "Is Your Doctor Certified?" lists doctors' names along with their specialty and their educational background. The directory is available in most libraries and online at https://www.abms.org/WC/login.aspxon the internet. Users must register to use this online self-serve resource, which allows users to conduct searches by a physician's name or area of certification and a state name.

- The American Medical Association (AMA) DoctorFinder database at http://webapps.ama-assn.org/doctorfinder/home.jsp provides basic information on licensed physicians in the United States. Users can search for physicians by name or by medical specialty.

- The American Society of Clinical Oncology (ASCO) provides an online list of doctors who are members of ASCO. The member database has the names and affiliations of over 27,000 oncologists worldwide. It can be searched by doctor's name, institution, location, oncology specialty, and/or type of board certification. This service is available at http://www.cancer.net/portal/site/patient (click on "Find an Oncologist").

- The American College of Surgeons (ACS) membership database is an online list of surgeons who are members of the ACS. The list can be searched by doctor's name, geographic location, or medical specialty. This service is located at http://web3.facs.org/acsdir/default_public.cfm on the internet. The ACS can be contacted by telephone at 800-621-4111.

- The American Osteopathic Association (AOA) Find a D.O. database provides an online list of practicing osteopathic physicians who are AOA members. The information can be searched by doctor's name, geographic location, or medical specialty. The database is available at http://www.osteopathic.org/directory.cfm on the internet. The AOA can be contacted by telephone at 800-621-1773.

- Local medical societies may maintain lists of doctors in each specialty.

- Public and medical libraries may have print directories of doctors' names listed geographically by specialty.

- Your local Yellow Pages or Yellow Book may have doctors listed by specialty under "Physicians."

- The Agency for Healthcare Research and Quality (AHRQ) offers "Your Guide to Choosing Quality Health Care," which has information for consumers on choosing a health plan, a doctor, a hospital, or a long-term care provider. The Guide includes suggestions and checklists that you can use to determine which doctor or hospital is best for you. This resource is available at http://www.ahrq.gov/consumer/qntool.htm on the internet. You can also order the Guide by calling the AHRQ Publications Clearinghouse at 800-358-9295 or 703-437-2078 if outside the United States.

If you are a member of a health insurance plan, your choice may be limited to doctors who participate in your plan. Your insurance company can provide you with a list of participating primary care doctors and specialists. It is important to ask your insurance company if the doctor you choose is accepting new patients through your health plan. You also have the option of seeing a doctor outside your health plan and paying the costs yourself. If you have a choice of health insurance plans, you may first wish to consider which doctor or doctors you would like to use, and then choose a plan that includes your chosen physician(s).

If you are using a federal or state health insurance program such as Medicare or Medicaid, you may want to ask the doctor about accepting patients who use these programs.

You will have many factors to consider when choosing a doctor. To make an informed decision, you may wish to speak with several doctors before choosing one. When you meet with each doctor, you might want to consider the following:

- Does the doctor have the education and training to meet my needs?

- Does the doctor use the hospital that I have chosen?

- Does the doctor listen to me and treat me with respect?

- Does the doctor explain things clearly and encourage me to ask questions?

- What are the doctor's office hours?

- Who covers for the doctor when he or she is unavailable? Will that person have access to my medical records?

- How long does it take to get an appointment with the doctor?

If you are choosing a surgeon, you may wish to ask additional questions about the surgeon's background and experience with specific procedures. These questions may include:

- Is the surgeon board-certified?

- Has the surgeon been evaluated by a national professional association of surgeons, such as the American College of Surgeons (ACS)?

- At which treatment facility or facilities does the surgeon practice?

- How often does the surgeon perform the type of surgery I need?

- How many of these procedures has the surgeon performed? What was the success rate?

It is important for you to feel comfortable with the specialist that you choose because you will be working closely with that person to make decisions about your cancer treatment. Trust your own observations and feelings when deciding on a doctor for your medical care.

Getting a Second Opinion

Once you receive your doctor's opinion about the diagnosis and treatment plan, you may want to get another doctor's advice before you begin treatment. This is known as getting a second opinion. You can do this by asking another specialist to review all of the materials related to your case. A second opinion can confirm or suggest modifications to your doctor's proposed treatment plan, provide reassurance that you have explored all of your options, and answer any questions you may have.

Getting a second opinion is done frequently, and most physicians welcome another doctor's views. In fact, your doctor may be able to recommend a specialist for this consultation. However, some people find it uncomfortable to request a second opinion. When discussing this issue with your doctor, it may be helpful to express satisfaction with your doctor's decision and care and to mention that you want

your decision about treatment to be as thoroughly informed as possible. You may also wish to bring a family member along for support when asking for a second opinion. It is best to involve your doctor in the process of getting a second opinion, because your doctor will need to make your medical records (such as your test results and x-rays) available to the specialist.

Some health care plans require a second opinion, particularly if a doctor recommends surgery. Other health care plans will pay for a second opinion if the patient requests it. If your plan does not cover a second opinion, you can still obtain one if you are willing to cover the cost.

If your doctor is unable to recommend a specialist for a second opinion, or if you prefer to choose one on your own, the following resources can help:

- Many of the resources listed above for finding a doctor can also help you find a specialist for a consultation.

- The National Institutes of Health (NIH) Clinical Center in Bethesda, Maryland, is the research hospital for the NIH, including the National Cancer Institute (NCI). Several branches of the NCI provide second opinion services. The NCI fact sheet "Cancer Clinical Trials at the National Institutes of Health Clinical Center: Questions and Answers" describes these NCI branches and their services, and is available at http://www.cancer.gov/cancertopics/factsheet/NCI/clinical-center on the internet.

- The R. A. Bloch Cancer Foundation, Inc., can refer cancer patients to institutions that are willing to provide multidisciplinary second opinions. A list of these institutions is available at http://blochcancer.org/2009/03/multidisciplinary-second-opinion-centers/ on the internet. You can also contact the R. A. Bloch Cancer Foundation, Inc., by telephone at 816-854-5050 or 800-433-0464.

Finding a Treatment Facility for Patients Living in the United States

Choosing a treatment facility is another important consideration for getting the best medical care possible. Although you may not be able to choose which hospital treats you in an emergency, you can choose a facility for scheduled and ongoing care. If you have already found a doctor for your cancer treatment, you may need to choose a facility based on where your doctor practices. Your doctor may be able to recommend a facility that provides quality care to meet your

needs. You may wish to ask the following questions when considering a treatment facility:

- Has the facility had experience and success in treating my condition?

- Has the facility been rated by state, consumer, or other groups for its quality of care?

- How does the facility check on and work to improve its quality of care?

- Has the facility been approved by a nationally recognized accrediting body, such as the American College of Surgeons (ACS) Commission on Cancer and/or The Joint Commission?

- Does the facility explain patients' rights and responsibilities? Are copies of this information available to patients?

- Does the treatment facility offer support services, such as social workers and resources, to help me find financial assistance if I need it?

- Is the facility conveniently located?

If you are a member of a health insurance plan, your choice of treatment facilities may be limited to those that participate in your plan. Your insurance company can provide you with a list of approved facilities. Although the costs of cancer treatment can be very high, you have the option of paying out-of-pocket if you want to use a treatment facility that is not covered by your insurance plan. If you are considering paying for treatment yourself, you may wish to discuss the possible costs with your doctor beforehand. You may also want to speak with the person who does the billing for the treatment facility. In some instances, nurses and social workers can provide you with more information about coverage, eligibility, and insurance issues.

The following resources may help you find a hospital or treatment facility for your care:

- The NCI-Designated Cancer Centers database provides contact information for NCI-designated cancer centers around the country.

- The ACS's Commission on Cancer (CoC) accredits cancer programs at hospitals and other treatment facilities. More than 1,433 programs in the United States have been designated by the CoC as Approved Cancer Programs. The ACS website offers a searchable database of these programs at http://web.facs.org/

cpm/CPMApprovedHospitals_Search.htm on the internet. The CoC can be contacted by telephone at 312-202-5085.

- The Joint Commission is an independent, not-for-profit organization that evaluates and accredits health care organizations and programs in the United States. It also offers information for the general public about choosing a treatment facility. The Joint Commission's website can be found at http://www.jointcommission .org. The Joint Commission can be contacted by telephone at 630-792-5000.

- The Joint Commission offers an online Quality Check™ service that patients can use to determine whether a specific facility has been accredited by the Joint Commission and to view the organization's performance reports. This service is located at http:// www.qualitycheck.org on the internet.

- The AHRQ publication "Your Guide to Choosing Quality Health Care" has suggestions and checklists for choosing the treatment facility that is right for you.

Finding a Treatment Facility for Patients Living Outside the United States

If you live outside the United States, facilities that offer cancer treatment may be located in or near your country. Cancer information services are available in many countries to provide information and answer questions about cancer; they may also be able to help you find a cancer treatment facility close to where you live. A list of these cancer information services is available on the International Cancer Information Service Group's (ICISG) website at http://www.icisg.org/ meet_memberslist.htm on the internet. A list may also be requested by writing to the NCI Public Inquiries Office at this address:

Cancer Information Service
Room 3036A, MSC 8322
6116 Executive Boulevard
Bethesda, MD 20892-8322
USA

The ICISG is an independent international organization composed of cancer information services. Their mission is to provide high-quality cancer information services and resources to those concerned about, or affected by, cancer throughout the world.

The International Union Against Cancer (UICC) is another resource for people living outside the United States who want to find a cancer treatment facility. The UICC consists of international cancer-related organizations devoted to the worldwide fight against cancer. UICC membership includes research facilities and treatment centers and, in some countries, ministries of health. Other members include volunteer cancer leagues, associations, and societies. These organizations serve as resources for the public and may have helpful information about cancer and treatment facilities. To find a resource in or near your country, contact the UICC at this address:

International Union Against Cancer (UICC)
62 route de Frontenex
1207 Geneva
Switzerland
Telephone: + 41 22 809 1811
Website: http://www.uicc.org

Some people living outside the United States may wish to obtain a second opinion or have their cancer treatment in this country. Many facilities in the United States offer these services to international cancer patients. These facilities may also provide support services, such as language interpretation, assistance with travel, and guidance in finding accommodations near the treatment facility for patients and their families.

If you live outside the United States and would like to obtain cancer treatment in this country, you should contact cancer treatment facilities directly to find out whether they have an international patient office.

Citizens of other countries who are planning to travel to the United States for cancer treatment generally must first obtain a nonimmigrant visa for medical treatment from the U.S. Embassy or Consulate in their home country. Visa applicants must demonstrate that the purpose of their trip is to enter the United States for medical treatment; that they plan to remain for a specific, limited period; that they have funds to cover expenses in the United States; that they have a residence and social and economic ties outside the United States; and that they intend to return to their home country.

To determine the specific fees and documentation required for the nonimmigrant visa and to learn more about the application process, contact the U.S. Embassy or Consulate in your home country. A list of links to the websites of U.S. Embassies and Consulates worldwide can be found at http://usembassy.gov on the internet.

More information about nonimmigrant visa services is available on the U.S. Department of State's website at http://travel.state.gov/visa/temp/temp_1305.html on the internet.

Section 27.2

How to Be a Proactive Patient

Everyone wants the best medical care possible. This involves more than scheduling a doctor's appointment. A proactive patient is an informed one who finds a good doctor and medical facility, does independent research using reliable sources, and asks detailed, relevant questions. Each of us is ultimately in charge of our own health. The following are some tips for becoming a more proactive patient.

This is a printable guide you can use as a reference and a questions checklist to bring with you to your doctor's appointment(s).

Find a Good Doctor and Medical Facility

As in every profession, there are doctors who excel in their specialty, doctors who perform average work, and doctors whose skills are less than desirable. Finding the best takes some effort on the part of the patient.

Get a recommendation from a friend, family member, healthcare professional, or neighbor. Many times, patients need to see physicians who participate in their health insurance's "network" of doctors. In this case, asking a co-worker who carries the same insurance can be a good approach. However, asking your general practitioner or another doctor or healthcare professional is often the best way to find experts in a particular field. Healthcare professionals network at medical conferences and other events and almost always know who "the top performers" are.

Do a background check: Once a doctor has been identified, visit the American Medical Association's (AMA) website and perform a

345

search. The AMA is the largest medical society in the United States. Its website provides useful information on 650,000 member and nonmember doctors of medicine (MD) and doctors of osteopathy or osteopathic medicine (DO). Note that it does not include other licensed healthcare professionals such as dentists, optometrists, chiropractors, nurses, or allied health personnel. Use the website to learn or verify a doctor's credentials, including specialty, where and when he/she attended medical or professional school, and whether the doctor is board-certified. Medical specialty boards determine whether candidates have received sufficient preparation in accordance with established educational standards, provide comprehensive examinations designed to assess knowledge, skills, and experience requisite to the provision of high quality patient care in that specialty, and certify those candidates who have satisfied the requirements. Many boards require recertification at periodic intervals.

All doctors must be licensed. Licensure requires medical school plus a minimum of one year of internship. Board certification comes from a specialty board usually after a minimum of three years postgraduate residency training. Many doctors are NOT board certified. Board certification is a minimum standard, and patients seeking the best care should always see a board certified physician whenever possible. Fellowship training is a level beyond basic residency training and usually implies expertise in a particular subspecialty field within a more general specialty.

Ask questions. Call the doctor's office and ask about the doctor's patient load, how long it generally takes to get an appointment, the average wait time at the office, etc. If health insurance is a concern, always verify that the doctor accepts a particular insurance prior to scheduling an appointment.

Consider the medical facility. If treatment requires time in a hospital or medical facility, it's important to research the facility as well. A doctor may be affiliated with or located in a hospital or other type of treatment facility. Some doctors treat patients in multiple hospitals. Ask the doctor for a recommendation of the best facility in the area for the specialty. The Joint Commission on Accreditation of Healthcare Organizations advises choosing a facility that performs a large number of the procedure(s) the patients will need. According to the American Cancer Society, hospitals with at least 500 beds typically offer more services. The best hospitals offer pathology labs, diagnostic labs, and blood banks; round-the-clock physician staffing; social work services; advanced diagnostic and therapeutic equipment; and an intensive care

unit. Teaching hospitals are often affiliated with reputable medical facilities. Before leaving a hospital or treatment facility, it is important to ask about follow-up care. Be prepared and ask questions.

Research, research, research: Research the health concern using reliable print or online sources prior to the doctor's appointment whenever possible. Contact non-profit organizations or governmental agencies for information or advice on credible resources. (Imaginis provides a list of resources for breast cancer and women's health issues at http://www.imaginis.com/breasthealth/menu-resources.asp). Don't rely on memory on the day of the appointment. Jot down questions and bring reference materials. If unsure of the diagnosis prior to the appointment, try searching by symptoms to get an idea of possible diagnoses. Read about various diagnostic tests and treatments for the condition. An informed patient asks more relevant information and often gets more detailed answers to her questions. After the appointment, performed more detailed research using the information the doctor has provided.

Try to bring past medical records to a new doctor whenever possible: If diagnostic tests (such as CAT scans, MRIs, mammograms, etc.) were performed, bring a copy of the films.

Ask questions, questions, and more questions. Being a proactive patient means asking a lot of questions. As described earlier, researching before and after appointments can help patients determine what questions to ask. Here are some suggestions:

- If a medicine is prescribed, try to ask detailed questions about the medicine. For example, ask the name of the medicine, how it works, when and how long to take it, what foods and drinks to avoid, what side effects are possible and if there are ways to deal with those side effects, how to know when the medicine is working or not working, and whether interactions are possible with other prescription or non-prescription drugs.

- If a medical test or procedure is needed, get a full explanation of what will happen. Ask the doctor to explain the procedure from start to finish. Ask why the doctor believes the procedure should be performed, whether it will require a hospital stay (and if so, for how long), what side effects are possible, the estimated length of recovery, what it will feel like after the procedure, whether follow-up care is necessary, when test results will be available, etc. Don't

forget to ask about the doctor's experience. Ask how many how many of the particular procedure the doctor has performed. The more the better. Ask about the alternatives and pros and cons of any recommended procedure/treatment.

- If a doctor won't answer your questions, ask one more: "Where's the door?"

Always get the test results: Never assume no news is good news. Ask for the results of all medical tests and for an explanation of what the results mean. Before the test, ask when to expect the results. Follow up with the doctor's office or medical facility if results don't come when expected.

Get a second opinion for any major procedure, such as surgery. Patients diagnosed with serious conditions (such as breast cancer) should not hesitate to get a second opinion before beginning treatment. The purpose of a second opinion is to obtain a comprehensive, independent review of the diagnosis and the planned course of treatment. It is essential that patients have confidence in their doctors and treatment teams before proceeding with treatment.

Follow the doctor's instructions: According to the Food and Drug Administration (FDA) and the National Council on Patient Information and Education, 14% to 21% of patients never even fill their original prescriptions. Many others fail to schedule follow-up appointments in a timely manner or conform to other doctor's instructions. Patients should never blindly follow advice that makes them uncomfortable. They should ask questions if a doctor's advice sounds out of the ordinary. If the answers aren't satisfactory, get a second opinion. However, patients satisfied with their doctor's answers should adhere to their advice to ensure the best medical care possible.

Section 27.3

How to Get a Second Opinion

Excerpted from "How to Get a Second Opinion," National Women's
Health Information Center (www.womenshealth.gov), 2008.

Even though doctors may get similar medical training, they can
have their own opinions and thoughts about how to practice medicine.
They can have different ideas about how to diagnose and treat conditions or diseases. Some doctors take a more conservative, or traditional,
approach to treating their patients. Other doctors are more aggressive
and use the newest tests and therapies. It seems like we learn about
new advances in medicine almost every day.

Many doctors specialize in one area of medicine, such as cardiology
or obstetrics or psychiatry. Not every doctor can be skilled in using all
the latest technology. Getting a second opinion from a different doctor might give you a fresh perspective and new information. It could
provide you with new options for treating your condition. Then you
can make more informed choices. If you get similar opinions from two
doctors, you can also talk with a third doctor.

Tips: What to Do

Ask your doctor for a recommendation: Ask for the name of another doctor or specialist, so you can get a second opinion. Don't worry
about hurting your doctor's feelings. Most doctors welcome a second
opinion, especially when surgery or long-term treatment is involved.

Ask someone you trust for a recommendation: If you don't
feel comfortable asking your doctor for a referral, then call another
doctor you trust. You can also call university teaching hospitals and
medical societies in your area for the names of doctors. Some of this
information is also available on the internet.

Check with your health insurance provider. Call your insurance
company before you get a second opinion. Ask if they will pay for this
office visit. Many health insurance providers do. Ask if there are any
special procedures you or your primary care doctor needs to follow.

Ask to have medical records sent to the second doctor. Ask your primary care doctor to send your medical records to the new doctor. You need to give written permission to your current doctor to send any records or test results to a new doctor. You can also ask for a copy of your own medical records for your files. Your new doctor can then examine these records before your office visit.

Learn as much as you can: Ask your doctor for information you can read. Go to a local library. Search the internet. Find a teaching hospital or university that has medical libraries open to the public. The information you find can be hard to understand, or just confusing. Make a list of your questions, and bring it with you when you see your new doctor.

Do not rely on the internet or a telephone conversation: When you get a second opinion, you need to be seen by a doctor. That doctor will perform a physical examination and perhaps other tests. The doctor will also thoroughly review your medical records, ask you questions, and address your concerns.

Chapter 28

Diagnosing Cancer

Chapter Contents

Section 28.1

Commonly Used Diagnostic Tests and Procedures

Doctors use many tests to diagnose cancer and determine if it has metastasized (spread). Some tests may also determine which treatments may be the most effective. Diagnostic tests may include a biopsy, imaging tests, endoscopic tests, and blood and urine tests; the most common diagnostic tests are described below. When choosing a diagnostic test(s), your doctor will consider the person's age and medical condition, the type of cancer that is suspected, the severity of the symptoms, and previous test results.

Biopsy

A biopsy is the removal of a small amount of tissue for examination under a microscope. For most types of cancer, a biopsy is the only way to make a definitive diagnosis of cancer. The sample removed from the biopsy is analyzed by a pathologist (a doctor who specializes in interpreting laboratory tests and evaluating cells, tissues, and organs to diagnose disease). There are different types of biopsies.

Fine needle aspiration biopsy: This test uses a thin, hollow needle in a syringe to collect a small amount of fluid and cells from the suspicious area.

Core needle biopsy: A core biopsy uses a slightly larger needle to obtain a cylinder of tissue. It is often done instead of a fine needle aspiration biopsy because it provides more tissue for the pathologist to review.

Vacuum-assisted biopsy: This type of biopsy uses vacuum pressure (suction) to collect the sample tissue through a specially designed hollow needle. This technique allows the doctor to collect multiple or

larger samples from the same biopsy site without having to insert the needle more than once.

Image-guided biopsy: An image-guided biopsy is a procedure in which the doctor uses imaging technology, such as ultrasound, fluoroscopy, a computed tomography (CT or CAT) scan, x-ray, or a magnetic resonance imaging (MRI) test, to determine the exact location where the tissue sample will be removed for analysis. (Find more information about these imaging tests is in the next section of this article.) An image-guided biopsy may be used when a suspected tumor appears on an imaging scan, such as an x-ray, but cannot be felt by the doctor, or when the area is located deeper inside the body. Once the area to biopsy is located, a needle is used to obtain a sample of the tissue from the site. The type of imaging technology used depends on the location of the biopsy site and other factors.

Surgical biopsy: In a surgical biopsy, a surgeon makes an incision in the skin and removes some or all of the suspicious tissue. It is often used after a needle biopsy shows cancer cells, or it can be used as the first method to obtain tissue for diagnosis. There are two types of surgical biopsies:

- An incisional biopsy removes a piece of the suspicious area for examination. An incisional biopsy may be used for soft tissue tumors, such as those from muscle or fat tissue, to distinguish between benign (noncancerous) lumps and cancerous tumors called sarcomas.

- An excisional biopsy removes the entire lump. An excisional biopsy, which was more common before the development of fine needle aspiration, may be used for enlarged lymph nodes or breast lumps, or in situations where the lump is small enough to be completely removed in one procedure.

Endoscopic biopsy: An endoscope is a tube with a camera that doctors use to view the inside of body, including the bladder, abdomen, joints, or gastrointestinal (GI) tract. An endoscope can be inserted through the mouth or a tiny surgical incision. Using an endoscope, the doctor can see any abnormal areas and remove tiny samples of the tissue using forceps that are part of the endoscope.

Bone marrow aspiration and biopsy: A bone marrow aspiration and biopsy is a diagnostic examination of the bone marrow, the spongy

tissue inside of bone that has both fluid and solid parts. The sample is usually collected from the back of the hipbone. For this test, the patient's skin is numbed with a local anesthetic, and a needle is inserted into a bone in the hip until it reaches the bone marrow. A small amount of bone marrow fluid is removed and examined under a microscope. This is called an aspirate. The doctor may also use a hollow needle in the same location to withdraw a solid core of bone marrow. This is called a biopsy. This test is used to determine if a person has a blood disorder or a blood cancer, such as leukemia or multiple myeloma. It can also be used to find out if a cancer that started in another part of the body has spread to the bone marrow. Learn what to expect during a bone marrow aspiration and biopsy.

Imaging Tests

Doctors use imaging tests to determine whether the cancer has spread to other areas in the body, and to evaluate the size and location of the tumor. Imaging tests alone are usually not specific enough to diagnose cancer.

X-ray: An x-ray is a picture of the inside of the body. For instance, a chest x-ray can help doctors determine if the cancer has spread to the lungs. Although an x-ray is not as sophisticated as other imaging tests, it is still useful for finding and monitoring some types of tumors. There can be specific types of x-rays, such as mammography (an x-ray of the breast) and a barium enema (which is used in the x-ray of the colon and rectum).

Bone scan: A bone scan uses a radioactive tracer to look at the inside of the bones. The tracer is injected into a patient's vein. It collects in areas of the bone and is detected by a special camera. Healthy bone appears gray to the camera, and areas of injury, such as those caused by cancer, appear dark.

CT or CAT scan: A CT scan creates a three-dimensional picture of the inside of the body with an x-ray machine. A computer then combines these images into a detailed, cross-sectional view that shows any abnormalities or tumors. Sometimes, a contrast medium (a special dye) is injected into a patient's vein to provide better detail.

Positron emission tomography (PET) scan: A PET scan is a way to create pictures of organs and tissues inside the body. A small amount of a radioactive substance is injected into a patient's body and absorbed

by the organs or tissues being studied. This substance gives off energy that is detected by a scanner, which produces the images.

MRI: An MRI uses magnetic fields, not x-rays, to produce detailed images of the body. A contrast medium (a special dye) may be injected into a patient's vein to create a clearer picture.

Ultrasound: An ultrasound uses sound waves to create a picture of the internal organs.

Endoscopic Tests

Any medical procedure performed with an endoscope is called an endoscopy. As explained above, an endoscope is a thin, flexible tube with a camera used to examine the inside of the body. The specific type of endoscope varies depending on what part of the body needs to be viewed. The following are some common examples of endoscopic tests.

- A bronchoscopy uses a bronchoscope to examine the lungs.

- A colonoscopy uses a colonoscope to examine the colon and rectum.

- A laparoscopy uses a laparoscope to examine the abdominal area.

Laboratory Tests

Laboratory tests involve testing a sample of blood, urine, and/or other body fluids to learn or confirm what is happening in the body. One of the most common tests is a complete blood count (CBC). A CBC measures the components of the blood, including white blood cells, red blood cells, and platelets. Blood tests are also used to monitor potential side effects of cancer treatment, such as anemia (low red blood cell count) or infection.

Some tests help with diagnosing a specific type of cancer, such as the test for prostate specific antigen (PSA) for prostate cancer, or the Pap test for the detection of cervical cancer. Other tests help doctors make treatment decisions. For example, the breast cells of women with breast cancer may be tested to determine whether the cells have the estrogen receptor, which lets doctors know whether hormone therapy can be used to treat the cancer. Or, the breast cells are tested for the human epidermal growth factor receptor 2 (HER2) to help the doctor know whether the cancer can be treated with drugs that target HER2.

Finally, other tests using tumor markers help the doctors figure out if cancer treatment is working. A tumor marker is a substance found in higher amounts in a person's blood, urine, or the tumor itself if the person has a specific type of cancer. It is produced by the tumor or the body in response to cancer, such as carcinoembryonic antigen (CEA) for colorectal cancer. However, these tests are only meaningful in specific situations.

Section 28.2

What to Expect During a Biopsy

A biopsy is a medical procedure that is almost always required to make a definitive cancer diagnosis; it provides the most accurate analysis of tissue. Often, doctors will recommend a biopsy after a physical examination or imaging study, such as an x-ray, has identified a tumor. During the biopsy, a doctor removes a sample of tissue, which is then specially processed and examined under a microscope by a pathologist. The pathologist (a doctor who specializes in interpreting laboratory tests and evaluating cells, tissues, and organs to diagnose disease) will determine if the sample is benign or cancerous.

About the Procedure

Because tissue samples can be taken from skin, areas just below the skin, or internal organs, a biopsy can be a simple procedure performed in a doctor's office, as an outpatient surgical procedure, or invasive surgery requiring hospitalization.

Types of biopsies include:

Fine needle aspiration biopsy: A fine needle biopsy may be the first type of biopsy done on tumors that can be felt by the doctor. The doctor uses a very thin, hollow needle in a syringe to gather a small amount of fluid and cells from the suspicious area.

Core needle biopsy: The size of the syringe needle used in a core needle biopsy is larger than the one in a fine needle biopsy, so that a cylinder of tissue can be obtained. If a fine needle biopsy cannot provide a definitive diagnosis, the doctor may want to do a core needle biopsy. Core biopsies are often performed instead of fine needle aspiration biopsies because they provide more tissue to review.

Vacuum-assisted biopsy: Vacuum pressure (suction) is used to pull the sample tissue through a specially designed hollow needle in this biopsy method. This gives the doctor the ability to collect multiple or larger samples from the same biopsy site without having to insert the needle more than once.

Image-guided biopsy: An image-guided biopsy is a procedure in which the doctor uses imaging technology, such as ultrasound, fluoroscopy, CT scan, x-ray, or MRI scan, to determine the exact location from which the tissue sample will be removed for analysis. A needle is used to obtain a sample of the tissue from the site; the needle type used may be a fine needle, core needle, or vacuum-assisted needle. An image-guided biopsy may be used when a tumor appears on an imaging scan, such as an x-ray, but cannot be felt by the doctor, or when the area is located deeper inside the body. The type of imaging technology used depends on the location of the biopsy site and other factors.

Surgical biopsy: Unlike the needle methods described above, in a surgical biopsy, a surgeon makes an incision in the skin and removes some or all of the suspicious tissue. It is often used after a needle biopsy shows cancer cells, or it can be used as the first method to obtain tissue for diagnosis. There are two main categories of surgical biopsies:

- Incisional biopsy removes a piece of the suspicious area for examination. An incisional biopsy may be used for soft tissue tumors, such as those arising from muscle or fat, to distinguish between benign lumps and cancerous tumors called sarcomas.

- Excisional biopsy removes the entire lump. An excisional biopsy, which was more common prior to the development of fine needle aspiration, may be used for enlarged lymph nodes or breast lumps or in situations where the lump is small enough to be easily completely removed in one procedure.

Endoscopic biopsy: Endoscopes are tubes with cameras that doctors use to view the inside of body, including the bladder, abdomen, joints,

or gastrointestinal (GI) tract. Endoscopes can be inserted through the mouth or a tiny surgical incision. Using an endoscope, the doctor can see any abnormal areas and pinch off tiny samples of the tissue using forceps that are part of the endoscope. Many common medical procedures, such as a cystoscopy to examine the bladder and colonoscopy to examine the colon, use endoscopic techniques.

Bone marrow biopsy: The doctor uses a large, rigid needle to go through a bone, often the back of the hipbone, and into the marrow in order to gather a sample. A core biopsy of the bone may also be performed at the same time. A bone marrow biopsy is used to determine if a person has a blood disorder or a blood cancer, including leukemia and multiple myeloma. It can also be used to find out if a cancer that originated in another part of the body has spread to the bone marrow.

The Medical Team

Because there are different types of biopsies, members of the medical team involved in the procedures may vary.

Most incisional and excisional biopsies are performed by surgeons. Less invasive biopsies, such as fine needle aspirations and endoscopic biopsies, can be performed by a surgeon, radiologist (a doctor who diagnoses diseases by obtaining and interpreting medical images), oncologist (a doctor who specializes in cancer), gastroenterologist (a doctor who specializes in the function and disorders of the gastrointestinal tract, including stomach, intestines, and associated organs), pathologist, or other specialist.

Questions to Ask Your Doctor

Before having a biopsy, consider asking your doctor the following questions:

- What will happen during the biopsy?
- Who will perform the biopsy, and who else will be in the room?
- How long will the procedure take?
- Will it be painful?
- Will I be given general or local anesthesia?
- Is there a risk of infection, bleeding, or other adverse effects after the biopsy?

- What are the risks of not having the test?
- Will the biopsy have a cosmetic effect on my body?
- Will I need to stay in the hospital after the biopsy?
- Will I need to avoid any activities after the biopsy?
- Will I need to have someone drive me home after the biopsy?
- When will I learn the results of the biopsy? How will they be communicated to me?
- What further tests will be necessary if the results are positive (indicates cancer)? What if they are negative?

Preparing for the Procedure

Preparation for a biopsy depends on the type of biopsy you will have. A fine needle biopsy, for example, may be performed in a doctor's office. An incisional or excisional biopsy, which involves surgery, will require more extensive preparations. Depending on the type of biopsy you will need to take off all or most of your clothing. You will be given a gown to wear during the biopsy.

Review with your doctor or nurse what you should or should not eat or drink before your biopsy, and whether you should take your regular medications that day. In addition, tell your doctor about all medications you are taking, as well as any drug allergies or other medical conditions you have.

You will have the procedure explained to you by your doctor or nurse. You will be asked to sign a consent form that states you understand the benefits and risks of the biopsy and agree to have the test done. Talk with your doctor about any concerns you have about the biopsy.

During the Procedure

Depending on the part of your body where the biopsy will be performed, you may be lying on your stomach or your back, or sitting up, for the procedure. You may be asked to hold your breath while a biopsy needle is inserted. You will need to be still for the duration of the procedure.

You may feel some amount of pain or discomfort during a biopsy, including slight, stinging pain when a local anesthetic is injected by needle, pressure and dull pain where the biopsy needle is inserted, discomfort from lying still for an extended period of time, and soreness at the biopsy site. If a general anesthetic is used, you will feel minimal pain during the procedure because you will be asleep.

After the Procedure

Your recovery period will depend on the type of biopsy performed. The least invasive procedures require no recovery; after the procedure, you will be able to resume your normal activities. If you have a surgical biopsy, you will be observed for a variable period after the procedure to be sure that you are fully awake and you may need to stay in the hospital to recover.

Following a biopsy, be aware of any symptoms that indicate a complication from the procedure. Severe pain, fever, or bleeding are signs that you should be seen by your doctor or nurse. Talk with your doctor or nurse about taking care of the area where the biopsy was performed.

Section 28.3

Colposcopy

What is colposcopy?

Colposcopy is a special visual examination of the cervix, vagina, and sometimes the outer lips or vulvar area. If you have an abnormal Pap smear, you may require a colposcopy. This requires your healthcare provider to look through an instrument called a "colposcope" which is a type of microscope mounted on a pole. The colposcope helps your healthcare provider check for problems, which are often very small, on the cervix and vagina and may not be seen during your regular exam. If abnormalities are seen, a small sample of tissue, called a biopsy, is usually done.

The biopsy gives your healthcare provider important information to decide if treatment would be necessary. Biopsies may cause mild cramping. The colposcopy exam takes about 10 to 20 minutes.

Who needs colposcopy?

Colposcopy is most often advised for women who have had an abnormal Pap smear. An abnormal Pap smear may be a sign of a precancerous condition that can then be successfully treated before turning into cancer. Occasionally, a patient may be referred for colposcopy because of some abnormal appearance of their cervix, noted during a pelvic examination.

How is colposcopy performed?

The colposcope used in colposcopy is instrument that looks like a pair of binoculars mounted on a pole. A speculum is placed in the vagina to hold the vaginal walls open, just as if you were having a Pap smear done, and remains in place until the exam is finished. The colposcope is placed a few inches in front of the vagina, but does not touch you. A repeat Pap smear may also be done at this time, in the same way it is collected during your prior exam. Your health care provider may place vinegar, and sometimes an iodine solution (notify your healthcare provider if you are allergic to iodine), directly onto the cervix and vagina to identify any abnormal areas.

You may have some mild burning or tingling, but most patients do not experience this. The provider might also adjust the colposcope by changing the magnification or looking through different colored filters. This helps in finding suspicious areas. Sometime photographs of your cervix, vagina, or vulva are taken during your exam and become part of your medical record.

Abnormal cells that cause cervical disease may extend up toward the lining of the uterus or womb through an opening called the endocervical canal. This is the same birth canal that dilates when women have vaginal childbirth. Sampling the endocervical canal may cause cramping or, rarely, light-headedness. If abnormal areas are seen on the cervix, they often require a biopsy to make a correct diagnosis. The biopsy takes a very small piece of tissue from the abnormal areas. If more than one area is abnormal, several different biopsies may be performed. Any bleeding from the biopsy sites can be stopped using silver nitrate or an iron-containing compound called Monsel's solution. A pathologist, who will tell your healthcare provider the final diagnosis, then sends the biopsy specimens that are collected to the

lab for processing and examination. This may take several days or even a few weeks.

What should you expect after the biopsy?

For about three to five days following a colposcopy with biopsies you may experience some spotting or a brown crumbly discharge, like coffee grounds, which may require you to use a mini-pad. There are few restrictions after the procedure and you may usually go about your daily routine. If biopsies are performed you may be restricted from certain activities until the spotting has stopped and your cervix has time to heal. These include:

- Sexual activity (vaginal intercourse)
- Putting tampons into your vagina
- Washing or douching inside your vagina

You should call your healthcare provider if you have:

- Fever
- Bright red, heavy bleeding which is more than what you have with your period
- Bad cramps or pain that do not improve with over-the-counter medications, such as ibuprofen

What is the treatment after a colposcopy?

The treatment following a colposcopy depends on the degree of abnormality reported on the biopsy. For minor or low-grade abnormalities, no treatment may be necessary and only a follow up Pap smear or HPV testing would be required. If there are greater or more severe abnormalities, other treatment may be required including destroying surface cells of the cervix with laser or freezing therapies. Another option includes a larger biopsy of the cervix called a "Loop" or loop electro excision procedure (LEEP), which may be performed in the healthcare provider's office. A surgical conization in the operating room is needed occasionally. Your healthcare provider will discuss these treatments with you, if any is needed.

Is colposcopy safe for pregnant women?

As with non-pregnant women any abnormal Pap smear in pregnancy needs further examination.

Looking through the colposcope is completely safe and biopsies may be performed in pregnancy if suspicious areas are identified. Sampling from the birth canal, such as by an endocervical curettage, should not be performed in pregnancy. Most of the treatment methods, which are used on non-pregnant patients are not recommended during pregnancy. These treatments can usually wait until after the pregnancy is finished. Often a repeat exam is done after the pregnancy to determine if treatment is still necessary.

What are the risks to colposcopy?

There are no serious risks to colposcopy, which is performed routinely in the healthcare provider's clinic. The most likely side effect is mild discomfort from the solutions used and cramping or pinching from the endocervical curettage or biopsies. There may be a small amount of spotting for a few days, but heavy bleeding is rare. The Monsel's solution or silver nitrate used to help stop bleeding may also cause a brown crumbly discharge for two to three days.

Is there anything I should or should not do before my colposcopy?

If your abnormal Pap test was done by another healthcare provider, it is useful to have a copy of the report at the time of your referral for a colposcopy. Undergoing colposcopy does not require any special preparation. You may take over-the-counter medications like ibuprofen or acetaminophen before the procedure to help reduce the cramping. To avoid obscuring the abnormal cells, it is best to avoid anything in the vagina for two days prior to the procedure such as sexual activity, intravaginal medications, tampons, or douching. Try to avoid having colposcopy during your period, but if the bleeding is light, the exam may still be satisfactory.

Section 28.4

Loop Electrosurgical Excision Procedure

What Is LEEP?

LEEP stands for loop electrosurgical excision procedure. This is a procedure designed to treat and/or diagnose pre-cancerous changes on the cervix (the portion of the uterus visible in the vagina) in women with an abnormal Pap tests. This procedure has several other names which have been used to describe the process, including LLETZ (large loop excision of the transformation zone), LLEC (large loop excision of the cervix), and loop cone biopsy of the cervix. A fine wire loop which is attached to a high-frequency electrical generator allows very precise removal of abnormal tissue from your cervix.

Because the procedure is so exact, and the loop very thin, there is very little damage to the tissue surrounding the area that needs to be removed, and the procedure allows for the blood vessels surrounding the area to be sealed.

The LEEP Procedure

The procedure should be done when you are not having your menstrual period, allowing for better view of the cervix. This also helps you determine if any post procedure bleeding you may have is abnormal. You may be given something for pain relief prior to the procedure.

- You will be placed in the room, with your legs in stirrups or supports.

- The speculum will be inserted as for a Pap test.

- A local anesthetic will be injected (similar to the anesthetic you would get at a dental office). At the time of the injection, you may experience stinging or cramping while the anesthesia is being injected. You may also experience some increase in your heart rate with some of the local anesthesia, and possibly some shakiness of your legs. These symptoms are normal and related to the medication.

- A solution is applied to the cervix to show the abnormal area that needs to be removed.

- You will hear the sound of a smoke evacuator (like a vacuum). You will also hear a humming sound when the electrosurgical generator is being used. It is VERY important that you do not move when the electrosurgical generator is making a sound.

- You may feel cramping, however if you feel anything sharp, you should let the person performing the procedure know immediately. The removal of the tissue is over within a few seconds. The cautery portion of the procedure (burning of vessels after the procedure to prevent bleeding) takes a few minutes.

- Monsel's solution (a green paste to assist in prevention of bleeding) is often applied, and the speculum is removed. The paste will cause a dark brown-black grainy vaginal discharge for several days after the procedure.

Risks of LEEP

Risks and complications from LEEP are very unlikely, however they include:

- Heavy bleeding (more than our normal period)
- Bleeding with clots
- Severe abdominal cramping
- Fever
- Foul-smelling discharge (other than the odor from the procedure and Monsel's solution)
- Incomplete removal of abnormal tissue
- Narrowing of the cervix (cervical stenosis)
- Infection

- Accidental cutting or burning of normal tissue (usually with patient movement during the procedure)

Benefits of LEEP

The major benefit to LEEP is that this outpatient procedure is minimally painful and minimally invasive yet allows removal of abnormal tissue that can be thoroughly evaluated by the pathologist. There are few risks, and generally, no in-patient time is required for the procedure.

Post LEEP Instructions

Follow-up after LEEP is very important. You should expect some bleeding after the procedure, as well as some mild cramping and a black-brown discharge.

General Instructions

- Do not lift anything over 15 pounds

- Do not have intercourse for four weeks after the procedure

- Do not put anything (including tampons, a douche, fingers, vibrators, etc.) in your vagina for four weeks after the procedure

- You may take ibuprofen (generic or Motrin or Advil) as needed for mild cramping

You should call the clinic immediately should any of the following occur:

- Bleeding heavier than a regular menstrual period, with excessive bleeding or excessive clots

- Any severe abdominal cramping

- Any temperature over 101 degrees Fahrenheit

- Discharge with an odor is not unusual, however if you have any pus from the vagina, or are concerned you should contact your health care provider

If the symptoms occur after clinic hours or on the weekend, please call or go to your local emergency department if you feel you have an emergency.

Section 28.5

Questions and Answers about Tumor Markers

"Tumor Markers: Questions and Answers,"
National Cancer Institute (www.cancer.gov), February 3, 2006.

What are tumor markers?

Tumor markers are substances produced by tumor cells or by other cells of the body in response to cancer or certain benign (noncancerous) conditions. These substances can be found in the blood, in the urine, in the tumor tissue, or in other tissues. Different tumor markers are found in different types of cancer, and levels of the same tumor marker can be altered in more than one type of cancer. In addition, tumor marker levels are not altered in all people with cancer, especially if the cancer is early stage. Some tumor marker levels can also be altered in patients with noncancerous conditions.

To date, researchers have identified more than a dozen substances that seem to be expressed abnormally when some types of cancer are present. Some of these substances are also found in other conditions and diseases. Scientists have not found markers for every type of cancer.

What are risk markers?

Some people have a greater chance of developing certain types of cancer because of a change, known as a mutation or alteration, in specific genes. The presence of such a change is sometimes called a risk marker. Tests for risk markers can help the doctor to estimate a person's chance of developing a certain cancer. Risk markers can indicate that cancer is more likely to occur, whereas tumor markers can indicate the presence of cancer.

How are tumor markers used in cancer care?

Tumor markers are used in the detection, diagnosis, and management of some types of cancer. Although an abnormal tumor marker level may suggest cancer, this alone is usually not enough to diagnose

cancer. Therefore, measurements of tumor markers are usually combined with other tests, such as a biopsy, to diagnose cancer.

Tumor marker levels may be measured before treatment to help doctors plan appropriate therapy. In some types of cancer, tumor marker levels reflect the stage (extent) of the disease.

Tumor marker levels also may be used to check how a patient is responding to treatment. A decrease or return to a normal level may indicate that the cancer is responding to therapy, whereas an increase may indicate that the cancer is not responding. After treatment has ended, tumor marker levels may be used to check for recurrence (cancer that has returned).

How and when are tumor markers measured?

The doctor takes a blood, urine, or tissue sample and sends it to the laboratory, where various methods are used to measure the level of the tumor marker.

If the tumor marker is being used to determine whether a treatment is working or if there is recurrence, the tumor marker levels are often measured over a period of time to see if the levels are increasing or decreasing. Usually these "serial measurements" are more meaningful than a single measurement. Tumor marker levels may be checked at the time of diagnosis; before, during, and after therapy; and then periodically to monitor for recurrence.

Does the NCI have guidelines for the use of tumor markers?

No, the National Cancer Institute (NCI) does not have such guidelines. However, some organizations do have these guidelines for some types of cancer.

The American Society of Clinical Oncology (ASCO), a nonprofit organization that represents more than 25,000 cancer professionals worldwide, has published clinical practice guidelines on a variety of topics, including tumor markers for breast and colorectal cancer. These guidelines, called "Patient Guides," are available on the ASCO website at http://www.cancer.net/patient/ASCO%2BResources/Patient%2BGuides on the internet.

The National Comprehensive Cancer Network® (NCCN), which is also a nonprofit organization, is an alliance of cancer centers. The NCCN provides Patient Guidelines, which include tumor marker information for several types of cancer. Most of the guidelines are available in English and Spanish versions. The "Patient Guidelines" are on the

NCCN's website at http://www.nccn.org/patients/patient_gls.asp on the internet.

The National Academy of Clinical Biochemistry (NACB) is a professional organization dedicated to advancing the science and practice of clinical laboratory medicine through research, education, and professional development. The Academy publishes "Practice Guidelines and Recommendations for Use of Tumor Markers in the Clinic," which focuses on the appropriate use of tumor markers for specific cancers. More information can be found at http://direct.aacc.org/ProductCatalog/Product.aspx?ID=2131 on the internet.

Can tumor markers be used as a screening test for cancer?

Screening tests are a way of detecting cancer early, before there are any symptoms. For a screening test to be helpful, it should have high sensitivity and specificity. Sensitivity refers to the test's ability to identify people who have the disease. Specificity refers to the test's ability to identify people who do not have the disease. Most tumor markers are not sensitive or specific enough to be used for cancer screening.

Even commonly used tests may not be completely sensitive or specific. For example, prostate-specific antigen (PSA) levels are often used to screen men for prostate cancer, but this is controversial. It is not yet known if early detection using PSA screening actually saves lives. Elevated PSA levels can be caused by prostate cancer or benign conditions, and most men with elevated PSA levels turn out not to have prostate cancer. Moreover, it is not clear if the benefits of PSA screening outweigh the risks of follow-up diagnostic tests and cancer treatments.

Another tumor marker, CA 125, is sometimes used to screen women who have an increased risk for ovarian cancer. Scientists are studying whether measurement of CA 125, along with other tests and exams, is useful to find ovarian cancer before symptoms develop. So far, CA 125 measurement is not sensitive or specific enough to be used to screen all women for ovarian cancer. Mostly, CA 125 is used to monitor response to treatment and check for recurrence in women with ovarian cancer.

What research is being done in this field?

Scientists continue to study tumor markers and their possible role in the early detection and diagnosis of cancer. The NCI is currently conducting the Prostate, Lung, Colorectal, and Ovarian Cancer screening trial, or PLCO trial, to determine if certain screening tests reduce

the number of deaths from these cancers. Along with other screening tools, PLCO researchers are studying the use of PSA to screen for prostate cancer and CA 125 to screen for ovarian cancer. Final results from this study are expected in several years.

Cancer researchers are turning to proteomics (the study of protein shape, function, and patterns of expression) in hopes of developing better cancer screening and treatment options. Proteomics technology is being used to search for proteins that may serve as markers of disease in its early stages or to predict the effectiveness of treatment or the chance of the disease returning after treatment has ended.

Scientists are also evaluating patterns of gene expression (the step required to translate what is in the genes to proteins) for their ability to predict a patient's prognosis (likely outcome or course of disease) or response to therapy. NCI's Early Detection Research Network is developing a number of genomic- and proteomic-based biomarkers, some of which are being validated. More information about this program can be found at http://edrn.nci.nih.gov/ on the internet.

Chapter 29

What Do Your Cancer Test Results Mean?

Chapter Contents

Section 29.1

Understanding a Pathology Report

All cancers are diagnosed by providing a sample of a patient's tumor to a specialized medical doctor called a pathologist. The pathologist microscopically examines the sample, or biopsy, and provides a written report to the oncologist or treating doctor. The pathologist provides a disease diagnosis, and this information forms the basis of cancer treatment.

Despite the complex medical language used in the pathology reports, the reports can be understood with help from the oncologist. A person is entitled by law to a copy of his or her pathology report, and this copy can be used when seeking a second opinion to develop treatment options. Ultimately, treatment of a patient's cancer depends on what he or she and the oncologist feel is the best interpretation of the pathology report.

The Pathologist

A pathologist is a doctor who microscopically examines tissue biopsies from the patient's body. Scientific analysis of the sample provides valuable information that forms the basis for the patient's treatment. To be a pathologist, a medical graduate completes a five-year residency training program before being eligible to take an examination given by the American Board of Pathology. Those who successfully complete the examination are then board certified.

What Is a Pathology Report?

The pathology report begins with an evaluation of the biopsy and may include additional tests to aid diagnosis. The information from the tests arrives as it becomes available, meaning that the full report may not be available for several weeks.

The report itself will be highly technical because it is mostly used as a communication between pathologists and oncologists. Help in

understanding the report for specific cancers can be found on patient advocacy websites, such as breastcancer.org. Most importantly, a patient should feel free to ask his or her oncologist for assistance in understanding the report. The oncologist knows his or her patients' medical background, their overall health, and other factors that personalize the pathologist's diagnosis and aid in developing appropriate treatments. Getting a second opinion can help identify additional treatment options, although this will rarely change the primary diagnosis. Agreement between pathologists on whether the tumor is benign (noncancerous) or malignant (cancerous) is high for most tumors.

Parts of the Pathology Report

The pathology report of the biopsy is often long and complex. Most pathology reports follow a particular form and use similar subheadings.

Patient, doctor, and specimen identification: This section provides information to identify the tissue specimen and includes the patient's name and other personal information, the name of the oncologist to whom the report will be issued, and details about the specimen, including the type of tissue obtained and the type of biopsy or surgery performed. The name of the pathologist who performed the examination will also be included, so that he or she can be contacted if there are questions.

Gross (obvious) description: This section of the pathology report describes the specimen as seen with the naked eye. For a small biopsy, the general color, weight, size, and consistency is described. For larger biopsies or tissue samples, such as a mastectomy for breast cancer, the description includes the size of the cancer, how close the cancer is to the margin (the edge of the specimen), and how many lymph nodes were present in the underarm area.

Microscopic description: This section details the appearance of the cancer cells when viewed under a microscope, discusses how the cells are physically arranged together, and describes the extent to which the cancer invades nearby tissues. For many tumors, special tests and stains are performed to further characterize the tumor. This is especially important in cases of lymphoma and leukemia where treatment may depend on the results of these tests. Often technical, this section provides the basis for the diagnosis section.

Diagnosis: This section provides the "bottom line" and may be found either at the beginning or the end of the report. If cancer is diagnosed, this section will identify the tumor type (carcinoma or sarcoma) and usually the organ from which the tumor arose. An important part of the report is whether cancer cells are present at the edges of the biopsy (stated as "positive" or "involved" margins). Such results may indicate the need for additional resection, to completely remove the tumor. In addition, specialized test results will be reported in this section. These tests may reveal the presence of hormone receptors and other special markers on the tumor cells or how rapidly the tumor cells are dividing.

This section details three fundamental and often critical characteristics of the tumor:

- **Histologic grade:** This refers to how closely the tumor resembles normal, noncancerous tissue. In some instances, the description may be listed as well differentiated, moderately differentiated, or poorly differentiated. In most instances, the more differentiated, the better the prognosis. For some tumors, the grade is provided in a numeric form and a higher number indicates greater aggressiveness of the tumor. An example of this is prostate cancer, which uses a system called the Gleason score. A low number, such as 4, means there is a more slowly growing tumor as opposed to an 8 or 9, which means the tumor may be growing fast. The grade of a tumor can be an important characteristic for some tumors, such as ovarian and sarcoma, and not as important in others, such as lung.

- **Tumor size, invasiveness, and spread:** The tumor size is measured, since size influences prognosis (chance of recovery). The pathologist also provides information about the invasion of the tumor into nearby tissues. Tumors may be classified as noninvasive (in-situ) or invasive. Invasive tumors have the capacity to metastasize (spread to other organs). Although noninvasive tumors do not metastasize, they can develop into or raise a patient's risk of more serious, invasive cancer in the future. For some tumors, such as colon and stomach cancers, an important question will be how far the tumor has invaded into the wall of the organ where it started. The pathology report will also document if there is spread into other nearby organs or into the lymph nodes in the region of the tumor. Positive lymph nodes indicate the spread of cancer; negative lymph nodes mean the pathologist has not detected any cancer cells in a particular sample. If the

tumor has invaded blood vessels or lymph vessels that feed into the lymph nodes, the likelihood of distant spread may be greater.

- **Tumor stage:** This measures the extent of disease by assessing tumor size and presence of spread. The tumor stage designation most often relies on a staging system developed by the America Joint Commission on Cancer (AJCC). Staging integrates laboratory test results showing tumor size, degree of invasion, lymph node involvement, and evidence of distant spread and labels cancer as stage I (minimal tumor spread) through stage IV (most advanced or distant spread) cancer.

Questions to Ask the Doctor

These questions can be used to start a dialogue between the patient and his or her doctor about his or her pathology report. The doctor will be able to address the real concern after each question, which can and should be asked each time: "What does the answer to this question mean for me?"

- What is the type of cancer, and from where did it originate?
- How large is the tumor?
- Is the cancer invasive or noninvasive?
- How fast are the cancer cells growing?
- What is the grade of the cancer?
- Does the cancer have hormone receptors or other markers to help define the outlook?
- Has the whole cancer been removed, or is there evidence of remaining tumor at the edges?
- Are there cancer cells in the lymph or blood vessels?
- What is the stage of the cancer?

Obtain a Second Opinion

Discussing one's medical situation with another doctor, or obtaining a second opinion, may be useful, especially in difficult cases. It is often recommended by the first doctor and may even be required by the health insurance company. If a patient is having a second opinion, obtain the pathology report and other medical records to share with the second doctor, but be aware that doctors work closely with their

own pathologists and may prefer to have their own pathologist's opinion, in addition to the original pathologist's opinion. Also, a patient can personally initiate the request for a second interpretation of the pathology report. Additional tests can be performed on the biopsy if deemed necessary; the tissue specimen is kept for a long time and is available upon request.

Sampling differences. In some cases, the report from an initial biopsy may differ from a later report when the entire tumor has been removed. This occurs because the characteristics of a tumor may vary in different areas so different samples yield different pictures of the tumor. An oncologist's final treatment plan will consider the findings in all of the reports in order to develop a plan that most closely addresses a patient's particular situation.

Section 29.2

Questions and Answers about Cancer Staging

Excerpted from "Staging: Question and Answers,"
National Cancer Institute (www.cancer.gov), 2004.

What is staging?

Staging describes the extent or severity of an individual's cancer based on the extent of the original (primary) tumor and the extent of spread in the body. Staging is important:

- Staging helps the doctor plan a person's treatment.

- The stage can be used to estimate the person's prognosis (likely outcome or course of the disease).

- Knowing the stage is important in identifying clinical trials (research studies) that may be suitable for a particular patient.

Staging helps researchers and health care providers exchange information about patients. It also gives them a common language for

evaluating the results of clinical trials and comparing the results of different trials.

What is the basis for staging?

Staging is based on knowledge of the way cancer develops. Cancer cells divide and grow without control or order to form a mass of tissue, called a growth or tumor. As the tumor grows, it can invade nearby organs and tissues. Cancer cells can also break away from the tumor and enter the bloodstream or lymphatic system. By moving through the bloodstream or lymphatic system, cancer can spread from the primary site to form new tumors in other organs. The spread of cancer is called metastasis.

What are the common elements of staging systems?

Staging systems for cancer have evolved over time. They continue to change as scientists learn more about cancer. Some staging systems cover many types of cancer; others focus on a particular type. The common elements considered in most staging systems are the following:

- Location of the primary tumor

- Tumor size and number of tumors

- Lymph node involvement (spread of cancer into lymph nodes)

- Cell type and tumor grade (how closely the cancer cells resemble normal tissue)

- Presence or absence of metastasis

What is the TNM system?

The TNM system is one of the most commonly used staging systems. This system has been accepted by the International Union Against Cancer (UICC) and the American Joint Committee on Cancer (AJCC). Most medical facilities use the TNM system as their main method for cancer reporting. PDQ®, the National Cancer Institute (NCI)'s comprehensive cancer database, also uses the TNM system.

The TNM system is based on the extent of the tumor (T), the extent of spread to the lymph nodes (N), and the presence of metastasis (M). A number is added to each letter to indicate the size or extent of the tumor and the extent of spread.

377

Primary Tumor (T)

- TX: Primary tumor cannot be evaluated

- T0: No evidence of primary tumor

- Tis: Carcinoma in situ (early cancer that has not spread to neighboring tissue)

- T1, T2, T3, T4: Size and/or extent of the primary tumor

Regional Lymph Nodes (N)

- NX: Regional lymph nodes cannot be evaluated

- N0: No regional lymph node involvement (no cancer found in the lymph nodes)

- N1, N2, N3: Involvement of regional lymph nodes (number and/or extent of spread)

Distant Metastasis (M)

- MX: Distant metastasis cannot be evaluated

- M0: No distant metastasis (cancer has not spread to other parts of the body)

- M1: Distant metastasis (cancer has spread to distant parts of the body)

For example, breast cancer T3 N2 M0 refers to a large tumor that has spread outside the breast to nearby lymph nodes, but not to other parts of the body. Prostate cancer T2 N0 M0 means that the tumor is located only in the prostate and has not spread to the lymph nodes or any other part of the body.

For many cancers, TNM combinations correspond to one of five stages. Criteria for stages differ for different types of cancer. For example, bladder cancer T3 N0 M0 is stage III; however, colon cancer T3 N0 M0 is stage II.

Stage Definition

- Stage 0: Carcinoma in situ (early cancer that is present only in the layer of cells in which it began).

- Stage I, Stage II, and Stage III: Higher numbers indicate more extensive disease, greater tumor size, and/or spread of the cancer

to nearby lymph nodes and/or organs adjacent to the primary tumor.

- Stage IV: The cancer has spread to another organ.

Are all cancers staged with TNM classifications?

Most types of cancer have TNM designations, but some do not. For example, cancers of the brain and spinal cord are classified according to their cell type and grade. Different staging systems are also used for many cancers of the blood or bone marrow, such as lymphoma. The Ann Arbor staging classification is commonly used to stage lymphomas and has been adopted by both the AJCC and the UICC. However, other cancers of the blood or bone marrow, including most types of leukemia, do not have a clear-cut staging system. Another staging system, developed by the International Federation of Gynecology and Obstetrics, is used to stage cancers of the cervix, uterus, ovary, vagina, and vulva. This system uses the TNM format. Additionally, childhood cancers are staged using either the TNM system or the staging criteria of the Children's Oncology Group, a group that conducts pediatric clinical trials.

Many cancer registries, such as the NCI's Surveillance, Epidemiology, and End Results Program (SEER), use summary staging. This system is used for all types of cancer. It groups cancer cases into five main categories:

- In situ is early cancer that is present only in the layer of cells in which it began.

- Localized is cancer that is limited to the organ in which it began, without evidence of spread.

- Regional is cancer that has spread beyond the original (primary) site to nearby lymph nodes or organs and tissues.

- Distant is cancer that has spread from the primary site to distant organs or distant lymph nodes.

- Unknown is used to describe cases for which there is not enough information to indicate a stage.

What types of tests are used to determine stage?

The types of tests used for staging depend on the type of cancer. Tests include the following:

379

- Physical exams are used to gather information about the cancer. The doctor examines the body by looking, feeling, and listening for anything unusual. The physical exam may show the location and size of the tumor(s) and the spread of the cancer to the lymph nodes and/or to other organs.

- Imaging studies produce pictures of areas inside the body. These studies are important tools in determining stage. Procedures such as x-rays, computed tomography (CT) scans, magnetic resonance imaging (MRI) scans, and positron emission tomography (PET) scans can show the location of the cancer, the size of the tumor, and whether the cancer has spread.

- Laboratory tests are studies of blood, urine, other fluids, and tissues taken from the body. For example, tests for liver function and tumor markers (substances sometimes found in increased amounts if cancer is present) can provide information about the cancer.

- Pathology reports may include information about the size of the tumor, the growth of the tumor into other tissues and organs, the type of cancer cells, and the grade of the tumor (how closely the cancer cells resemble normal tissue). A biopsy (the removal of cells or tissues for examination under a microscope) may be performed to provide information for the pathology report. Cytology reports also describe findings from the examination of cells in body fluids.

- Surgical reports tell what is found during surgery. These reports describe the size and appearance of the tumor and often include observations about lymph nodes and nearby organs.

Section 29.3

Questions and Answers about Tumor Grades

Excerpted from "Tumor Grade: Questions and Answers,"
National Cancer Institute, 2004.

What is a tumor?

In order to understand tumor grade, it is helpful to know how tumors form. The body is made up of many types of cells. Normally, cells grow and divide to produce new cells in a controlled and orderly manner. Sometimes, however, new cells continue to be produced when they are not needed. As a result, a mass of extra tissue called a tumor may develop. A tumor can be benign (not cancerous) or malignant (cancerous). Cells in malignant tumors are abnormal and divide without control or order. These cancerous cells can invade and damage nearby tissue, and spread to other parts of the body (metastasize).

What is tumor grade?

Tumor grade is a system used to classify cancer cells in terms of how abnormal they look under a microscope and how quickly the tumor is likely to grow and spread. Many factors are considered when determining tumor grade, including the structure and growth pattern of the cells. The specific factors used to determine tumor grade vary with each type of cancer.

Histologic grade, also called differentiation, refers to how much the tumor cells resemble normal cells of the same tissue type. Nuclear grade refers to the size and shape of the nucleus in tumor cells and the percentage of tumor cells that are dividing.

Tumor grade should not be confused with the stage of a cancer. Cancer stage refers to the extent or severity of the cancer, based on factors such as the location of the primary tumor, tumor size, number of tumors, and lymph node involvement (spread of cancer into lymph nodes).

How is tumor grade determined?

If a tumor is suspected to be malignant, a doctor removes a sample of tissue or the entire tumor in a procedure called a biopsy. A pathologist (a doctor who identifies diseases by studying cells under a microscope) examines the tissue to determine whether the tumor is benign or malignant. The pathologist can also determine the tumor grade and identify other characteristics of the tumor cells.

What do the different tumor grades signify?

Based on the microscopic appearance of cancer cells, pathologists commonly describe tumor grade by four degrees of severity: Grades 1, 2, 3, and 4. The cells of Grade 1 tumors resemble normal cells, and tend to grow and multiply slowly. Grade 1 tumors are generally considered the least aggressive in behavior.

Conversely, the cells of Grade 3 or Grade 4 tumors do not look like normal cells of the same type. Grade 3 and 4 tumors tend to grow rapidly and spread faster than tumors with a lower grade.

The American Joint Commission on Cancer recommends the following guidelines for grading tumors (1):

- GX Grade cannot be assessed (Undetermined grade)

- G1 Well-differentiated (Low grade)

- G2 Moderately differentiated (Intermediate grade)

- G3 Poorly differentiated (High grade)

- G4 Undifferentiated (High grade)

Does the same grading scale apply to all tumors?

Grading systems are different for each type of cancer. For example, pathologists use the Gleason system to describe the degree of differentiation of prostate cancer cells. The Gleason system uses scores ranging from Grade 2 to Grade 10. Lower Gleason scores describe well-differentiated, less aggressive tumors. Higher scores describe poorly differentiated, more aggressive tumors. Other grading systems include the Bloom-Richardson system for breast cancer and the Fuhrman system for kidney cancer.

Does tumor grade affect a patient's treatment options?

Doctors use tumor grade and many other factors, such as cancer stage, to develop an individual treatment plan for the patient and to

predict the patient's prognosis. Generally, a lower grade indicates a better prognosis (the likely outcome or course of a disease; the chance of recovery or recurrence). However, the importance of tumor grade in planning treatment and estimating a patient's prognosis is greater for certain types of cancers, such as soft tissue sarcoma, primary brain tumors, lymphomas, and breast and prostate cancer. Patients should speak with their doctor about tumor grade and how it relates to their diagnosis and treatment.

Chapter 30

Commonly Used Surgical Procedures for Women with Cancer

Chapter Contents

Section 30.1

Hysterectomy

Hysterectomy (his"ter-ek'to-me) is the surgical removal of the uterus, or womb. This text will explain:

- Why you may need to have a hysterectomy

- How hysterectomy is performed

- What to expect before and after the operation

Remember, no two women undergoing a hysterectomy are alike. The reasons for and the outcome of any surgical procedure depend on your age, the severity of your problem, and your general health. This information is not intended to take the place of your surgeon's professional opinion. Rather, it is intended to help you understand the basic elements of this surgical procedure. Read this information carefully. If you have questions after reading this material, discuss them openly and honestly with your surgeon.

Why are hysterectomies performed?

Hysterectomy may be performed to treat a variety of gynecological (female reproductive system) problems. It is an elective procedure 90 percent of the time.

Today most hysterectomies are done to treat benign (non-cancerous) fibroid tumors of the uterus. While not life-threatening, these growths cause pelvic pain, excessive bleeding, or pain during sexual intercourse. Fibroid tumors are common and usually do not require surgery. Other forms of treatment which preserve the uterus and childbearing capacity are also available. You should discuss these options with your surgeon.

Endometriosis is a condition in which the tissue lining the uterus becomes displaced and grows in other parts of the abdomen, where

it can cause pain. Endometriosis is the second most common reason for a woman to have a hysterectomy. However, the practice of treating endometriosis by performing hysterectomy has been declining in the last decade because other treatments have evolved. You should discuss these other options with your surgeon first to see if another treatment for endometriosis may be effective for you.

Prolapse of the uterus is another reason why some women decide to undergo a hysterectomy. In this condition, the uterus descends or sags into the vagina due to stretching of the ligaments and fibrous tissue that usually hold it in place.

Women with cancer of the uterus or cancer of the cervix require special types of treatment which may include a simple or radical hysterectomy. These women should seek the counsel of a gynecologic oncologist.

Are all hysterectomies the same?

You may hear different names used to refer to this type of operation. That is because there are different types of hysterectomies. A total hysterectomy or panhysterectomy applies only to the removal of the uterus and cervix. When the ovaries and fallopian tubes on both sides of the uterus are also removed, the procedure is called a hysterectomy and bilateral salpingo-oophorectomy ("salpingo" is from the Greek word for "tube," while "oophor" is from the Greek word for "bearing eggs," that is, the ovaries). A radical hysterectomy is a much more extensive procedure and is only performed in special situations such as cancer of the uterus or cervix. It includes removal of the uterus, cervix, and surrounding tissue, the upper vagina, and usually the pelvic lymph nodes. A surgeon with special training in gynecologic oncology performs this type of procedure.

Is hysterectomy mainly for older women?

You may be surprised to know that 42, a relatively young age, is the average age of women undergoing hysterectomy. More than three-fourths of all women who have a hysterectomy are between 20 and 49 years of age.

Is there any reason to avoid or delay hysterectomy?

It is not sensible to have a hysterectomy in order to prevent cancer of the cervix or uterus.

In this case, the risks of having a major operation outweigh any supposed cancer-protection benefits. Furthermore, hysterectomy is

not considered to be the first choice for sterilization in most healthy women. Another procedure, tubal ligation, is a cheaper, easier, and safer method for most women.

Hysterectomy may not be advisable if your problem has not been adequately diagnosed.

For instance, if you have pelvic pain that is not specifically caused by the uterus, a hysterectomy may not relieve your pain. The pain may be due to problems in your digestive, urinary, or skeletal systems. In these cases, your doctor will want to do the proper tests and x-rays to locate the exact source of your pain. In addition to the tests and x-rays indicated, a diagnostic laparoscopy may be helpful in selecting the appropriate treatment.

Similarly, most women with abnormal bleeding, especially menopausal or post-menopausal women, should have an endometrial biopsy (EMB) or a dilatation and curettage (D&C) procedure to rule out uterine cancer before undergoing a hysterectomy. Hysteroscopy (a surgical procedure in which a gynecologist uses a small lighted telescopic instrument to view the inside of the uterus) should not be performed until uterine cancer has been ruled out by D&C or EMB. If cancer is present within the uterus, the hysteroscope has the potential to push it out through the fallopian tubes into the abdominal cavity.

Finally, women who are obese, who have diabetes, high blood pressure, or some other chronic conditions, are at increased risk during any type of operation. For these women, hysterectomy should only be considered if reasonable alternatives have been exhausted.

If you have any questions about hysterectomy, ask your doctor. If it would make you feel more confident about your medical treatment, get a second opinion from another physician who is qualified to diagnose and treat your condition. Unless you have a severe pelvic infection, or uncontrollable bleeding, you do not have to rush into having a hysterectomy. Even with a diagnosis of cancer, a short delay to seek another qualified opinion is usually safe and worthwhile.

How do I decide if I should have a hysterectomy?

You will no longer be able to get pregnant after a hysterectomy. Thus, before you choose elective hysterectomy, you must consider both the severity of your problem and your desire to have children in the future. Although this operation may improve your quality of life by relieving chronic symptoms such as pain or bleeding, some women are willing to tolerate these conditions.

Ask Yourself

- Do I want to become pregnant in the future?

- How do I feel about not having a uterus?

- What is my husband's (or partner's) attitude toward this operation?

Ask Your Surgeon

- What will happen if I don't have a hysterectomy?

- What are the risks of a hysterectomy in my particular case?

- Is my condition likely to improve on its own, stay the same, or get worse?

- Is a hysterectomy medically necessary or recommended to relieve my particular symptoms?

Before your operation, you will be asked to sign a document giving your "informed consent" to the operation. This form lets you know any risks or possible complications that can be caused by the surgical procedure. Some states have specific laws that pertain to hysterectomies. These laws require surgeons to explain the alternatives and the risks of the procedure and are intended to make sure you understand the potential after-effects of the operation.

How is hysterectomy performed?

The surgeon can remove the uterus through a surgical incision made either inside the vagina or in the abdomen. In both the vaginal and abdominal approaches, the surgeon detaches the uterus from the fallopian tubes and ovaries as well as from the upper vagina.

Abdominal Hysterectomy

When a hysterectomy is performed through an incision in the abdomen, it allows the surgeon to see the pelvic organs easily and gives him or her more operating space than is permitted in a vaginal hysterectomy. Thus, for large pelvic tumors or suspected cancer, your surgeon may decide to do the procedure abdominally. Patients who have an abdominal hysterectomy require a longer hospital stay than those who have a vaginal hysterectomy. In addition, they may experience greater discomfort immediately following the operation, and will have a visible scar.

However, the surgeon often can make a less-noticeable horizontal incision, called a bikini-cut, that extends along the top of the pubic hairline.

Vaginal Hysterectomy

The vaginal approach to hysterectomy is ideal when the uterus is not enlarged or when the uterus has dropped as a result of the weakening of surrounding muscles. This approach is technically more difficult than the abdominal procedure because it offers the surgeon less operating space and less opportunity to view the pelvic organs. However, it may be preferred if a patient has a prolapsed uterus, if the patient is obese, or in some cases has early cervical or uterine cancer. A vaginal hysterectomy leaves no external scar.

A variation on vaginal hysterectomy is LAVH (laparoscopic-assisted vaginal hysterectomy). A laparoscope is a device the surgeon can use to examine the inside of the pelvis. LAVH is an alternative for women who have ovarian disease but previously had only one choice: an abdominal hysterectomy that leaves a long incision. With LAVH, much of the procedure is done through tiny incisions using a laparoscope. The rest of the procedure then can be finished vaginally.

Stages of Recovery

After the operation, you will likely remain in the recovery room for one to three hours. You may be given pain medication, and possibly antibiotics to prevent infection.

You will probably be able to walk around your room the day after your operation, depending on the type of procedure you underwent. Most patients go home the third day following an abdominal hysterectomy and by the first or second day after a vaginal hysterectomy or LAVH.

Complete recovery from abdominal hysterectomy usually takes six to eight weeks because the incision is typically five inches long. During your recovery, you can expect a gradual increase in activities. Avoid all lifting during the first two weeks of your recovery period and get plenty of rest. In the weeks following the surgical procedure, you can begin to do light chores, some driving, and even return to work, provided your occupation does not involve too much physical activity.

Around the sixth week following the operation, you can take tub baths and resume sexual activity. Women who have had vaginal hysterectomies generally recover more quickly.

Risks or Complications?

Hysterectomy is regarded as one of the safest operations. Nevertheless, no operation is without risk. Severe complications and even death occasionally occur with this operation. The uterus is located between the ureters (small tubes which transport urine from the kidneys to the bladder) on each side, the urinary bladder in front, and the rectum behind. All of these structures are subject to injury, especially if the operation is difficult, as can occur with large fibroids, endometriosis, or cancer. Bleeding and infection can also occur, but most infections are now avoided by using antibiotics. Blood clots in the legs (DVT-deep vein thromboses) sometimes occur postoperatively and can break off and travel to the lungs causing a sometimes fatal pulmonary embolism (blood clot). These clots largely can be avoided in high-risk patients by using special stockings during the operation or by using blood thinners.

Long-Term Effects

After having a hysterectomy, you will no longer be able to get pregnant and will no longer have menstrual periods. If you were premenopausal (still menstruating) before the operation and have your fallopian tubes and ovaries removed, you will experience all of the symptoms of menopause as your body gets used to different hormone levels. These symptoms may include hot flashes and perhaps irritability and depression. If the symptoms are severe, your doctor may prescribe hormone replacement medication. Hysterectomy usually has no physical effect on your ability to experience sexual pleasure or orgasm.

Following hysterectomy, the ovaries will continue to function; however, the actual occurrence of menopause will be difficult to determine since the uterus has been removed and the patient will no longer have periods. As the age of menopause, approximately age 50, is approached, symptoms such as hot flashes may warrant testing to see if hormone replacement therapy is indicated.

If you experience vaginal dryness, it can be remedied by using prescription hormone creams or pills or water-soluble lubricants that you can purchase at the pharmacy.

A sense of loss following the removal of any organ is normal and takes time for adjustment. While depression following hysterectomy does not happen to everyone, it is more common if the operation was done because of cancer or severe illness, rather than as an elective operation. Additionally, if you are under age 40 or the operation interfered with your plans to have children, depression is more likely to

occur. This depression can be temporary, depending on your general outlook on life, and the availability of a good support group of family and friends.

Most women experience an improvement of mood and increased sense of well-being following hysterectomy. For many, relief from fear of pregnancy results in heightened sexual enjoyment following the procedure.

—*Reviewed by Conley G. Lacey, MD, FACS Clinical Professor of Gynecology University of Southern California Los Angeles, CA*

Surgery by Surgeons

A fully trained surgeon is a physician who, after medical school, has gone through years of training in an accredited residency program to learn the specialized skills of a surgeon. One good sign of a surgeon's competence is certification by a national surgical board approved by the American Board of Medical Specialities. All such board-certified surgeons have satisfactorily completed an approved residency training program and have passed a rigorous specialty examination.

The letters F.A.C.S. (Fellow of the American College of Surgeons) after a surgeon's name are a further indication of a physician's qualifications. Surgeons who become Fellows of the College have passed a comprehensive evaluation of their education, training, and professional qualifications, and their credentials have been found to be consistent with the standards established and demanded by the College.

The text in this section was prepared as a public service by the American College of Surgeons, 633 N. Saint Clair St., Chicago, IL 60611-3211. Visit the ACS website at www.facs.org.

Section 30.2

Mastectomy

Mastectomy

Mastectomy is the surgical removal of a breast. Surgery is presently the most common treatment for breast cancer. Following mastectomy, immediate or delayed breast reconstruction is possible in many instances.

Types of Mastectomy

There are several different types of surgical procedures used to treat breast cancer. Depending on the location or surgeon who performs the procedure, different terms may be used.

Surgical procedures for breast cancer include:

- **Simple or total mastectomy:** Removal of the breast, with its skin and nipple, but no lymph nodes. In some cases, a separate sentinel node biopsy is performed to remove only the first one to three axillary (armpit) lymph nodes.

- **Modified radical mastectomy:** Removal of the entire breast, nipple/areolar region, and often the axillary lymph nodes. This is the most common form of mastectomy performed today.*

- **Radical mastectomy:** Removal of the entire breast, nipple/areolar region, the pectoral (chest) major and minor muscles, and lymph nodes. This procedure is rarely performed today.*

- **Quadrantectomy:** Removal of a quarter of the breast, including the skin and breast fascia (connective tissues). The surgeon may also perform a separate procedure to remove some or all of the axillary (armpit) lymph nodes, either an axillary node dissection or a sentinel node biopsy.

- **Partial or segmental mastectomy:** Removal of a portion of the breast tissue and a margin of normal breast tissue. This procedure

usually involves removing less tissue than a quadrantectomy but more than a lumpectomy or wide excision.

- **Lumpectomy or wide excision:** Removal of the breast cancer tumor and a surrounding margin of normal breast tissue. [Lumpectomies are discussed in greater detail later in this section.]

- **Excisional biopsy:** Also the removal of the breast tumor and a surrounding margin of normal breast tissue. Sometimes further surgery is not needed if an excisional biopsy successfully removes the entire breast cancer tumor. This is most likely to occur if the breast tumor is very small. An excisional biopsy may be performed with "needle" or "wire" localization.

*In the past, radical mastectomy was the frequently performed on women with breast cancer. However, experts have found that modified radical mastectomy is equally effective in most cases, and therefore, it has become the most common type procedure for removing the entire breast.

Axillary Node Dissection

Axillary node dissection, the surgical removal of the axillary (armpit) lymph nodes, is usually performed on patients with invasive cancers. A radical mastectomy, modified radical mastectomy, or lumpectomy operation often includes axillary node dissection (this involves a separate incision for lumpectomy patients). After surgery, the axillary lymph nodes are examined under a microscope to determine whether the cancer has spread past the breast and to evaluate treatment options.

The most common side effect of axillary node dissection is lymphedema: chronic swelling of the arm. Approximately 10% to 20% of patients typically experience lymphedema when axillary node dissection is combined with radiation therapy. Patients are encouraged to report any tightness or swelling of the arm to their physicians as soon as symptoms occur to prevent possible long-term suffering. Other side effects of axillary node dissection include temporary to permanent limitations of arm and shoulder movement and numbness in the upper-arm skin.

Side effects of axillary node dissection:

- Lymphedema (swelling of the arm)

- Limitations of arm/shoulder movement

- Numbness of upper-arm skin

Sentinel Lymph Node Biopsy

Sentinel lymph node biopsy is a procedure that involves removing only one to three sentinel lymph nodes (the first nodes in the lymphatic chain). To perform sentinel node biopsy, a radioactive tracer and/or blue dye is injected into a region of a tumor. The dye is then carried to the sentinel node (the lymph node most likely to be cancerous if the disease has spread from its original origin). If the surgeon determines that the sentinel node contains cancer, more lymph nodes are removed and examined. Surgeons detect the sentinel lymph node by either spotting the blue dye or by measuring a node's radioactivity with a Geiger counter. If the removed sentinel node is cancer-free, additional lymph node surgery may be avoided. Research has shown that sentinel lymph node biopsy may safely eliminate the need to remove many lymph nodes and reduce the chances of lymphedema (chronic arm swelling). However, the procedure may not be appropriate for all patients.

Choosing Mastectomy as Breast Cancer Treatment

Breast cancer is often first detected by an abnormality on a mammogram (an x-ray examination of soft breast tissues used to identify lumps, cysts, tumors, and other abnormalities). Patients are urged to receive a mammogram if they notice any suspicious lumps during breast self-examination (BSE). If an abnormality is seen on the mammogram then additional breast imaging is usually ordered. Breast cancer is confirmed by biopsy.

After biopsy, several factors are evaluated when determining how to treat breast cancer including the following:

- Tumor size
- Tumor type
- Cancer stage
- Histologic grade
- Lymph node status
- Estrogen and progesterone receptors
- Her-2-neu receptors

While some patients will be clear candidates for mastectomy, other women are faced with the choice between mastectomy or breast conserving therapy (lumpectomy, usually followed by radiation therapy). Though

both mastectomy and lumpectomy have equal survival rates, there are advantages and disadvantages to both procedures. Lumpectomy may preserve the physical appearance of the breast but usually requires six to seven weeks of radiation therapy. Mastectomy may reduce local recurrence of breast cancer, but additional decisions about breast reconstruction are introduced. Patients are encouraged to educate themselves on all possible options and to thoroughly discuss treatment and reconstruction with their physicians before deciding on a course of treatment.

Mastectomy and Breast Reconstruction

It is important for women to realize that breast reconstruction is possible for the majority of breast cancer patients after mastectomy. Often modified radical mastectomy patients may undergo breast reconstructive surgery during the same operation to remove the breast.

Advantages to immediate breast reconstruction:

- Patients do not wake up to the "shock" of losing a breast.

- Patients may avoid additional reconstructive surgery.

Disadvantages to immediate breast reconstruction:

- Patients may find it emotionally difficult to weigh all of their reconstructive options while also dealing with their recent breast cancer diagnosis and treatment alternatives.

- Occasionally there may be complications with reconstructive healing that interfere with chemotherapy or radiation treatment, if needed.

Reconstructive surgery usually involves insertion of breast implant or a muscle flap.

Women who do not wish to have further surgery may be fitted with an external prosthesis (an artificial breast) after healing from mastectomy. Most prostheses are made to resemble the body's own weight and touch. According to the American Cancer Society, it is essential for women to have their prostheses properly weighed to balance the body and anchor their bra. Women should take their time in determining which prosthesis is right for them as prices vary considerably. Several manufacturers also make special mastectomy bras that have breast pockets sewn into them.

Before Surgery

Most mastectomy patients will meet with their surgeon a few days prior to surgery to ask any questions they may have about the procedure and its risks. Patients must also sign a consent form which they should review carefully. It may also be necessary for patients to donate blood for a possible blood transfusion during surgery.

Patients are encouraged to discuss any medications they may be taking that could interfere with surgery. Patients will typically be instructed not to have any food or drink at least eight hours before surgery.

The Mastectomy Procedure

General anesthesia is administered during mastectomy, and an EKG monitor (electrocardiogram) is connected to the patient to monitor heart rates. Blood pressure and vital signs are also monitored throughout the surgery.

To perform a simple mastectomy, a surgeon makes an incision along the perimeter of the breast (closest to the tumor area), leaving most of the skin intact. Typically, the nipple is not removed during simple mastectomy, although milk ducts leading to the nipple are cut. The underlying tissue is gently cut free and removed. Often a plastic or rubber drainage tube is inserted in the affected area. The skin is carefully closed with stitches or clips, which are usually removed within a week, and a dressing (bandage) normally covers the site. Mastectomy with axillary (armpit) lymph node dissection usually lasts between two to three hours. Immediate breast reconstruction will increase the duration of surgery.

The drainage tube placed in the breast or under the arm removes blood and lymph node fluid accumulated during the healing process. Drainage tubes are usually removed within two weeks, when the drainage is reduced to less than 30 ccs (one fluid ounce) per day.

Possible effects of mastectomy include the following:

- Wound infection

- Hematoma (blood trapped in the wound)

- Seroma (clear fluid trapped in the wound)

- Lymphedema: Temporary to permanent limitations of arm/shoulder movement (if lymph nodes are removed during the operation)

- Numbness in the upper-arm skin

- Phantom breast pain

After Surgery

After mastectomy, patients generally spend two to three days in the hospital, although some may stay up to eight days. Most modified radical mastectomy patients spend an average of three days at the hospital, and those who have breast reconstruction in addition to mastectomy may spend three to six days, depending on the body's rate of healing.

Major soreness from mastectomy usually lasts two to three days, although many mastectomy patients do not experience soreness after surgery. A linear scar at the mastectomy site is probable. Many patients do experience a pulling sensation near or under their arm after mastectomy.

Patients should receive instructions before leaving the hospital concerning these topics:

- Care of the wound and dressing

- Type of pain/sensations to expect

- Use of pain medications

- How to monitor the drainage tube

- How to recognize signs of infection

- Any restricted activities

- Emotional feelings to expect

- Proper diet

- When to begin arm exercises to reduce stiffness

- When to wear a bra

- When to begin wearing a prosthesis (if chosen)

Source of information: American Cancer Society Online: Surgery: What to Expect

Physicians will normally schedule follow up exams seven to 14 days after mastectomy. At the follow up exam, the results of the pathology report are usually shared with patients. Radiation treatment may or may not be necessary after mastectomy. Patients with problems or concerns after surgery should contact their surgeon right away.

Phantom Breast Pain

Studies have shown that many women experience phantom breast sensations after mastectomy. In a recent study conducted at Johns Hopkins Hospital, more than one third of 279 mastectomy patients experienced phantom breast pain after mastectomy. The incidence of phantom breast pain was similar, regardless of whether or not the women had breast reconstruction after breast cancer surgery. Symptoms of phantom breast pain may include the following:

- Unpleasant itching
- Pins and needles
- Pressure
- Throbbing

Physicians believe that phantom breast pain occurs after mastectomy for the same reasons as phantom pains occur after limb amputations. According to Srinivasa Raja, MD of Johns Hopkins, during mastectomy, small nerves are cut between the breast tissue and skin area. This causes the neural connections in the brain to undergo neural plasticity (reorganization). This process, as well as the spontaneous firing of electrical signals from the ends of cut or injured nerves, causes phantom sensations, said Dr. Raja. Women who experience breast pain prior to mastectomy are most likely to have sensations of pain in the breast area after surgery.

Physicians recommend that patients who experience phantom sensations in the breast area after surgery report their symptoms to their physicians immediately so that the pain can be properly managed. In some cases, exercise or breast massage may help alleviate phantom breast pain, although patients should first discuss these options with their physicians. In more severe cases, medications may be prescribed to reduce phantom breast pain. Phantom breast pain does not indicate that cancer cells are still present in the breast area or that cancer may return.

Exercising after Mastectomy and Lymph Node Removal

It is important that a patient ask her physician when it is safe to begin exercising and using the surgery-side arm again after a mastectomy. While there are no contraindications to performing any number of exercises after full recovery from mastectomy, there are certain precautions that should be taken by any person who has undergone

a mastectomy, especially those who have had accompanying lymph node dissection.

Any minor injury to the skin on the side of the mastectomy may become infected more easily than an injury on the other arm. This is because the lymphatics have been disrupted and lymph nodes have been removed, leaving the arm more vulnerable to invading organisms such as bacteria. The lymphatics normally serve to drain fluids from the limb and the lymph nodes act, in some sense, as a filter, removing harmful substances from the lymph fluid.

Up to 20% of women who have undergone mastectomy and axillary lymph node dissection experience some edema (swelling) in the arm and report a higher incidence of irritation to minor skin trauma for this reason.

In addition, there may be a higher chance of axillary vein thrombosis (a clot in the deep vein in the armpit) in women who have undergone surgery in that area; especially if a more complete axillary dissection with the removal of 30 or more lymph nodes is performed. This is because the lymph nodes are normally located near blood vessels, and (unavoidable) scarring at or near the axillary vein may result from surgery. This scarring may tether, kink, or narrow the blood vessel and make it more susceptible to further injury.

While an increased incidence of deep vein thrombosis has not been reported in the medical literature after axillary surgery, it has been, in rare cases, associated with strenuous upper body exercise, since overdeveloped musculature may affect nearby nerves, veins, and arteries (thoracic outlet syndrome). Therefore, many physicians recommend tempering upper extremity exercise after surgery with periods of rest, and keeping the arm elevated above the level of the heart for a few hours, to avoid undue swelling. Mastectomy patients should be careful not to exercise too intensely in order to avoid preventable injury.

On a positive note, regular use of the muscles after mastectomy will keep joints limber, stretch and soften scar tissue, help recruit (open up) new lymphatics, and promote blood flow and actually help reduce clot formation. These benefits generally outweigh the risks of a careful exercise program after mastectomy.

Recurrence of Breast Cancer

Occasionally breast cancer can return (recur) after mastectomy or other treatment. There are three types of breast cancer recurrence: local, regional, and distant. With local recurrence, cancerous tumor cells remain in the original site, and over time, they grow back. A regional

recurrence of breast cancer is more serious than local recurrence because it usually indicates that the cancer has spread past the breast and the axillary (underarm) lymph nodes. A distant breast cancer recurrence, also known as a metastasis (spread), is the most dangerous type of recurrence. With this type of recurrence, breast cancer spreads to distant regions of the body, such as the bone, lung, liver, or brain.

Treatment will depend on the type and severity of the breast cancer recurrence. Breast cancer recurrences may be treated with additional surgery, chemotherapy, radiation, or other drug therapies (such as tamoxifen).

Lumpectomy

Lumpectomy, also known as breast-conserving surgery, is the surgical removal of a cancerous lump (or tumor) in the breast, along with a small margin of the surrounding normal breast tissue. Lumpectomy may also be called wide excision biopsy, breast conserving therapy, or quadrantectomy (this latter term is used when up to one fourth of the breast is removed). The procedure is often performed on women with small or localized breast cancers and can be an attractive surgical treatment option for breast cancer because it allows women to maintain most of their breast after surgery. Several studies have shown that women with small breast tumors have an equal chance of surviving breast cancer regardless of whether they have a lumpectomy, followed by a full course of radiation therapy, or mastectomy (complete breast removal, which generally does not require post-operative radiation treatment).

Who Is/Is Not a Candidate for Lumpectomy?

After a patient has been diagnosed with breast cancer, physicians will stage the cancer to determine the extent of the disease and help decide the most appropriate course of treatment. Lumpectomy is often a suitable treatment option for patients with the following breast cancers:

- Ductal carcinoma in situ (DCIS)
- Stage I
- Stage II
- Stage III

Lumpectomy involves removing the cancerous breast lump and a surrounding margin of normal breast tissue. In addition to the lumpectomy,

a separate incision may be required to include a sampling or removal of the axillary (underarm) lymph nodes. This part of the surgery, which may be a sentinel node biopsy, an axillary lymph node sampling, or an axillary lymph node dissection, is performed to determine whether the cancer has begun to spread out of the breast itself (see the section below on lymph node removal for more information).

After the lumpectomy is performed, the pathologist will check to make sure the surgeon removed the entire cancerous tumor by seeing if the tissue margins are "clear" (in other words, if there is no cancer present in the outermost edges of the breast tissue sample). A preliminary check of the tissue margins may be performed while the patient is still in the operating room and may allow the surgeon to obtain "clear margins" during the same operation. However, this is only a preliminary reading, and the final results, available over the course of a few days, may reveal residual cancer cells (known as a "positive" margin). If the margins of the removed breast tissue do contain cancer cells, then additional surgery (re-excision) is usually necessary to attempt to remove the remaining cancer. If it is not possible to clear the margins on re-excision, then a mastectomy is usually offered as an alternative.

Lumpectomy is often combined with adjuvant (additional) therapy, either local or systemic. Most commonly, lumpectomy is followed by at least six weeks of radiation therapy to ensure that all cancer cells in the remaining breast have been destroyed. Newer studies are beginning to show that shorter radiation times may be equally effective in preventing local tumor recurrence for many patients after lumpectomy; however, this is still under investigation. Other types of adjuvant therapy that may be given in addition to lumpectomy include agents designed to help control the systemic spread of breast cancer. These agents include chemotherapy, the drug tamoxifen (brand name, Nolvadex), or a combination of hormonal or drug therapies.

Several studies have shown that lumpectomy is a viable treatment option for most women with small, localized breast cancers. In fact, there is no statistically significant difference in overall survival rates between women who undergo lumpectomy (and radiation) and those who undergo mastectomy, although a slightly higher local recurrence rate was reported in some larger studies in women who undergo lumpectomy instead of mastectomy. More recently, a large study conducted by Yale researchers found that women with very early-stage breast cancers who undergo lumpectomy followed by radiation therapy are no more likely to develop a second cancer than women who undergo mastectomy, as long as candidates are selected appropriately and the edges of the surgical sample are free of cancer cells.

There are some women who are not good candidates for lumpectomy. The American Cancer Society suggests that women who have already undergone radiation in the breast/chest area, women with two or more areas of cancer in the same breast (known as multicentric disease), women whose previous lumpectomy did not completely remove the cancer, women with connective tissue diseases such as scleroderma (which make tissue sensitive to radiation), or women who would be pregnant at the time of radiation therapy (possibly harming the fetus) should not consider lumpectomy as advisable treatment. In addition, women with cancers more than five centimeters in diameters (two inches) or women with larger cancers within relatively small breasts may not be suitable candidates for lumpectomy. Table 30.1 summarizes conditions for which lumpectomy may not be the most suitable choice.

Women who have been diagnosed with breast cancer should carefully discuss their treatment options with their surgeon and other members of their cancer treatment team. Lumpectomy is becoming an increasingly suitable option for many women with early stage breast cancers. While some women are clearly not candidates for lumpectomy (and would benefit more from mastectomy), studies have shown that the type of breast cancer surgery a patient receives is sometimes influenced by her surgeon's personal preference, geographical location, age, or insurance coverage. It is very common and usually recommended that patients seek a second opinion before undergoing any type of surgery.

How Is Lumpectomy Performed?

Lumpectomy may be performed using a local anesthetic, sedation, or general anesthesia, depending on the extent of the surgery needed.

Table 30.1. Poor Candidates for Lumpectomy

- Previously underwent radiation therapy in breast/chest
- Previous lumpectomy did not completely remove tumor
- Have two or more cancerous areas within the same breast
- Have connective tissue disease(s)
- Would be pregnant at the time of radiation after surgery
- Tumor larger than five centimeters (two inches)
- Cancer large relative to small size of breast

Source of information: American Cancer Society

The surgeon makes a small incision over or near the breast tumor and excises (cuts free) the lump or abnormality along with a margin of at least one centimeter (approximately one half inch) of normal surrounding breast tissue (see the section above for information on margins). Unlike after mastectomy, a drainage tube is usually not necessary after lumpectomy.

A seroma (clear fluid trapped in the wound) usually fills the surgical cavity after the operation and helps to naturally remold the breast's shape. Gradually, the seroma is absorbed and the body replaces it with scar tissue. This natural healing process and formation of scar tissue occurs over a period of months, so that the final results of the surgery may not be apparent for some time. Depending on such factors as the location of the mass, its initial size, the type of incision used, etc., the final result will be different for each person. Possible side effects of lumpectomy include temporary swelling of the breast, breast tenderness, and hardness due to scar tissue that forms in the surgical site.

Patients are usually able to go home the same day or one to two days following lumpectomy. Most women are able to resume normal activities within two weeks. Wound infection or bleeding is not common with lumpectomy. The extent of breast soreness correlates with the amount and location of tissue removed during surgery, whether axillary (underarm) lymph node surgery was performed, and an individual's tolerance to pain. Major soreness usually ceases after two to three days and should be checked by a physician if there is any increase in pain over time. Because lumpectomy is usually intended to preserve the cosmetic appearance of the breast, surgeons generally do not recommend lumpectomy when over one fourth of the breast must be removed. In these cases, mastectomy, along with the option of reconstruction, may be preferable.

In rare instances, women may experience recurring seromas after lumpectomy. Seromas are collections of fluid in the cavity (empty space) left behind by the surgery. These collections are easily drained (aspirated) in the surgeon's office. If a seroma recurs, surgeons may

Table 30.2. Rates of Breast-Conserving Surgery by U.S. Region

Northeast	60.5%
North Central	51.1%
West	50.2%
South	48.0%

use several methods including compression or sclerosis (the injection of ethanol, autologous fibrin clot, or fibrin sealant) to fill and harden the space in the breast. At times, these treatments can be uncomfortable, but they are rarely needed.

Radiation Therapy after Lumpectomy

Lumpectomy (and sometimes mastectomy) is typically followed by six to seven weeks of radiation therapy immediately following surgery to help ensure that any remaining cancer cells are destroyed and to help prevent the chance of a cancer recurrence. Treatment with radiation usually begins one month after surgery, allowing the breast tissue adequate time to heal. Treatments are given daily and each treatment generally lasts a few minutes; the entire radiation session after machine set-up typically lasts 15 to 30 minutes. The procedure itself is pain-free. While the radiation is being administered, the technologist will leave the room to monitor the patient on a closed-circuit television. However, patients should be able to communicate with the technologist at any time over an intercom system.

Common side effects of radiation therapy include hair loss to the area being treated, fatigue, skin reactions (such as rash or redness) in the treated area, loss of appetite, and nausea. Most of the side effects associated with radiation therapy are temporary, and many patients do not experience significant discomfort after radiation sessions.

Researchers have been investigating whether a shorter duration, higher dose of radiation may be as effective as the conventional six to seven week regimen. Recent research suggests that limiting radiation therapy to four weeks at a higher dose may be as effective as the traditional regimen and could reduce side effects. IMRT (intensity-modulated radiation therapy) uses a highly sophisticated system of delivering external-beam radiation. According to recent research, this system uses advanced computer optimized planning and radiation delivery techniques that create more optimal dose distributions, greater sparing of the skin and lower doses to organs such as lung and heart—thus reducing potential side effects. However, there may be patients who are uncomfortable with the idea of an accelerated treatment and want to be treated with a more conventional six to seven week course of treatment. "In addition, we need more research to determine which women are ideal candidates for this treatment because of differences in anatomy or other treatments for their breast cancer." Women are encouraged to talk to their cancer treatment team about their radiation therapy options.

Lumpectomy and Lymph Node Removal

When breast cancer cells begin to escape from the primary tumor site in the breast, they first travel to the lymph nodes under the upper arm. Therefore, it is often necessary to remove some or all of the axillary (underarm) lymph nodes during lumpectomy or mastectomy to determine if or to what extent the cancer has spread.

Lymph node removal usually requires a separate incision when it is performed during the same procedure as lumpectomy. There are two procedures for removing lymph nodes in breast cancer patients: axillary node dissection and sentinel node biopsy.

- **Axillary node dissection:** This is the standard way to remove axillary lymph nodes. Typically, between 10 to 30 lymph nodes are removed and examined in a pathology laboratory to determine whether they contain cancer cells.

- **Sentinel lymph node biopsy:** This is a technique that involves the injection of a blue dye, radioactive tracer, or both, to identify the "sentinel" lymph nodes (first nodes) draining the breast. Using this method, only the first one to three lymph nodes in the lymphatic chain are removed. Research has shown that checking the sentinel lymph nodes allows physicians to accurately determine whether the axillary (armpit) lymph nodes contains cancer while causing fewer side effects such as lymphedema (chronic swelling) of the arm. If the sentinel nodes are positive (contain cancer cells), then additional surgery is performed to remove (dissect) the remaining axillary lymph nodes. If the removed axillary lymph nodes are negative (do not contain cancer cells), then no additional lymph nodes are removed, reducing the side effects of axillary dissection. Sentinel lymph node biopsy has become more common in recent years. However, it is not always appropriate.

The most common side effect of lymph node removal is lymphedema (chronic swelling) of the arm. Between 10% and 20% of patients who have lymph nodes removed develop lymphedema, including some patients who only have a sentinel lymph node biopsy. The risk of lymphedema is greater if the patient also undergoes radiation therapy and/or the lymph nodes contained cancer cells upon final examination. To help manage lymphedema and prevent long-term suffering, patients should report symptoms as soon as they occur. In addition, special exercises should be performed shortly after recovering from surgery to help encourage and maintain lymphatic flow of the affected side of surgery.

Early Signs of Lymphedema

- Feeling of tightness in the arm

- Pain, aching or heaviness in the arm

- Swelling and redness of the arm

- Less movement/flexibility in the arm, hand, wrist

- Rings, bracelets or sleeves do not fit

In addition to lymphedema, other common side effects of lymph node removal include limitations of arm/shoulder movement, and numbness of the upper arm skin.

Section 30.3

Oophorectomy

This section begins with "Medical Procedures That Cause Menopause" © 2010 The Cleveland Clinic Foundation, 9500 Euclid Avenue, Cleveland, OH 44195. All rights reserved. Reprinted with permission. Additional information is available from the Cleveland Clinic Health Information Center, 216-444-3771, toll-free 800-223-2273 extension 43771, or at http://my.clevelandclinic.org/health. Additional information under the heading "Ovary Removal Linked to Cognitive Problems, Dementia" is excerpted from "Cancer Research Highlights," *NCI Cancer Bulletin*, National Cancer Institute (www.cancer.gov), September 2007.

Medical Procedures that Cause Menopause

Natural menopause is the permanent ending of menstruation that is not brought on by any type of medical treatment. For women undergoing natural menopause, the process is described in three stages: perimenopause, menopause, and postmenopause.

Perimenopause may begin in a woman's 40s. During this time, she may experience hot flashes and irregular periods due to declining ovarian function. Menopause is defined as the absence of a menstrual period for 12 consecutive months. However, not all women undergo

natural menopause. Some women experience induced menopause as a result of surgery or medical treatments, such as chemotherapy and pelvic radiation therapy.

What is surgical menopause?

Surgical menopause occurs when a premenopausal woman has her ovaries surgically removed in a procedure called a bilateral oophorectomy. This causes an abrupt menopause, with women often experiencing more severe menopausal symptoms than if they were to experience menopause naturally.

Why would someone have a bilateral oophorectomy?

In most cases, bilateral oophorectomy is performed because of cancer, including cervical, endometrial (cancer of the uterus), and ovarian cancer. Prophylactic bilateral oophorectomy may be performed in patients who are at increased risk for breast and ovarian cancer who carry a mutation in the BRCA gene. Occasionally, however, it may be done to treat non-cancerous conditions such as uterine fibroids, endometriosis, or infections.

Which surgical procedures involve bilateral oophorectomy?

Hysterectomy (the surgical removal of the uterus) can sometimes, though not always, include bilateral oophorectomy. Hysterectomy that does not involve removal of the ovaries usually does not result in menopause (although women who undergo a hysterectomy may experience menopause a few years earlier).

Other surgeries that may involve the removal of both ovaries include:

- **Abdominal resection:** This is a surgical procedure done to treat colon and rectal cancer. While this surgery usually involves the removal of the lower colon and rectum, it can also include partial or total removal of the uterus and ovaries, as well as the rear wall of the vagina.

- **Total pelvic exenteration:** This procedure is usually only performed in cases of genitourinary cancers, such as cervical cancer, that recur despite treatment with surgery and radiation. It involves the removal of most pelvic organs, including the following:

  - Uterus
  - Cervix

- Ovaries
- Fallopian tubes
- Vagina
- bladder
- Urethra
- Part of the rectum

What medical treatments can cause menopause?

Medical treatments such as chemotherapy and radiation therapy can cause menopause by damaging the ovaries. However, not all pre-menopausal women undergoing these procedures will experience induced menopause. Additionally, even if the ovaries are damaged, the damage is not always permanent.

Ovary Removal Linked to Cognitive Problems, Dementia

Women who had one or both ovaries removed before menopause for noncancer reasons faced an increased risk of developing cognitive problems or dementia later in life, according to a new study. But women who underwent estrogen replacement therapy until at least age 50 after having their ovaries removed were not at increased risk. The study supports the hypothesis that there may be a "critical age window for the protective effects of estrogen on the brain," the researchers write in the September 11, 2007 issue of *Neurology*.

The study included nearly 3,000 women, who were followed for more than 25 years. Dr. Walter Rocca of the Mayo Clinic and his colleagues studied 813 women who had one ovary removed, 676 women who had both ovaries removed, and a comparison group of women who did not have their ovaries removed when the study began. About half the women had their ovaries removed because of a benign condition, such as cysts or inflammation; the others had their ovaries removed prophylactically to prevent ovarian cancer. Women who had the procedure for ovarian cancer or another estrogen-related cancer (usually breast cancer) were excluded because of their high risk of death shortly after surgery.

The researchers suggest three possible mechanisms to explain the association they observed. First, ovary removal may cause an estrogen deficiency that initiates biological changes leading to the elevated risk. Second, the association may involve a deficit of progesterone or testosterone rather than estrogen secreted by the ovaries. Third, the

association may be caused by susceptibility genes that independently increase both the risk of ovary removal and cognitive impairment or dementia.

The study's strengths include the long follow-up and the fact that the women were representative of the general population. Its limitations include the use of telephone interviews to assess cognitive abilities and an overall interview participation rate of 62 percent. In addition, the surgeries were done between 1950 and 1987, when surgical practices and estrogen use may have differed from today.

Nevertheless, the findings should lead to a reassessment of prophylactic removal of the ovaries in premenopausal women and of the use of estrogen treatment following ovary removal, the researchers say. "The results of this study are important for the majority of women who do not have an increased risk of ovarian cancer," says Dr. Rocca. "Women should consult with their physicians when considering the risks and benefits of prophylactic removal of the ovaries, and when considering treatment afterwards."

Section 30.4

Laparoscopy

"Laparoscopic Surgery," by Marelyn Medina, MD. © 2004 Society of Laparoendoscopic Surgeons (www.sls.org). Reprinted with permission.

The second millennium has brought with it a new era of modern surgery. The creation of video surgery is as revolutionary to this century as the development of anesthesia and sterile technique was to the last one. With ten years of solid experience behind them, surgeons can now confidently approach almost every part of the human body with cameras and video monitors. First they make a small cut in the skin and then introduce a harmless gas, such as carbon dioxide, into the body cavity to expand it and create a large working space. Through additional small cuts, a rod shaped telescope, attached to a camera, and other long and narrow surgical instruments are placed into the newly formed space. By this means, under high magnification diseased organs are able to be examined with minimal trauma to the patient.

Instead of making a large cut into the skin and underlying muscles, surgeons are now able to make small entry ports into the area of interest and perform all the major maneuvers previously done when a large opening was present.

Almost every organ in the human body has become accessible to the surgeon's camera and scalpel. Gall stones can now be removed with the gallbladder by laparoscopic surgery in over 90% of patients presenting with this disorder. Instead of months of bed rest and limited activities, which was associated with the old method of removing the gallbladder, patients can now usually resume their normal activities in several weeks.

Many other organs can now also be approached in a similar manner. These include the stomach, intestines, pancreas and spleen, kidneys and all the females organs. More recently operations have also been developed for diseases of the bladder and the prostate in men.

As new surgical instruments and better cameras and video display systems are developed, the frontiers for laparoscopic surgery will expand even further. Hopefully, in time the cost of this impressive technology should decrease—allowing surgeons in all corners of the global community to practice it.

The advantages of this method of operating are several. First, since the overall trauma to the skin and muscles is reduced, post operative pain is less—allowing patients to get out of bed sooner. They are often able then to walk and move around within a few short hours following their operations.

The second advantage is a reduced infection rate. This is because delicate tissues are not exposed to the air of the operating room over long periods of time—as they are when the body is wide open in traditional operations. Video magnification also offers surgeons better exposure of the diseased organ and its surrounding vessels and nerves. As a result, delicate maneuvers can be performed to protect these vital structures during the removal or repair of target organs.

The disadvantages of laparoscopy include the expensive equipment involved in performing it. Not all hospital operating rooms can afford to offer it because of cost containment. The other major issue is the need for surgeons to take special training in performing the many operations that are available by this means. Even surgeons that are brilliant in open techniques need special training to transfer their excellent surgical skills to the video monitor and display.

The need for additional training is because laparoscopic surgeons leave the familiar territory of a three dimensional operating field to working on a two dimensional flat video display. The shift is a critical

411

one, and requires some degree of practice moving around long laparoscopic instruments while handling delicate tissues. Despite these temporary disadvantages, with the proper training, surgeons are able to adapt to this means of operating.

Finally, laparoscopy cannot always be performed on everyone. Some patients with many prior operations may have so much scar tissue within the body that a safe operation cannot be done. In time, what disadvantages exist may be overcome with continued laparoscopic research and development. The future is still wide open for this new and revolutionary way of performing surgery. As new generations of surgeons come into training with solid computer and video skills established since childhood—only time will tell what wonderful innovations lie in store for all of us.

Section 30.5

Cryosurgery

Excerpted from "Cryosurgery in Cancer Treatment: Questions and Answers," National Cancer Institute (www.cancer.gov), September 2003.

What is cryosurgery?

Cryosurgery (also called cryotherapy) is the use of extreme cold produced by liquid nitrogen (or argon gas) to destroy abnormal tissue. Cryosurgery is used to treat external tumors, such as those on the skin. For external tumors, liquid nitrogen is applied directly to the cancer cells with a cotton swab or spraying device.

Cryosurgery is also used to treat tumors inside the body (internal tumors and tumors in the bone). For internal tumors, liquid nitrogen or argon gas is circulated through a hollow instrument called a cryoprobe, which is placed in contact with the tumor. The doctor uses ultrasound or magnetic resonance imaging (MRI) to guide the cryoprobe and monitor the freezing of the cells, thus limiting damage to nearby healthy tissue. (In ultrasound, sound waves are bounced off organs and other tissues to create a picture called a sonogram.) A ball of ice crystals forms around the probe, freezing nearby cells. Sometimes more than

one probe is used to deliver the liquid nitrogen to various parts of the tumor. The probes may be put into the tumor during surgery or through the skin (percutaneously). After cryosurgery, the frozen tissue thaws and is either naturally absorbed by the body (for internal tumors), or it dissolves and forms a scab (for external tumors).

What types of cancer can be treated with cryosurgery?

Cryosurgery is used to treat several types of cancer, and some pre-cancerous or noncancerous conditions. In addition to prostate and liver tumors, cryosurgery can be an effective treatment for the following:

- Retinoblastoma (a childhood cancer that affects the retina of the eye). Doctors have found that cryosurgery is most effective when the tumor is small and only in certain parts of the retina.

- Early-stage skin cancers (both basal cell and squamous cell carcinomas).

- Precancerous skin growths known as actinic keratosis.

- Precancerous conditions of the cervix known as cervical intraepithelial neoplasia (abnormal cell changes in the cervix that can develop into cervical cancer).

Cryosurgery is also used to treat some types of low-grade cancerous and noncancerous tumors of the bone. It may reduce the risk of joint damage when compared with more extensive surgery and help lessen the need for amputation. The treatment is also used to treat AIDS-related Kaposi sarcoma when the skin lesions are small and localized.

Researchers are evaluating cryosurgery as a treatment for a number of cancers, including breast, colon, and kidney cancer. They are also exploring cryotherapy in combination with other cancer treatments, such as hormone therapy, chemotherapy, radiation therapy, or surgery.

Does cryosurgery have any complications or side effects?

Cryosurgery does have side effects, although they may be less severe than those associated with surgery or radiation therapy. The effects depend on the location of the tumor. Cryosurgery for cervical intraepithelial neoplasia has not been shown to affect a woman's fertility, but it can cause cramping, pain, or bleeding. When used to treat skin cancer (including Kaposi sarcoma), cryosurgery may cause scarring and swelling; if nerves are damaged, loss of sensation may occur, and, rarely, it

may cause a loss of pigmentation and loss of hair in the treated area. When used to treat tumors of the bone, cryosurgery may lead to the destruction of nearby bone tissue and result in fractures, but these effects may not be seen for some time after the initial treatment and can often be delayed with other treatments. In rare cases, cryosurgery may interact badly with certain types of chemotherapy. Although the side effects of surgery may be less severe than those associated with conventional surgery or radiation, more studies are needed to determine the long-term effects.

What are the advantages of cryosurgery?

Cryosurgery offers advantages over other methods of cancer treatment. It is less invasive than surgery, involving only a small incision or insertion of the cryoprobe through the skin. Consequently, pain, bleeding, and other complications of surgery are minimized. Cryosurgery is less expensive than other treatments and requires shorter recovery time and a shorter hospital stay, or no hospital stay at all. Sometimes cryosurgery can be done using only local anesthesia.

Because physicians can focus cryosurgical treatment on a limited area, they can avoid the destruction of nearby healthy tissue. The treatment can be safely repeated and may be used along with standard treatments such as surgery, chemotherapy, hormone therapy, and radiation. Cryosurgery may offer an option for treating cancers that are considered inoperable or that do not respond to standard treatments. Furthermore, it can be used for patients who are not good candidates for conventional surgery because of their age or other medical conditions.

What are the disadvantages of cryosurgery?

The major disadvantage of cryosurgery is the uncertainty surrounding its long-term effectiveness. While cryosurgery may be effective in treating tumors the physician can see by using imaging tests (tests that produce pictures of areas inside the body), it can miss microscopic cancer spread. Furthermore, because the effectiveness of the technique is still being assessed, insurance coverage issues may arise.

What does the future hold for cryosurgery?

Additional studies are needed to determine the effectiveness of cryosurgery in controlling cancer and improving survival. Data from these studies will allow physicians to compare cryosurgery with standard treatment options such as surgery, chemotherapy, and radiation.

Moreover, physicians continue to examine the possibility of using cryosurgery in combination with other treatments.

Where is cryosurgery currently available?

Cryosurgery is widely available in gynecologists' offices for the treatment of cervical neoplasias. A limited number of hospitals and cancer centers throughout the country currently have skilled doctors and the necessary technology to perform cryosurgery for other noncancerous, precancerous, and cancerous conditions. Individuals can consult with their doctors or contact hospitals and cancer centers in their area to find out where cryosurgery is being used.

Chapter 31

Chemotherapy

What is chemotherapy?

Chemotherapy (also called chemo) is a type of cancer treatment that uses drugs to destroy cancer cells.

How does chemotherapy work?

Chemotherapy works by stopping or slowing the growth of cancer cells, which grow and divide quickly. But it can also harm healthy cells that divide quickly, such as those that line your mouth and intestines or cause your hair to grow. Damage to healthy cells may cause side effects. Often, side effects get better or go away after chemotherapy is over.

What does chemotherapy do?

Depending on your type of cancer and how advanced it is, chemotherapy can:

Cure cancer: When chemotherapy destroys cancer cells to the point that your doctor can no longer detect them in your body and they will not grow back.

Control cancer: When chemotherapy keeps cancer from spreading, slows its growth, or destroys cancer cells that have spread to other parts of your body.

Excerpted from "Chemotherapy and You: Support for People with Cancer," National Cancer Institute (www.cancer.gov), 2007.

Ease cancer symptoms (also called palliative care): When chemotherapy shrinks tumors that are causing pain or pressure.

How is chemotherapy used?

Sometimes, chemotherapy is used as the only cancer treatment. But more often, you will get chemotherapy along with surgery, radiation therapy, or biological therapy.

- Chemotherapy can make a tumor smaller before surgery or radiation therapy. This is called neoadjuvant chemotherapy.

- Chemotherapy can destroy cancer cells that may remain after surgery or radiation therapy. This is called adjuvant chemotherapy.

- Chemotherapy can help radiation therapy and biological therapy work better.

- Chemotherapy can destroy cancer cells that have come back (recurrent cancer) or spread to other parts of your body (metastatic cancer).

How does my doctor decide which chemotherapy drugs to use?

This choice depends on the type of cancer you have. Some types of chemotherapy drugs are used for many types of cancer. Other drugs are used for just one or two types of cancer. The decision also depends on whether you have had chemotherapy before and whether you have other health problems, such as diabetes or heart disease.

Where do I go for chemotherapy?

You may receive chemotherapy during a hospital stay, at home, or in a doctor's office, clinic, or outpatient unit in a hospital (which means you do not have to stay overnight). No matter where you go for chemotherapy, your doctor and nurse will watch for side effects and make any needed drug changes.

How often will I receive chemotherapy?

Treatment schedules for chemotherapy vary widely. How often and how long you get chemotherapy depends on your type of cancer and how advanced it is and the goals of treatment (whether chemotherapy is used to cure your cancer, control its growth, or ease the symptoms). It also depends on the type of chemotherapy and how your body reacts to chemotherapy.

You may receive chemotherapy in cycles. A cycle is a period of chemotherapy treatment followed by a period of rest. For instance, you might receive one week of chemotherapy followed by three weeks of rest. These four weeks make up one cycle. The rest period gives your body a chance to build new healthy cells.

Can I miss a dose of chemotherapy?

It is not good to skip a chemotherapy treatment. But sometimes your doctor or nurse may change your chemotherapy schedule. This can be due to side effects you are having. If this happens, your doctor or nurse will explain what to do and when to start treatment again.

How is chemotherapy given?

Chemotherapy may be given in many ways:

- **Injection:** The chemotherapy is given by a shot in a muscle in your arm, thigh, or hip or right under the skin in the fatty part of your arm, leg, or belly.
- **Intra-arterial (IA):** The chemotherapy goes directly into the artery that is feeding the cancer.
- **Intraperitoneal (IP):** The chemotherapy goes directly into the peritoneal cavity (the area that contains organs such as your intestines, stomach, liver, and ovaries).
- **Intravenous (IV):** The chemotherapy goes directly into a vein.
- **Topically:** The chemotherapy comes in a cream that you rub onto your skin.
- **Orally:** The chemotherapy comes in pills, capsules, or liquids that you swallow.

What techniques are used for IV chemotherapy?

Chemotherapy is often given through a thin needle that is placed in a vein on your hand or lower arm. Your nurse will put the needle in at the start of each treatment and remove it when treatment is over. Let your doctor or nurse know right away if you feel pain or burning while you are getting IV chemotherapy.

IV chemotherapy is often given through catheters or ports, sometimes with the help of a pump.

Catheters: A catheter is a soft, thin tube. A surgeon places one end of the catheter in a large vein, often in your chest area. The other end

of the catheter stays outside your body. Most catheters stay in place until all your chemotherapy treatments are done. Catheters can also be used for drugs other than chemotherapy and to draw blood. Be sure to watch for signs of infection around your catheter.

Ports: A port is a small, round disc made of plastic or metal that is placed under your skin. A catheter connects the port to a large vein, most often in your chest. Your nurse can insert a needle into your port to give you chemotherapy or draw blood. This needle can be left in place for chemotherapy treatments that are given for more than one day. Be sure to watch for signs of infection around your port.

Pumps: Pumps are often attached to catheters or ports. They control how much and how fast chemotherapy goes into a catheter or port. Pumps can be internal or external. External pumps remain outside your body. Most people can carry these pumps with them. Internal pumps are placed under your skin during surgery.

How will I feel during chemotherapy?

Chemotherapy affects people in different ways. How you feel depends on how healthy you are before treatment, your type of cancer, how advanced it is, the kind of chemotherapy you are getting, and the dose. Doctors and nurses cannot know for certain how you will feel during chemotherapy.

Some people do not feel well right after chemotherapy. The most common side effect is fatigue, feeling exhausted and worn out. You can prepare for fatigue by asking someone to drive you to and from chemotherapy, planning time to rest on the day of and day after chemotherapy, and getting help with meals and childcare the day of and at least one day after chemotherapy.

Can I work during chemotherapy?

Many people can work during chemotherapy, as long as they match their schedule to how they feel. Whether or not you can work may depend on what kind of work you do. If your job allows, you may want to see if you can work part-time or work from home on days you do not feel well.

Many employers are required by law to change your work schedule to meet your needs during cancer treatment. Talk with your employer about ways to adjust your work during chemotherapy. You can learn more about these laws by talking with a social worker.

Can I take over-the-counter and prescription drugs while I get chemotherapy?

This depends on the type of chemotherapy you get and the other types of drugs you plan to take. Take only drugs that are approved by your doctor or nurse. Tell your doctor or nurse about all the over-the-counter and prescription drugs you take, including laxatives, allergy medicines, cold medicines, pain relievers, aspirin, and ibuprofen.

One way to let your doctor or nurse know about these drugs is by bringing in all your pill bottles. Your doctor or nurse needs to know the name of each drug, the reason you take it, how much you take, and how often you take it.

Talk to your doctor or nurse before you take any over-the-counter or prescription drugs, vitamins, minerals, dietary supplements, or herbs.

Can I take vitamins, minerals, dietary supplements, or herbs while I get chemotherapy?

Some of these products can change how chemotherapy works. For this reason, it is important to tell your doctor or nurse about all the vitamins, minerals, dietary supplements, and herbs that you take before you start chemotherapy. During chemotherapy, talk with your doctor before you take any of these products.

How will I know if my chemotherapy is working?

Your doctor will give you physical exams and medical tests (such as blood tests and x-rays). He or she will also ask you how you feel.

You cannot tell if chemotherapy is working based on its side effects. Some people think that severe side effects mean that chemotherapy is working well. Or that no side effects mean that chemotherapy is not working. The truth is that side effects have nothing to do with how well chemotherapy is fighting your cancer.

How much does chemotherapy cost?

It is hard to say how much chemotherapy will cost. It depends on several factors:

- The types and doses of chemotherapy used
- How long and how often chemotherapy is given

- Whether you get chemotherapy at home, in a clinic or office, or during a hospital stay

- The part of the country where you live

Does my health insurance pay for chemotherapy?

Talk with your health insurance plan about what costs it will pay for. Questions to ask include:

- What will my insurance pay for?

- Do I or does the doctor's office need to call my insurance company before each treatment for it to be paid for?

- What do I have to pay for?

- Can I see any doctor I want or do I need to choose from a list of preferred providers?

- Do I need a written referral to see a specialist?

- Is there a co-pay (money I have to pay) each time I have an appointment?

- Is there a deductible (certain amount I need to pay) before my insurance pays?

- Where should I get my prescription drugs?

- Does my insurance pay for all my tests and treatments, whether I am an inpatient or outpatient?

How can I best work with my insurance plan?

- Read your insurance policy before treatment starts to find out what your plan will and will not pay for.

- Keep records of all your treatment costs and insurance claims.

- Send your insurance company all the paperwork it asks for. This may include receipts from doctors' visits, prescriptions, and lab work. Be sure to also keep copies for your own records.

- As needed, ask for help with the insurance paperwork. You can ask a friend, family member, social worker, or local group such as a senior center.

- If your insurance does not pay for something you think it should, find out why the plan refused to pay. Then talk with your doctor or nurse about what to do next. He or she may suggest ways to appeal the decision or other actions to take.

Chapter 32

Radiation Therapy

Questions and Answers about Radiation Therapy

What is radiation therapy?

Radiation therapy (also called radiotherapy) is a cancer treatment that uses high doses of radiation to kill cancer cells and stop them from spreading. At low doses, radiation is used as an x-ray to see inside your body and take pictures, such as x-rays of your teeth or broken bones. Radiation used in cancer treatment works in much the same way, except that it is given at higher doses.

How is radiation therapy given?

Radiation therapy can be external beam (when a machine outside your body aims radiation at cancer cells) or internal (when radiation is put inside your body, in or near the cancer cells). Sometimes people get both forms of radiation therapy.

Who gets radiation therapy?

Many people with cancer need radiation therapy. In fact, more than half (about 60 percent) of people with cancer get radiation therapy. Sometimes, radiation therapy is the only kind of cancer treatment people need.

Excerpted from "Radiation Therapy and You: Support for People with Cancer," National Cancer Institute (www.cancer.gov), 2007.

What does radiation therapy do to cancer cells?

Given in high doses, radiation kills or slows the growth of cancer cells. Radiation therapy is used to treat cancer or reduce symptoms:

- **Treat cancer:** Radiation can be used to cure, stop, or slow the growth of cancer.

- **Reduce symptoms:** When a cure is not possible, radiation may be used to shrink cancer tumors in order to reduce pressure. Radiation therapy used in this way can treat problems such as pain, or it can prevent problems such as blindness or loss of bowel and bladder control.

How long does radiation therapy take to work?

Radiation therapy does not kill cancer cells right away. It takes days or weeks of treatment before cancer cells start to die. Then, cancer cells keep dying for weeks or months after radiation therapy ends.

What does radiation therapy do to healthy cells?

Radiation not only kills or slows the growth of cancer cells, it can also affect nearby healthy cells. The healthy cells almost always recover after treatment is over. But sometimes people may have side effects that do not get better or are severe. Doctors try to protect healthy cells during treatment by:

Using as low a dose of radiation as possible: The radiation dose is balanced between being high enough to kill cancer cells yet low enough to limit damage to healthy cells.

Spreading out treatment over time: You may get radiation therapy once a day for several weeks or in smaller doses twice a day. Spreading out the radiation dose allows normal cells to recover while cancer cells die.

Aiming radiation at a precise part of your body: New techniques, such as IMRT and 3-D conformal radiation therapy, allow your doctor to aim higher doses of radiation at your cancer while reducing the radiation to nearby healthy tissue.

Using medicines: Some drugs can help protect certain parts of your body, such as the salivary glands that make saliva (spit).

Does radiation therapy hurt?

No, radiation therapy does not hurt while it is being given. But the side effects that people may get from radiation therapy can cause pain or discomfort. Part VI of this book has a lot of information about ways that you, your doctor, and your nurse can help manage side effects.

Is radiation therapy used with other types of cancer treatment?

Yes, radiation therapy is often used with other cancer treatments. Here are some examples:

Radiation therapy and surgery: Radiation may be given before, during, or after surgery. Doctors may use radiation to shrink the size of the cancer before surgery, or they may use radiation after surgery to kill any cancer cells that remain. Sometimes, radiation therapy is given during surgery so that it goes straight to the cancer without passing through the skin. This is called intraoperative radiation.

Radiation therapy and chemotherapy: Radiation may be given before, during, or after chemotherapy. Before or during chemotherapy, radiation therapy can shrink the cancer so that chemotherapy works better. Sometimes, chemotherapy is given to help radiation therapy work better. After chemotherapy, radiation therapy can be used to kill any cancer cells that remain.

Is radiation therapy expensive?

Yes, radiation therapy costs a lot of money. It uses complex machines and involves the services of many health care providers. The exact cost of your radiation therapy depends on the cost of health care where you live, what kind of radiation therapy you get, and how many treatments you need.

Talk with your health insurance company about what services it will pay for. Most insurance plans pay for radiation therapy for their members. To learn more, talk with the business office where you get treatment.

Should I follow a special diet while I am getting radiation therapy?

Your body uses a lot of energy to heal during radiation therapy. It is important that you eat enough calories and protein to keep your

weight the same during this time. Ask your doctor or nurse if you need a special diet while you are getting radiation therapy. You might also find it helpful to speak with a dietitian.

Ask your doctor, nurse, or dietitian if you need a special diet while you are getting radiation therapy.

Can I go to work during radiation therapy?

Some people are able to work full-time during radiation therapy. Others can only work part-time or not at all. How much you are able to work depends on how you feel. Ask your doctor or nurse what you may expect based on the treatment you are getting.

You are likely to feel well enough to work when you start radiation therapy. As time goes on, do not be surprised if you are more tired, have less energy, or feel weak. Once you have finished your treatment, it may take a few weeks or many months for you to feel better.

You may get to a point during your radiation therapy when you feel too sick to work. Talk with your employer to find out if you can go on medical leave. Make sure that your health insurance will pay for treatment when you are on medical leave.

What happens when radiation therapy is over?

Once you have finished radiation therapy, you will need follow-up care for the rest of your life. Follow-up care refers to checkups with your radiation oncologist or nurse practitioner after your course of radiation therapy is over. During these checkups, your doctor or nurse will see how well the radiation therapy worked, check for other signs of cancer, look for late side effects, and talk with you about your treatment and care.

Your doctor or nurse will examine you and review how you have been feeling. Your doctor or nurse practitioner can prescribe medicine or suggest other ways to treat any side effects you may have. Your doctor or nurse may also order lab and imaging tests. These may include blood tests, x-rays, or CT, MRI, or PET scans. Your doctor or nurse practitioner may suggest that you have more treatment, such as extra radiation treatments, chemotherapy, or both. Your doctor or nurse will also answer your questions and respond to your concerns. It may be helpful to write down your questions ahead of time and bring them with you.

After radiation therapy is over, what symptoms should I look for?

You have gone through a lot with cancer and radiation therapy. Now you may be even more aware of your body and how you feel each

day. Pay attention to changes in your body and let your doctor or nurse know if you have any of the following symptoms:

- A pain that does not go away
- New lumps, bumps, swellings, rashes, bruises, or bleeding
- Appetite changes, nausea, vomiting, diarrhea, or constipation
- Weight loss that you cannot explain
- A fever, cough, or hoarseness that does not go away
- Any other symptoms that worry you

Make a list of questions and problems you want to discuss with your doctor or nurse. Be sure to bring this list to your follow-up visits.

External Beam Radiation Therapy

What is external beam radiation therapy?

External beam radiation therapy comes from a machine that aims radiation at your cancer. The machine is large and may be noisy. It does not touch you, but rotates around you, sending radiation to your body from many directions.

External beam radiation therapy is a local treatment, meaning that the radiation is aimed only at a specific part of your body. For example, if you have lung cancer, you will get radiation to your chest only and not the rest of your body.

External beam radiation therapy comes from a machine that aims radiation at your cancer.

How often will I get external beam radiation therapy?

Most people get external beam radiation therapy once a day, five days a week, Monday through Friday. Treatment lasts for two to 10 weeks, depending on the type of cancer you have and the goal of your treatment. The time between your first and last radiation therapy sessions is called a course of treatment.

Radiation is sometimes given in smaller doses twice a day (hyper-fractionated radiation therapy). Your doctor may prescribe this type of treatment if he or she feels that it will work better. Although side effects may be more severe, there may be fewer late side effects. Doctors are doing research to see which types of cancer are best treated this way.

427

Where do I go for external beam radiation therapy?

Most of the time, you will get external beam radiation therapy as an outpatient. This means that you will have treatment at a clinic or radiation therapy center and will not have to stay in the hospital.

What happens before my first external beam radiation treatment?

If you are getting radiation to the head, you may need a mask. You will have a one-to-two hour meeting with your doctor or nurse before you begin radiation therapy. At this time, you will have a physical exam, talk about your medical history, and maybe have imaging tests. Your doctor or nurse will discuss external beam radiation therapy, its benefits and side effects, and ways you can care for yourself during and after treatment. You can then choose whether to have external beam radiation therapy.

If you agree to have external beam radiation therapy, you will be scheduled for a treatment planning session called a simulation. At this time the following steps will be taken:

- A radiation oncologist and radiation therapist will define your treatment area (also called a treatment port or treatment field). This refers to the places in your body that will get radiation. You will be asked to lie very still while x-rays or scans are taken to define the treatment area.

- The radiation therapist will then put small marks (tattoos or dots of colored ink) on your skin to mark the treatment area. You will need these marks throughout the course of radiation therapy. The radiation therapist will use them each day to make sure you are in the correct position. Tattoos are about the size of a freckle and will remain on your skin for the rest of your life. Ink markings will fade over time. Be careful not to remove them and make sure to tell the radiation therapist if they fade or lose color.

- You may need a body mold. This is a plastic or plaster form that helps keep you from moving during treatment. It also helps make sure that you are in the exact same position each day of treatment.

- If you are getting radiation to the head, you may need a mask. The mask has air holes, and holes can be cut for your eyes, nose, and mouth. It attaches to the table where you will lie to receive your treatments. The mask helps keep your head from moving so that you are in the exact same position for each treatment.

t should I wear when I get external beam radiation rapy?

Wear clothes that are comfortable and made of soft fabric, such as cotton. Choose clothes that are easy to take off, since you may need to change into a hospital gown or show the area that is being treated. Do not wear clothes that are tight, such as close-fitting collars or waist-bands, near your treatment area. Also, do not wear jewelry, BAND-AIDS®, powder, lotion, or deodorant in or near your treatment area, and do not use deodorant soap before your treatment.

What happens during treatment sessions?

- You may be asked to change into a hospital gown or robe.

- You will go to a treatment room where you will receive radiation.

- Depending on where your cancer is, you will either sit in a chair or lie down on a treatment table. The radiation therapist will use your body mold and skin marks to help you get into position.

- You may see colored lights pointed at your skin marks. These lights are harmless and help the therapist position you for treatment each day.

- You will need to stay very still so the radiation goes to the exact same place each time. You can breathe as you always do and do not have to hold your breath.

- The radiation therapist will leave the room just before your treatment begins. He or she will go to a nearby room to control the radiation machine and watch you on a TV screen or through a window. You are not alone, even though it may feel that way. The radiation therapist can see you on the screen or through the window. He or she can hear and talk with you through a speaker in your treatment room. Make sure to tell the therapist if you feel sick or are uncomfortable. He or she can stop the radiation machine at any time. You cannot feel, hear, see, or smell radiation.

- Your entire visit may last from 30 minutes to one hour. Most of that time is spent setting you in the correct position. You will get radiation for only one to five minutes. If you are getting IMRT, your treatment may last longer. Your visit may also take longer if your treatment team needs to take and review x-rays.

429

Your radiation therapist can see, hear, and talk with you at all times while you are getting external beam radiation therapy.

Will external beam radiation therapy make me radioactive?

No, external beam radiation therapy does not make people radioactive. You may safely be around other people, even babies and young children.

How can I relax during my treatment sessions?

- Bring something to read or do while in the waiting room.

- Ask if you can listen to music or books on tape.

- Meditate, breathe deeply, use imagery, or find other ways to relax.

Internal Radiation Therapy

What is internal radiation therapy?

Internal radiation therapy is a form of treatment where a source of radiation is put inside your body. One form of internal radiation therapy is called brachytherapy. In brachytherapy, the radiation source is a solid in the form of seeds, ribbons, or capsules, which are placed in your body in or near the cancer cells. This allows treatment with a high dose of radiation to a smaller part of your body. Internal radiation can also be in a liquid form. You receive liquid radiation by drinking it, by swallowing a pill, or through an IV. Liquid radiation travels throughout your body, seeking out and killing cancer cells.

Brachytherapy may be used with people who have cancers of the head, neck, breast, uterus, cervix, prostate, gall bladder, esophagus, eye, and lung. Liquid forms of internal radiation are most often used with people who have thyroid cancer or non-Hodgkin lymphoma. You may also get internal radiation along with other types of treatment, including external beam radiation, chemotherapy, or surgery.

What happens before my first internal radiation treatment?

You will have a one-to-two hour meeting with your doctor or nurse before you begin internal radiation therapy. At this time, you will have

a physical exam, talk about your medical history, and maybe have imaging tests. Your doctor will discuss the type of internal radiation therapy that is best for you, its benefits and side effects, and ways you can care for yourself during and after treatment. You can then choose whether to have internal radiation therapy.

How is brachytherapy put in place?

Most brachytherapy is put in place through a catheter, which is a small, stretchy tube. Sometimes, it is put in place through a larger device called an applicator. When you decide to have brachytherapy, your doctor will place the catheter or applicator into the part of your body that will be treated.

What happens when the catheter or applicator is put in place?

You will most likely be in the hospital when your catheter or applicator is put in place. Here is what to expect:

- You will either be put to sleep or the area where the catheter or applicator goes will be numbed. This will help prevent pain when it is put in.

- Your doctor will place the catheter or applicator in your body.

If you are awake, you may be asked to lie very still while the catheter or applicator is put in place. If you feel any discomfort, tell your doctor or nurse so he or she can give you medicine to help manage the pain. Tell your doctor or nurse if you are in pain.

What happens after the catheter or applicator is placed in my body?

Once your treatment plan is complete, radiation will be placed inside the catheter or applicator. The radiation source may be kept in place for a few minutes, many days, or the rest of your life. How long the radiation is in place depends on which type of brachytherapy you get, your type of cancer, where the cancer is in your body, your health, and other cancer treatments you have had.

What are the types of brachytherapy?

There are three types of brachytherapy:

431

Low-dose rate (LDR) implants: In this type of brachytherapy, radiation stays in place for one to seven days. You are likely to be in the hospital during this time. Once your treatment is finished, your doctor will remove the radiation sources and your catheter or applicator.

High-dose rate (HDR) implants: In this type of brachytherapy, the radiation source is in place for 10 to 20 minutes at a time and then taken out. You may have treatment twice a day for two to five days or once a week for two to five weeks. The schedule depends on your type of cancer. During the course of treatment, your catheter or applicator may stay in place, or it may be put in place before each treatment. You may be in the hospital during this time, or you may make daily trips to the hospital to have the radiation source put in place. Like LDR implants, your doctor will remove your catheter or applicator once you have finished treatment.

Permanent implants: After the radiation source is put in place, the catheter is removed. The implants always stay in your body, while the radiation gets weaker each day. You may need to limit your time around other people when the radiation is first put in place. Be extra careful not to spend time with children or pregnant women. As time goes by, almost all the radiation will go away, even though the implant stays in your body.

What happens while the radiation is in place?

Your body will give off radiation once the radiation source is in place. With brachytherapy, your body fluids (urine, sweat, and saliva) will not give off radiation. With liquid radiation, your body fluids will give off radiation for a while.

Your doctor or nurse will talk with you about safety measures that you need to take. If the radiation you receive is a very high dose, safety measures may include the following:

- Staying in a private hospital room to protect others from radiation coming from your body

- Being treated quickly by nurses and other hospital staff. They will provide all the care you need, but they may stand at a distance and talk with you from the doorway to your room.

Your visitors will also need to follow safety measures, which may include the following:

- Not being allowed to visit when the radiation is first put in

- Needing to check with the hospital staff before they go to your room

- Keeping visits short (30 minutes or less each day). The length of visits depends on the type of radiation being used and the part of your body being treated.

- Standing by the doorway rather than going into your hospital room

- Not having visits from children younger than 18 and pregnant women

You may also need to follow safety measures once you leave the hospital, such as not spending much time with other people. Your doctor or nurse will talk with you about the safety measures you should follow when you go home.

What happens when the catheter is taken out after treatment with LDR or HDR implants?

- You will get medicine for pain before the catheter or applicator is removed.

- The area where the catheter or applicator was might be tender for a few months.

- There is no radiation in your body after the catheter or applicator is removed. It is safe for people to be near you—even young children and pregnant women.

For one to two weeks, you may need to limit activities that take a lot of effort. Ask your doctor what kinds of activities are safe for you.

Chapter 33

Bone Marrow and Peripheral Blood Stem Cell Transplantation

What are bone marrow and hematopoietic stem cells?

Bone marrow is the soft, sponge-like material found inside bones. It contains immature cells known as hematopoietic or blood-forming stem cells. (Hematopoietic stem cells are different from embryonic stem cells. Embryonic stem cells can develop into every type of cell in the body.) Hematopoietic stem cells divide to form more blood-forming stem cells, or they mature into one of three types of blood cells: White blood cells, which fight infection; red blood cells, which carry oxygen; and platelets, which help the blood to clot. Most hematopoietic stem cells are found in the bone marrow, but some cells, called peripheral blood stem cells (PBSCs), are found in the bloodstream. Blood in the umbilical cord also contains hematopoietic stem cells. Cells from any of these sources can be used in transplants.

What are bone marrow transplantation and peripheral blood stem cell transplantation?

Bone marrow transplantation (BMT) and peripheral blood stem cell transplantation (PBSCT) are procedures that restore stem cells that have been destroyed by high doses of chemotherapy and/or radiation therapy. There are three types of transplants:

"Bone Marrow Transplantation and Peripheral Blood Stem Cell Transplantation," National Cancer Institute (www.cancer.gov), October 2008.

- In autologous transplants, patients receive their own stem cells.

- In syngeneic transplants, patients receive stem cells from their identical twin.

- In allogeneic transplants, patients receive stem cells from their brother, sister, or parent. A person who is not related to the patient (an unrelated donor) also may be used.

Why are BMT and PBSCT used in cancer treatment?

One reason BMT and PBSCT are used in cancer treatment is to make it possible for patients to receive very high doses of chemotherapy and/or radiation therapy. To understand more about why BMT and PBSCT are used, it is helpful to understand how chemotherapy and radiation therapy work.

Chemotherapy and radiation therapy generally affect cells that divide rapidly. They are used to treat cancer because cancer cells divide more often than most healthy cells. However, because bone marrow cells also divide frequently, high-dose treatments can severely damage or destroy the patient's bone marrow. Without healthy bone marrow, the patient is no longer able to make the blood cells needed to carry oxygen, fight infection, and prevent bleeding. BMT and PBSCT replace stem cells destroyed by treatment. The healthy, transplanted stem cells can restore the bone marrow's ability to produce the blood cells the patient needs.

In some types of leukemia, the graft-versus-tumor (GVT) effect that occurs after allogeneic BMT and PBSCT is crucial to the effectiveness of the treatment. GVT occurs when white blood cells from the donor (the graft) identify the cancer cells that remain in the patient's body after the chemotherapy and/or radiation therapy (the tumor) as foreign and attack them.

What types of cancer are treated with BMT and PBSCT?

BMT and PBSCT are most commonly used in the treatment of leukemia and lymphoma. They are most effective when the leukemia or lymphoma is in remission (the signs and symptoms of cancer have disappeared). BMT and PBSCT are also used to treat other cancers such as neuroblastoma (cancer that arises in immature nerve cells and affects mostly infants and children) and multiple myeloma. Researchers are evaluating BMT and PBSCT in clinical trials (research studies) for the treatment of various types of cancer.

How are the donor's stem cells matched to the patient's stem cells in allogeneic or syngeneic transplantation?

To minimize potential side effects, doctors most often use transplanted stem cells that match the patient's own stem cells as closely as possible. People have different sets of proteins, called human leukocyte-associated (HLA) antigens, on the surface of their cells. The set of proteins, called the HLA type, is identified by a special blood test.

In most cases, the success of allogeneic transplantation depends in part on how well the HLA antigens of the donor's stem cells match those of the recipient's stem cells. The higher the number of matching HLA antigens, the greater the chance that the patient's body will accept the donor's stem cells. In general, patients are less likely to develop a complication known as graft-versus-host disease (GVHD) if the stem cells of the donor and patient are closely matched.

Close relatives, especially brothers and sisters, are more likely than unrelated people to be HLA-matched. However, only 25 to 35 percent of patients have an HLA-matched sibling. The chances of obtaining HLA-matched stem cells from an unrelated donor are slightly better, approximately 50 percent. Among unrelated donors, HLA-matching is greatly improved when the donor and recipient have the same ethnic and racial background. Although the number of donors is increasing overall, individuals from certain ethnic and racial groups still have a lower chance of finding a matching donor. Large volunteer donor registries can assist in finding an appropriate unrelated donor.

Because identical twins have the same genes, they have the same set of HLA antigens. As a result, the patient's body will accept a transplant from an identical twin. However, identical twins represent a small number of all births, so syngeneic transplantation is rare.

How is bone marrow obtained for transplantation?

The stem cells used in BMT come from the liquid center of the bone, called the marrow. In general, the procedure for obtaining bone marrow, which is called "harvesting," is similar for all three types of BMTs (autologous, syngeneic, and allogeneic). The donor is given either general anesthesia, which puts the person to sleep during the procedure, or regional anesthesia, which causes loss of feeling below the waist. Needles are inserted through the skin over the pelvic (hip) bone or, in rare cases, the sternum (breastbone), and into the bone marrow to draw the marrow out of the bone. Harvesting the marrow takes about an hour.

The harvested bone marrow is then processed to remove blood and bone fragments. Harvested bone marrow can be combined with

a preservative and frozen to keep the stem cells alive until they are needed. This technique is known as cryopreservation. Stem cells can be cryopreserved for many years.

How are PBSCs obtained for transplantation?

The stem cells used in PBSCT come from the bloodstream. A process called apheresis or leukapheresis is used to obtain PBSCs for transplantation. For four or five days before apheresis, the donor may be given a medication to increase the number of stem cells released into the bloodstream. In apheresis, blood is removed through a large vein in the arm or a central venous catheter (a flexible tube that is placed in a large vein in the neck, chest, or groin area). The blood goes through a machine that removes the stem cells. The blood is then returned to the donor and the collected cells are stored. Apheresis typically takes four to six hours. The stem cells are then frozen until they are given to the recipient.

How are umbilical cord stem cells obtained for transplantation?

Stem cells also may be retrieved from umbilical cord blood. For this to occur, the mother must contact a cord blood bank before the baby's birth. The cord blood bank may request that she complete a questionnaire and give a small blood sample.

Cord blood banks may be public or commercial. Public cord blood banks accept donations of cord blood and may provide the donated stem cells to another matched individual in their network. In contrast, commercial cord blood banks will store the cord blood for the family, in case it is needed later for the child or another family member.

After the baby is born and the umbilical cord has been cut, blood is retrieved from the umbilical cord and placenta. This process poses minimal health risk to the mother or the child. If the mother agrees, the umbilical cord blood is processed and frozen for storage by the cord blood bank. Only a small amount of blood can be retrieved from the umbilical cord and placenta, so the collected stem cells are typically used for children or small adults.

Are any risks associated with donating bone marrow?

Because only a small amount of bone marrow is removed, donating usually does not pose any significant problems for the donor. The most serious risk associated with donating bone marrow involves the use of anesthesia during the procedure.

The area where the bone marrow was taken out may feel stiff or sore for a few days, and the donor may feel tired. Within a few weeks, the donor's body replaces the donated marrow; however, the time required for a donor to recover varies. Some people are back to their usual routine within two or three days, while others may take up to three to four weeks to fully recover their strength.

Are any risks associated with donating PBSCs?

Apheresis usually causes minimal discomfort. During apheresis, the person may feel lightheadedness, chills, numbness around the lips, and cramping in the hands. Unlike bone marrow donation, PBSC donation does not require anesthesia. The medication that is given to stimulate the release of stem cells from the marrow into the bloodstream may cause bone and muscle aches, headaches, fatigue, nausea, vomiting, and/or difficulty sleeping. These side effects generally stop within two to three days of the last dose of the medication.

How does the patient receive the stem cells during the transplant?

After being treated with high-dose anticancer drugs and/or radiation, the patient receives the stem cells through an intravenous (IV) line just like a blood transfusion. This part of the transplant takes one to five hours.

Are any special measures taken when the cancer patient is also the donor (autologous transplant)?

The stem cells used for autologous transplantation must be relatively free of cancer cells. The harvested cells can sometimes be treated before transplantation in a process known as "purging" to get rid of cancer cells. This process can remove some cancer cells from the harvested cells and minimize the chance that cancer will come back. Because purging may damage some healthy stem cells, more cells are obtained from the patient before the transplant so that enough healthy stem cells will remain after purging.

What happens after the stem cells have been transplanted to the patient?

After entering the bloodstream, the stem cells travel to the bone marrow, where they begin to produce new white blood cells, red blood

cells, and platelets in a process known as "engraftment." Engraftment usually occurs within about two to four weeks after transplantation. Doctors monitor it by checking blood counts on a frequent basis. Complete recovery of immune function takes much longer, however—up to several months for autologous transplant recipients and one to two years for patients receiving allogeneic or syngeneic transplants. Doctors evaluate the results of various blood tests to confirm that new blood cells are being produced and that the cancer has not returned. Bone marrow aspiration (the removal of a small sample of bone marrow through a needle for examination under a microscope) can also help doctors determine how well the new marrow is working.

What are the possible side effects of BMT and PBSCT?

The major risk of both treatments is an increased susceptibility to infection and bleeding as a result of the high-dose cancer treatment. Doctors may give the patient antibiotics to prevent or treat infection. They may also give the patient transfusions of platelets to prevent bleeding and red blood cells to treat anemia. Patients who undergo BMT and PBSCT may experience short-term side effects such as nausea, vomiting, fatigue, loss of appetite, mouth sores, hair loss, and skin reactions.

Potential long-term risks include complications of the pretransplant chemotherapy and radiation therapy, such as infertility (the inability to produce children); cataracts (clouding of the lens of the eye, which causes loss of vision); secondary (new) cancers; and damage to the liver, kidneys, lungs, and/or heart.

With allogeneic transplants, a complication known as graft-versus-host disease (GVHD) sometimes develops. GVHD occurs when white blood cells from the donor (the graft) identify cells in the patient's body (the host) as foreign and attack them. The most commonly damaged organs are the skin, liver, and intestines. This complication can develop within a few weeks of the transplant (acute GVHD) or much later (chronic GVHD). To prevent this complication, the patient may receive medications that suppress the immune system. Additionally, the donated stem cells can be treated to remove the white blood cells that cause GVHD in a process called "T-cell depletion." If GVHD develops, it can be very serious and is treated with steroids or other immunosuppressive agents. GVHD can be difficult to treat, but some studies suggest that patients with leukemia who develop GVHD are less likely to have the cancer come back. Clinical trials are being conducted to find ways to prevent and treat GVHD.

The likelihood and severity of complications are specific to the patient's treatment and should be discussed with the patient's doctor.

What is a "mini-transplant"?

A "mini-transplant" (also called a non-myeloablative or reduced-intensity transplant) is a type of allogeneic transplant. This approach is being studied in clinical trials for the treatment of several types of cancer, including leukemia, lymphoma, multiple myeloma, and other cancers of the blood.

A mini-transplant uses lower, less toxic doses of chemotherapy and/or radiation to prepare the patient for an allogeneic transplant. The use of lower doses of anticancer drugs and radiation eliminates some, but not all, of the patient's bone marrow. It also reduces the number of cancer cells and suppresses the patient's immune system to prevent rejection of the transplant.

Unlike traditional BMT or PBSCT, cells from both the donor and the patient may exist in the patient's body for some time after a mini-transplant. Once the cells from the donor begin to engraft, they may cause the graft-versus-tumor (GVT) effect and work to destroy the cancer cells that were not eliminated by the anticancer drugs and/or radiation. To boost the GVT effect, the patient may be given an injection of the donor's white blood cells. This procedure is called a "donor lymphocyte infusion."

What is a "tandem transplant"?

A "tandem transplant" is a type of autologous transplant. This method is being studied in clinical trials for the treatment of several types of cancer, including multiple myeloma and germ cell cancer. During a tandem transplant, a patient receives two sequential courses of high-dose chemotherapy with stem cell transplant. Typically, the two courses are given several weeks to several months apart. Researchers hope that this method can prevent the cancer from recurring (coming back) at a later time.

How do patients cover the cost of BMT or PBSCT?

Advances in treatment methods, including the use of PBSCT, have reduced the amount of time many patients must spend in the hospital by speeding recovery. This shorter recovery time has brought about a reduction in cost. However, because BMT and PBSCT are complicated technical procedures, they are very expensive. Many health insurance

companies cover some of the costs of transplantation for certain types of cancer. Insurers may also cover a portion of the costs if special care is required when the patient returns home.

There are options for relieving the financial burden associated with BMT and PBSCT. A hospital social worker is a valuable resource in planning for these financial needs. Federal Government programs and local service organizations may also be able to help.

What are the costs of donating bone marrow, PBSCs, or umbilical cord blood?

Persons willing to donate bone marrow or PBSCs must have a sample of blood drawn to determine their HLA type. This blood test usually costs $65 to $96. The donor may be asked to pay for this blood test, or the donor center may cover part of the cost. Community groups and other organizations may also provide financial assistance. Once a donor is identified as a match for a patient, all of the costs pertaining to the retrieval of bone marrow or PBSCs is covered by the patient or the patient's medical insurance.

A woman can donate her baby's umbilical cord blood to public cord blood banks at no charge. However, commercial blood banks do charge varying fees to store umbilical cord blood for the private use of the patient or his or her family.

Where can people get more information about potential donors and transplant centers?

The National Marrow Donor Program® (NMDP), a federally funded nonprofit organization, was created to improve the effectiveness of the search for donors. The NMDP maintains an international registry of volunteers willing to be donors for all sources of blood stem cells used in transplantation: Bone marrow, peripheral blood, and umbilical cord blood.

The NMDP Web site contains a list of participating transplant centers at http://www.marrow.org/PATIENT/Plan_for_Tx/Choosing_a_TC/US_NMDP_Transplant_Centers/tc_list_by_state.pl on the internet. The list includes descriptions of the centers, as well as their transplant experience, survival statistics, research interests, pretransplant costs, and contact information.

National Marrow Donor Program
3001 Broadway Street, NE, Suite 100
Minneapolis, MN 55413-1753

Telephone 612-627-5800
800-627-7692 (800-MARROW-2)
888-999-6743 (Office of Patient Advocacy)
E-mail: patientinfo@nmdp.org
Website: http://www.marrow.org

Where can people get more information about clinical trials of BMT and PBSCT?

Clinical trials that include BMT and PBSCT are a treatment option for some patients. Information about ongoing clinical trials is available from National Cancer Institute (NCI)'s Cancer Information Service, or from the NCI's website at http://www.cancer.gov/clinicaltrials on the internet.

Chapter 34

Biological Therapies for Cancer

What is biological therapy?

Biological therapy (sometimes called immunotherapy, biotherapy, or biological response modifier therapy) is a relatively new addition to the family of cancer treatments that also includes surgery, chemotherapy, and radiation therapy. Biological therapies use the body's immune system, either directly or indirectly, to fight cancer or to lessen the side effects that may be caused by some cancer treatments.

What is the immune system and what are its components?

The immune system is a complex network of cells and organs that work together to defend the body against attacks by "foreign" or "non-self" invaders. This network is one of the body's main defenses against infection and disease. The immune system works against diseases, including cancer, in a variety of ways. For example, the immune system may recognize the difference between healthy cells and cancer cells in the body and works to eliminate cancerous cells. However, the immune system does not always recognize cancer cells as "foreign." Also, cancer may develop when the immune system breaks down or does not function adequately. Biological therapies are designed to repair, stimulate, or enhance the immune system's responses.

Immune system cells include the following:

"Biological Therapies for Cancer: Questions and Answers," National Cancer Institute (www.cancer.gov), June 2006.

- Lymphocytes are a type of white blood cell found in the blood and many other parts of the body. Types of lymphocytes include B cells, T cells, and Natural Killer cells.

- B cells (B lymphocytes) mature into plasma cells that secrete proteins called antibodies (immunoglobulins). Antibodies recognize and attach to foreign substances known as antigens, fitting together much the way a key fits a lock. Each type of B cell makes one specific antibody, which recognizes one specific antigen.

- T cells (T lymphocytes) work primarily by producing proteins called cytokines. Cytokines allow immune system cells to communicate with each other and include lymphokines, interferons, interleukins, and colony-stimulating factors. Some T cells, called cytotoxic T cells, release pore-forming proteins that directly attack infected, foreign, or cancerous cells. Other T cells, called helper T cells, regulate the immune response by releasing cytokines to signal other immune system defenders.

- Natural killer cells (NK cells) produce powerful cytokines and pore-forming proteins that bind to and kill many foreign invaders, infected cells, and tumor cells. Unlike cytotoxic T cells, they are poised to attack quickly, upon their first encounter with their targets.

- Phagocytes are white blood cells that can swallow and digest microscopic organisms and particles in a process known as phagocytosis. There are several types of phagocytes, including monocytes, which circulate in the blood, and macrophages, which are located in tissues throughout the body.

What are biological response modifiers, and how can they be used to treat cancer?

Some antibodies, cytokines, and other immune system substances can be produced in the laboratory for use in cancer treatment. These substances are often called biological response modifiers (BRMs). They alter the interaction between the body's immune defenses and cancer cells to boost, direct, or restore the body's ability to fight the disease. BRMs include interferons, interleukins, colony-stimulating factors, monoclonal antibodies, vaccines, gene therapy, and nonspecific immunomodulating agents.

Researchers continue to discover new BRMs, to learn more about how they function, and to develop ways to use them in cancer therapy. Biological therapies may be used for the following purposes:

- Stop, control, or suppress processes that permit cancer growth.

- Make cancer cells more recognizable and, therefore, more susceptible to destruction by the immune system.

- Boost the killing power of immune system cells, such as T cells, NK cells, and macrophages.

- Alter the growth patterns of cancer cells to promote behavior like that of healthy cells.

- Block or reverse the process that changes a normal cell or a precancerous cell into a cancerous cell.

- Enhance the body's ability to repair or replace normal cells damaged or destroyed by other forms of cancer treatment, such as chemotherapy or radiation.

- Prevent cancer cells from spreading to other parts of the body.

Some BRMs are a standard part of treatment for certain types of cancer, while others are being studied in clinical trials (research studies). BRMs are being used alone or in combination with each other. They are also being used with other treatments, such as radiation therapy and chemotherapy.

What are interferons?

Interferons (IFNs) are types of cytokines that occur naturally in the body. They were the first cytokines produced in the laboratory for use as BRMs. There are three major types of interferons—interferon alpha, interferon beta, and interferon gamma; interferon alpha is the type most widely used in cancer treatment.

Researchers have found that interferons can improve the way a cancer patient's immune system acts against cancer cells. In addition, interferons may act directly on cancer cells by slowing their growth or promoting their development into cells with more normal behavior. Researchers believe that some interferons may also stimulate NK cells, T cells, and macrophages, boosting the immune system's anticancer function.

The U.S. Food and Drug Administration (FDA) has approved the use of interferon alpha for the treatment of certain types of cancer, including hairy cell leukemia, melanoma, chronic myeloid leukemia, and AIDS-related Kaposi sarcoma. Studies have shown that interferon alpha may also be effective in treating other cancers such as kidney cancer and non-Hodgkin lymphoma. Researchers are exploring combinations of

interferon alpha and other BRMs or chemotherapy in clinical trials to treat a number of cancers.

What are interleukins?

Like interferons, interleukins (ILs) are cytokines that occur naturally in the body and can be made in the laboratory. Many interleukins have been identified; interleukin-2 (IL-2 or aldesleukin) has been the most widely studied in cancer treatment. IL-2 stimulates the growth and activity of many immune cells, such as lymphocytes, that can destroy cancer cells. The FDA has approved IL-2 for the treatment of metastatic kidney cancer and metastatic melanoma.

Researchers continue to study the benefits of interleukins to treat a number of other cancers, including leukemia, lymphoma, and brain, colorectal, ovarian, breast, and prostate cancers.

What are colony-stimulating factors?

Colony-stimulating factors (CSFs) (sometimes called hematopoietic growth factors) usually do not directly affect tumor cells; rather, they encourage bone marrow stem cells to divide and develop into white blood cells, platelets, and red blood cells. Bone marrow is critical to the body's immune system because it is the source of all blood cells.

Stimulation of the immune system by CSFs may benefit patients undergoing cancer treatment. Because anticancer drugs can damage the body's ability to make white blood cells, red blood cells, and platelets, patients receiving anticancer drugs have an increased risk of developing infections, becoming anemic, and bleeding more easily. By using CSFs to stimulate blood cell production, doctors can increase the doses of anticancer drugs without increasing the risk of infection or the need for transfusion with blood products. As a result, researchers have found CSFs particularly useful when combined with high-dose chemotherapy.

Some examples of CSFs and their use in cancer therapy are as follows:

- G-CSF (filgrastim) and GM-CSF (sargramostim) can increase the number of white blood cells, thereby reducing the risk of infection in patients receiving chemotherapy. G-CSF and GM-CSF can also stimulate the production of stem cells in preparation for stem cell or bone marrow transplants.

- Erythropoietin (epoetin) can increase the number of red blood cells and reduce the need for red blood cell transfusions in patients receiving chemotherapy.

- Interleukin-11 (oprelvekin) helps the body make platelets and can reduce the need for platelet transfusions in patients receiving chemotherapy.

Researchers are studying CSFs in clinical trials to treat a large variety of cancers, including lymphoma, leukemia, multiple myeloma, melanoma, and cancers of the brain, lung, esophagus, breast, uterus, ovary, prostate, kidney, colon, and rectum.

What are monoclonal antibodies?

Researchers are evaluating the effectiveness of certain antibodies made in the laboratory called monoclonal antibodies (MOABs or MoABs). These antibodies are produced by a single type of cell and are specific for a particular antigen. Researchers are examining ways to create MOABs specific to the antigens found on the surface of various cancer cells.

To create MOABs , scientists first inject human cancer cells into mice. In response, the mouse immune system makes antibodies against these cancer cells. The scientists then remove the mouse plasma cells that produce antibodies, and fuse them with laboratory-grown cells to create "hybrid" cells called hybridomas. Hybridomas can indefinitely produce large quantities of these pure antibodies, or MOABs.

MOABs may be used in cancer treatment in a number of ways:

- MOABs that react with specific types of cancer may enhance a patient's immune response to the cancer.

- MOABs can be programmed to act against cell growth factors, thus interfering with the growth of cancer cells.

- MOABs may be linked to anticancer drugs, radioisotopes (radioactive substances), other BRMs, or other toxins. When the antibodies latch onto cancer cells, they deliver these poisons directly to the tumor, helping to destroy it.

- MOABs carrying radioisotopes may also prove useful in diagnosing certain cancers, such as colorectal, ovarian, and prostate.

What are cancer vaccines?

Cancer vaccines are another form of biological therapy currently under study. Vaccines for infectious diseases, such as measles, mumps, and tetanus, are injected into a person before the disease develops. These vaccines are effective because they expose the body's immune

cells to weakened forms of antigens that are present on the surface of the infectious agent. This exposure causes the immune system to increase production of plasma cells that make antibodies specific to the infectious agent. The immune system also increases production of T cells that recognize the infectious agent. These activated immune cells remember the exposure, so that the next time the agent enters the body, the immune system is already prepared to respond and stop the infection.

Researchers are developing vaccines that may encourage the patient's immune system to recognize cancer cells. Cancer vaccines are designed to treat existing cancers (therapeutic vaccines) or to prevent the development of cancer (prophylactic vaccines). Therapeutic vaccines are injected in a person after cancer is diagnosed. These vaccines may stop the growth of existing tumors, prevent cancer from recurring, or eliminate cancer cells not killed by prior treatments. Cancer vaccines given when the tumor is small may be able to eradicate the cancer. On the other hand, prophylactic vaccines are given to healthy individuals before cancer develops. These vaccines are designed to stimulate the immune system to attack viruses that can cause cancer. By targeting these cancer-causing viruses, doctors hope to prevent the development of certain cancers.

Early cancer vaccine clinical trials involved mainly patients with melanoma. Therapeutic vaccines are also being studied in the treatment of many other types of cancer, including lymphoma, leukemia, and cancers of the brain, breast, lung, kidney, ovary, prostate, pancreas, colon, and rectum. Researchers are also studying prophylactic vaccines to prevent cancers of the cervix and liver. Moreover, scientists are investigating ways that cancer vaccines can be used in combination with other BRMs.

What is gene therapy?

Gene therapy is an experimental treatment that involves introducing genetic material into a person's cells to fight disease. Researchers are studying gene therapy methods that can improve a patient's immune response to cancer. For example, a gene may be inserted into an immune cell to enhance its ability to recognize and attack cancer cells. In another approach, scientists inject cancer cells with genes that cause the cancer cells to produce cytokines and stimulate the immune system. A number of clinical trials are currently studying gene therapy and its potential application to the biological treatment of cancer.

What are nonspecific immunomodulating agents?

Nonspecific immunomodulating agents are substances that stimulate or indirectly augment the immune system. Often, these agents target key immune system cells and cause secondary responses such as increased production of cytokines and immunoglobulins. Two nonspecific immunomodulating agents used in cancer treatment are bacillus Calmette-Guerin (BCG) and levamisole.

BCG, which has been widely used as a tuberculosis vaccine, is used in the treatment of superficial bladder cancer following surgery. BCG may work by stimulating an inflammatory, and possibly an immune, response. A solution of BCG is instilled in the bladder and stays there for about two hours before the patient is allowed to empty the bladder by urinating. This treatment is usually performed once a week for six weeks.

Levamisole is sometimes used along with fluorouracil (5-FU) chemotherapy in the treatment of stage III (Dukes-C) colon cancer following surgery. Levamisole may act to restore depressed immune function.

Do biological therapies have any side effects?

Like other forms of cancer treatment, biological therapies can cause a number of side effects, which can vary widely from agent to agent and patient to patient. Rashes or swelling may develop at the site where the BRMs are injected. Several BRMs, including interferons and interleukins, may cause flu-like symptoms including fever, chills, nausea, vomiting, and appetite loss. Fatigue is another common side effect of some BRMs. Blood pressure may also be affected. The side effects of IL-2 can often be severe, depending on the dosage given. Patients need to be closely monitored during treatment with high doses of IL-2. Side effects of CSFs may include bone pain, fatigue, fever, and appetite loss. The side effects of MOABs vary, and serious allergic reactions may occur. Cancer vaccines can cause muscle aches and fever.

Chapter 35

Laser Treatment and Photodynamic Therapy

Lasers in Cancer Treatment

What is laser light?

The term "laser" stands for light amplification by stimulated emission of radiation. Ordinary light, such as that from a light bulb, has many wavelengths and spreads in all directions. Laser light, on the other hand, has a specific wavelength. It is focused in a narrow beam and creates a very high-intensity light. This powerful beam of light may be used to cut through steel or to shape diamonds. Because lasers can focus very accurately on tiny areas, they can also be used for very precise surgical work or for cutting through tissue (in place of a scalpel).

What is laser therapy, and how is it used in cancer treatment?

Laser therapy uses high-intensity light to treat cancer and other illnesses. Lasers can be used to shrink or destroy tumors. Lasers are most commonly used to treat superficial cancers (cancers on the surface of the body or the lining of internal organs) such as basal cell skin cancer and the very early stages of some cancers, such as cervical, penile, vaginal, vulvar, and non-small cell lung cancer.

This chapter includes "Lasers in Cancer Treatment: Questions and Answers," National Cancer Institute (NCI), August 10, 2004, and "Photodynamic Therapy for Cancer," NCI, May 23, 2004.

Lasers also may be used to relieve certain symptoms of cancer, such as bleeding or obstruction. For example, lasers can be used to shrink or destroy a tumor that is blocking a patient's trachea (windpipe) or esophagus. Lasers also can be used to remove colon polyps or tumors that are blocking the colon or stomach.

Laser therapy can be used alone, but most often it is combined with other treatments, such as surgery, chemotherapy, or radiation therapy. In addition, lasers can seal nerve endings to reduce pain after surgery and seal lymph vessels to reduce swelling and limit the spread of tumor cells.

How is laser therapy given to the patient?

Laser therapy is often given through a flexible endoscope (a thin, lighted tube used to look at tissues inside the body). The endoscope is fitted with optical fibers (thin fibers that transmit light). It is inserted through an opening in the body, such as the mouth, nose, anus, or vagina. Laser light is then precisely aimed to cut or destroy a tumor.

Laser-induced interstitial thermotherapy (LITT) (or interstitial laser photocoagulation) also uses lasers to treat some cancers. LITT is similar to a cancer treatment called hyperthermia, which uses heat to shrink tumors by damaging or killing cancer cells. During LITT, an optical fiber is inserted into a tumor. Laser light at the tip of the fiber raises the temperature of the tumor cells and damages or destroys them. LITT is sometimes used to shrink tumors in the liver.

Photodynamic therapy (PDT) is another type of cancer treatment that uses lasers. In PDT, a certain drug, called a photosensitizer or photosensitizing agent, is injected into a patient and absorbed by cells all over the patient's body. After a couple of days, the agent is found mostly in cancer cells. Laser light is then used to activate the agent and destroy cancer cells. Because the photosensitizer makes the skin and eyes sensitive to light for approximately six weeks, patients are advised to avoid direct sunlight and bright indoor light during that time.

What types of lasers are used in cancer treatment?

Three types of lasers are used to treat cancer: carbon dioxide ($CO2$) lasers, argon lasers, and neodymium:yttrium-aluminum-garnet (Nd:YAG) lasers. Each of these can shrink or destroy tumors and can be used with endoscopes. $CO2$ and argon lasers can cut the skin's surface without going into deeper layers. Thus, they can be used to remove superficial cancers, such as skin cancer. In contrast, the Nd:YAG laser is more commonly applied through an endoscope to treat internal organs,

such as the uterus, esophagus, and colon. Nd:YAG laser light can also travel through optical fibers into specific areas of the body during LITT. Argon lasers are often used to activate the drugs used in PDT.

What are the advantages of laser therapy?

Lasers are more precise than standard surgical tools (scalpels), so they do less damage to normal tissues. As a result, patients usually have less pain, bleeding, swelling, and scarring. With laser therapy, operations are usually shorter. In fact, laser therapy can often be done on an outpatient basis. It takes less time for patients to heal after laser surgery, and they are less likely to get infections. Patients should consult with their health care provider about whether laser therapy is appropriate for them.

What are the disadvantages of laser therapy?

Laser therapy also has several limitations. Surgeons must have specialized training before they can do laser therapy, and strict safety precautions must be followed. Also, laser therapy is expensive and requires bulky equipment. In addition, the effects of laser therapy may not last long, so doctors may have to repeat the treatment for a patient to get the full benefit.

What does the future hold for laser therapy?

In clinical trials (research studies), doctors are using lasers to treat cancers of the brain and prostate, among others.

Photodynamic Therapy for Cancer

Photodynamic therapy (PDT) is a treatment that uses a drug, called a photosensitizer or photosensitizing agent, and a particular type of light. When photosensitizers are exposed to a specific wavelength of light, they produce a form of oxygen that kills nearby cells.

Each photosensitizer is activated by light of a specific wavelength. This wavelength determines how far the light can travel into the body. Thus, doctors use specific photosensitizers and wavelengths of light to treat different areas of the body with PDT.

How is PDT used to treat cancer?

In the first step of PDT for cancer treatment, a photosensitizing agent is injected into the bloodstream. The agent is absorbed by cells all over

the body but stays in cancer cells longer than it does in normal cells. Approximately 24 to 72 hours after injection, when most of the agent has left normal cells but remains in cancer cells, the tumor is exposed to light. The photosensitizer in the tumor absorbs the light and produces an active form of oxygen that destroys nearby cancer cells.

In addition to directly killing cancer cells, PDT appears to shrink or destroy tumors in two other ways. The photosensitizer can damage blood vessels in the tumor, thereby preventing the cancer from receiving necessary nutrients. In addition, PDT may activate the immune system to attack the tumor cells.

The light used for PDT can come from a laser or other sources of light. Laser light can be directed through fiber optic cables (thin fibers that transmit light) to deliver light to areas inside the body. For example, a fiber optic cable can be inserted through an endoscope (a thin, lighted tube used to look at tissues inside the body) into the lungs or esophagus to treat cancer in these organs. Other light sources include light-emitting diodes (LEDs), which may be used for surface tumors, such as skin cancer.

PDT is usually performed as an outpatient procedure. PDT may also be repeated and may be used with other therapies, such as surgery, radiation, or chemotherapy.

What types of cancer are currently treated with PDT?

To date, the U.S. Food and Drug Administration (FDA) has approved the photosensitizing agent called porfimer sodium, or Photofrin®, for use in PDT to treat or relieve the symptoms of esophageal cancer and non-small cell lung cancer. Porfimer sodium is approved to relieve symptoms of esophageal cancer when the cancer obstructs the esophagus or when the cancer cannot be satisfactorily treated with laser therapy alone. Porfimer sodium is used to treat non-small cell lung cancer in patients for whom the usual treatments are not appropriate, and to relieve symptoms in patients with non-small cell lung cancer that obstructs the airways. In 2003, the FDA approved porfimer sodium for the treatment of precancerous lesions in patients with Barrett esophagus (a condition that can lead to esophageal cancer).

What are the limitations of PDT?

The light needed to activate most photosensitizers cannot pass through more than about one-third of an inch of tissue (one centimeter). For this reason, PDT is usually used to treat tumors on or just under the skin or on the lining of internal organs or cavities. PDT is

also less effective in treating large tumors, because the light cannot pass far into these tumors. PDT is a local treatment and generally cannot be used to treat cancer that has spread (metastasized).

Does PDT have any complications or side effects?

Porfimer sodium makes the skin and eyes sensitive to light for approximately six weeks after treatment. Thus, patients are advised to avoid direct sunlight and bright indoor light for at least six weeks.

Photosensitizers tend to build up in tumors and the activating light is focused on the tumor. As a result, damage to healthy tissue is minimal. However, PDT can cause burns, swelling, pain, and scarring in nearby healthy tissue. Other side effects of PDT are related to the area that is treated. They can include coughing, trouble swallowing, stomach pain, painful breathing, or shortness of breath; these side effects are usually temporary.

What does the future hold for PDT?

Researchers continue to study ways to improve the effectiveness of PDT and expand it to other cancers. Clinical trials (research studies) are under way to evaluate the use of PDT for cancers of the brain, skin, prostate, cervix, and peritoneal cavity (the space in the abdomen that contains the intestines, stomach, and liver). Other research is focused on the development of photosensitizers that are more powerful, more specifically target cancer cells, and are activated by light that can penetrate tissue and treat deep or large tumors. Researchers are also investigating ways to improve equipment and the delivery of the activating light.

Chapter 36

If You Are Considering Complementary and Alternative Medicine Treatments for Cancer

Many Choices

You have many choices to make before, during, and after your cancer treatment. One choice you may be thinking about is complementary and alternative medicine. We call this CAM, for short. People with cancer may use CAM for several reasons:

- Help cope with the side effects of cancer treatments, such as nausea, pain, and fatigue

- Comfort themselves and ease the worries of cancer treatment and related stress

- Feel that they are doing something more to help with their own care

- Try to treat or cure their cancer

It's natural to want to fight your cancer in any way you can. There is a lot of information available, and new methods for treating cancer are always being tested, so it may be hard to know where to start.

This chapter may help you understand what you find and make it easier to decide whether CAM is right for you. Many people try CAM therapies during cancer care. CAM does not work for everyone, but

---

"Thinking about Complementary and Alternative Medicine," National Cancer Institute (www.cancer.gov), June 2005.

some methods may help you manage stress, nausea, pain, or other symptoms or side effects.

The most important message of this chapter is to talk to your doctor before you try anything new. This will help ensure that nothing gets in the way of your cancer treatment.

What Is (CAM)?

CAM is any medical system, practice, or product that is not thought of as standard care. Standard medical care is care that is based on scientific evidence. For cancer, it includes chemotherapy, radiation, biological therapy, and surgery.

Complementary Medicine

Complementary medicine is used along with standard medical treatments. One example is using acupuncture to help with side effects of cancer treatment.

Alternative Medicine

Alternative medicine is used in place of standard medical treatments. One example is using a special diet to treat cancer instead of a method that a cancer specialist (an oncologist) suggests.

Integrative Medicine

Integrative medicine is a total approach to care that involves the patient's mind, body, and spirit. It combines standard medicine with the CAM practices that have shown the most promise. For example, some people learn to use relaxation as a way to reduce stress during chemotherapy.

Types of CAM

We are learning about CAM therapies every day, but there is still more to learn. Consumers may use the terms "natural," "holistic," "home remedy," or "Eastern medicine" to refer to CAM. However, experts use five categories to describe it. These are listed below with a few examples for each.

Mind-Body Medicines

These are based on the belief that your mind is able to affect your body. Some examples include the following:

- **Meditation:** Focused breathing or repetition of words or phrases to quiet the mind

- **Biofeedback:** Using simple machines, the patient learns how to affect certain body functions that are normally out of one's awareness (such as heart rate)

- **Hypnosis:** A state of relaxed and focused attention in which the patient concentrates on a certain feeling, idea, or suggestion to aid in healing

- **Yoga:** Systems of stretches and poses, with special attention given to breathing

- **Imagery:** Imagining scenes, pictures, or experiences to help the body heal

- **Creative outlets:** Such as art, music, or dance

Biologically Based Practices

This type of CAM uses things found in nature. This includes dietary supplements and herbal products. Some examples are vitamins, herbs, foods, and special diets.

A note about nutrition: It's common for people with cancer to have questions about different foods to eat during treatment. Yet it's important to know that there is no one food or special diet that has been proven to control cancer. Too much of any one food is not helpful, and may even be harmful. Because of nutrition needs you may have, it's best to talk with the doctor in charge of your treatment about the foods you should be eating.

Manipulative and Body-Based Practices

These are based on working with one or more parts of the body. Some examples include the following:

- **Massage:** Manipulation of tissues with hands or special tools

- **Chiropractic care:** A type of manipulation of the joints and skeletal system

- **Reflexology:** Using pressure points in the hands or feet to affect other parts of the body

Energy Medicine

Energy medicine involves the belief that the body has energy fields that can be used for healing and wellness. Therapists use pressure or

move the body by placing their hands in or through these fields. Some examples include the following:

- **Tai chi:** Involves slow, gentle movements with a focus on the breath and concentration

- **Reiki:** Balancing energy either from a distance or by placing hands on or near the patient

- **Therapeutic touch:** Moving hands over energy fields of the body

Whole Medical Systems

These are healing systems and beliefs that have evolved over time in different cultures and parts of the world. Some examples include the following:

- **Ayurvedic medicine:** A system from India emphasizing balance among body, mind, and spirit

- **Chinese medicine:** Based on the view that health is a balance in the body of two forces called yin and yang. Acupuncture is a common practice in Chinese medicine that involves stimulating specific points on the body to promote health, or to lessen disease symptoms and treatment side effects

- **Homeopathy:** Uses very small doses of substances to trigger the body to heal itself

- **Naturopathic medicine:** Uses different methods that help the body naturally heal itself

Talk with Your Doctor Before You Use CAM

Some people with cancer are afraid that their doctor won't understand or approve of the use of CAM. But doctors know that people with cancer want to take an active part in their care. They want the best for their patients and often are willing to work with them.

Talk to your doctor to make sure that all aspects of your cancer care work together. This is important because things that seem safe, such as certain foods or pills, may interfere with your cancer treatment.

Questions to Ask Your Doctor about CAM

- What types of CAM might help me cope, reduce my stress, and feel better?

- What types of CAM might help me feel less tired?
- What types of CAM might help me deal with cancer symptoms, such as pain, or side effects of treatment, such as nausea?

If you decide to try a CAM therapy, ask your doctor about the following

- Will it interfere with my treatment or medicines?
- Can you help me understand these articles I found about CAM?
- Can you suggest a CAM practitioner for me to talk to?
- Will you work with my CAM practitioner?

"Natural" Does Not Mean "Safe"

Here are some important facts about dietary supplements such as herbs and vitamins.

They may affect how well other medicines work in your body. Herbs and some plant-based products may keep medicines from doing what they are supposed to do. These medicines can be ones your doctor prescribes for you, or even ones you buy off the shelf at the store. For example, the herb St. John's wort, which some people with cancer use for depression, may cause certain anticancer drugs not to work as well as they should.

Herbal supplements can act like drugs in your body. They may be harmful when taken by themselves, with other substances, or in large doses. For example, some studies have shown that kava, an herb that has been used to help with stress and anxiety, may cause liver damage.

Vitamins can also take strong action in your body. For example, high doses of vitamins, even vitamin C, may affect how chemotherapy and radiation work. Too much of any vitamin is not safe—even in a healthy person.

Tell your doctor if you are taking any dietary supplements, no matter how safe you think they are. This is very important. Even though there are ads or claims that something has been used for years, they do not prove that it is safe or effective. It is still important to be careful.

Supplements do not have to be approved by the federal government before being sold to the public. Also, a prescription is not needed to buy them. Therefore, it's up to consumers to decide what is best for them.

Choose Practitioners with Care

CAM practitioners are people who have training in CAM therapies. Choosing one should be done with the same care as choosing a doctor. Here are some things to remember when choosing a practitioner:

- Ask your doctor or nurse to suggest someone or speak with someone who knows about CAM.

- Ask whether someone at your cancer center or doctor's office can help you find a CAM practitioner. There may be a social worker or physical therapist who can help you.

- Ask whether your hospital keeps lists of centers or has staff who can suggest people.

- Contact CAM professional organizations to get names of practitioners who are certified. This means that they have proper training in their field.

- Contact local health and wellness organizations.

- Ask about each practitioner's training and experience.

- Ask whether the practitioner has a license to practice in your state. If you want to confirm the answer, ask what organization gives out the licenses. Then, you may choose to follow up with a phone call.

- Call your health care plan to see if it covers this therapy.

General Questions to Ask the CAM Practitioner

- What types of CAM do you practice?

- What are your training and qualifications?

- Do you see other patients with my type of cancer?

- Will you work with my doctor?

Questions to Ask about the Therapy

- How can this help me?

- Do you know of studies that prove it helps?

- What are the risks and side effects?

- Will this interfere with my cancer treatment?

- How long will I be on the therapy?
- What will it cost?
- Do you have information that I can read about it?
- Are there any reasons why I should not use it?

Other Questions to Ask Yourself

- Do I feel comfortable with this person?
- Do I like how the office looks and feels?
- Do I like the staff?
- Does this person support standard cancer treatments?
- How far am I willing to travel for treatment?
- Is it easy to get an appointment?
- Are the hours good for me?
- Will insurance cover the cost of CAM?

Call your health plan or insurer to see whether they cover CAM therapies. Many are not covered.

Getting Information from Trusted Sources

Government Agencies

There is a lot of information on CAM, so it's important to go to sources you can trust. Good places to start are the government agencies listed in the back of this booklet. They offer lots of information about CAM that might be helpful to you. They may also know of universities or hospitals that have CAM resources.

Be careful of products advertised by people or companies with these characteristics:

- Make claims that they have a "cure"
- Do not give specific information about how well their product works
- Make claims only about positive results that have few side effects
- Say they have clinical studies, but provide no proof or copies of the studies

Just remember, if it sounds too good to be true, it probably is. For ways to find out more about CAM, see the resources section.

Websites

Patients and families have been able to find answers to many of their questions about CAM on the internet. Many websites are good resources for CAM information. However, some may be unreliable or misleading. Here are some questions to ask about a website:

- Who runs and pays for the site?

- Does it list any credentials?

- Does it represent an organization that is well-known and respected?

- What is the purpose of the site, and who is it for?

- Is the site selling or promoting something?

- Where does the information come from?

- Is the information based on facts or only on someone's feelings or opinions?

- How is the information chosen? Is there a review board or is the content reviewed by experts?

- How current is the information?

- Does the site tell when it was last updated?

- How does the site choose which other sites to link you to?

Books

A number of books have been written about different CAM therapies. Some books are better than others and contain trustworthy content, while others do not.

If you go to the library, ask the staff for suggestions. Or if you live near a college or university, there may be a medical library available. Local bookstores may also have people on staff who can help you.

It's important to know that information is always changing and that new research results are reported every day. Be aware that if a book is written by only one person, you may only be getting that one person's view.

Here are some questions to ask about books:

- Is the author an expert on this subject?

- Do you know anyone else who has read the book?
- Has the book been reviewed by other experts?
- Was it published in the past five years?
- Does the book offer different points of view, or does it seem to hold one opinion?
- Has the author researched the topic in full?
- Are the references listed in the back?

Magazine Articles

If you want to look for articles you can trust, ask your librarian to help you look for medical journals, books, and other research that has been done by experts.

Articles in popular magazines are usually not written by experts. Rather, the authors speak with experts, gather information, and then write the article. If claims about CAM are made in magazine articles, remember the following points:

- The authors may not have expert knowledge in this area.
- They may not say where they found their information.
- The articles have not been reviewed by experts.
- The publisher may have ties to advertisers or other organizations. Therefore, the article may be one-sided.

When you read these articles, you can use the same process that the magazine writer uses:

- Speak with experts.
- Ask lots of questions.
- Then decide if the therapy is right for you.

Chapter 37

Cancer Clinical Trials

What Is a Clinical Trial?

Clinical trials are research studies in which people help doctors find ways to improve health and cancer care. Each study tries to answer scientific questions and to find better ways to prevent, diagnose, or treat cancer.

A clinical trial is one of the final stages of a long and careful cancer research process. Studies are done with cancer patients to find out whether promising approaches to cancer prevention, diagnosis, and treatment are safe and effective.

Treatment trials test new treatments (like a new cancer drug, new approaches to surgery or radiation therapy, new combinations of treatments, or new methods such as gene therapy). Prevention trials test new approaches, such as medicines, vitamins, minerals, or other supplements that doctors believe may lower the risk of a certain type of cancer. These trials look for the best way to prevent cancer in people who have never had cancer or to prevent cancer from coming back or a new cancer occurring in people who have already had cancer. Screening trials test the best way to find cancer, especially in its early stages. Quality of life trials (also called supportive care trials) explore ways to improve comfort and quality of life for cancer patients.

From "What Is a Clinical Trial?" National Cancer Institute (NCI), April 8, 2008, and "How to Find a Cancer Treatment Trial: A 10-Step Guide," NCI, May 8, 2009.

Phases of Clinical Trials

Most clinical research that involves the testing of a new drug progresses in an orderly series of steps, called phases. This allows researchers to ask and answer questions in a way that results in reliable information about the drug and protects the patients. Most clinical trials are classified into one of three phases:

- **Phase I trials:** These first studies in people evaluate how a new drug should be given (by mouth, injected into the blood, or injected into the muscle), how often, and what dose is safe. A phase I trial usually enrolls only a small number of patients, sometimes as few as a dozen.

- **Phase II trials:** A phase II trial continues to test the safety of the drug, and begins to evaluate how well the new drug works. Phase II studies usually focus on a particular type of cancer.

- **Phase III trials:** These studies test a new drug, a new combination of drugs, or a new surgical procedure in comparison to the current standard. A participant will usually be assigned to the standard group or the new group at random (called randomization). Phase III trials often enroll large numbers of people and may be conducted at many doctors' offices, clinics, and cancer centers nationwide.

In addition, after a treatment has been approved and is being marketed, the drug's maker may study it further in a phase IV trial. The purpose of phase IV trials is to evaluate the side effects, risks, and benefits of a drug over a longer period of time and in a larger number of people than in phase III clinical trials. Thousands of people are involved in a phase IV trial.

How to Find a Cancer Treatment Trial

This information will help you to look for a cancer treatment clinical trial that might benefit you. It will help you to gather the information you need to begin your search for a clinical trial, identify sources of clinical trial listings, learn about clinical trials that may be of benefit to you, and ask questions that will help you decide whether or not to participate in a particular trial. It is not intended to provide medical advice. You, your health care team, and your loved ones are in the best position to decide whether a clinical trial is right for you.

A Word about Timing

Many treatment trials will only take patients who have not yet been treated for their condition. Researchers conducting these trials are hoping to find an improved "first-line" treatment option for that type of cancer.

If you are newly diagnosed with cancer, the time to consider joining a clinical trial is before you've had surgery, chemotherapy, radiation, or other forms of treatment (tests to diagnose your cancer are okay). However, don't delay treatment if waiting could harm you. Talk with your doctor about how quickly you need to make a treatment decision.

If you have received one or more forms of treatment and are looking for a new treatment option, there also are many clinical trial options for you. You may want to look for trials that are testing a new follow-up treatment that may prevent the return of your cancer. Or, if your first treatment failed to work, you may want to look for trials of new "second-line" or even "third-line" treatments.

Step 1: Before You Start

This guide assumes you already know what clinical trials are and why you might want to join one. If you need to, review your understanding of clinical trials before you continue the steps in this guide.

Step 2: Talk with Your Doctor

When considering clinical trials, your best starting point is your doctor and other members of your health care team. Your primary care physician, cancer doctor (oncologist), surgeon, or other health care provider might know about a clinical trial you should consider. He or she can help you determine whether a clinical trial might be a good option.

In some cases, your doctor may be reluctant to discuss clinical trials as a treatment option for you. Some doctors are unfamiliar with clinical trials, cautious about turning your care over to another medical team, or wary of the extra time that joining a clinical trial might require of them and their staff. If so, you may wish to get a second opinion about your treatment options and clinical trials. Remember, you do not always need a referral from your doctor to join a clinical trial.

If you are eligible to join a trial (discussed in Step 3), the final decision is up to you. However, be sure to consider the professional opinions of your doctor. He or she may present very specific reasons why a clinical trial may not be beneficial for you right now.

471

Step 3: Complete the Diagnosis Checklist

Before you begin looking for a clinical trial, you must know certain details about your cancer diagnosis. You will need to compare these details with the eligibility criteria of any trial in which you are interested. Eligibility criteria are the guidelines for who can and cannot participate in a particular study.

To help you gather the details of your diagnosis so you will know which trials you may be eligible to join, complete the "Diagnosis Checklist" found at the end of this chapter. The checklist asks questions about your diagnosis. [If you would rather print out a version of the form that has the questions with space for your answers, you can go to the website www.cancer.gov/clinicaltrials/finding/treatment-trial-guide/page15 and click on the print link. Or, if you prefer, you can download a print version of this entire guide from http://www.cancer.gov/clinical-trials/finding/treatment-trial-guide-pdf.] After you have written down the answers to the questions, keep this information with you during your search for a clinical trial.

To get the information you need to answer the questions ask a nurse or social worker at your doctor's office for help. Explain to them that you are interested in looking for a clinical trial that may benefit you and that you need these details before starting to look. They will be able to review your medical records and help you.

Step 4: Search the PDQ® Clinical Trials Database

There are many nonprofit and for-profit resources in the United States that offer lists of cancer clinical trials. Unfortunately, no single list is complete. Clinical trials are run by many different organizations, so it is hard to collect information about all of them in one place. Furthermore, it is important to understand the possible biases and limitations of any clinical trials website.

However, the majority of trials listed in most resources are obtained from the Physician Data Query (PDQ) clinical trials database, which is maintained by the U.S. National Cancer Institute (NCI). The NCI is the U.S. government's chief agency for cancer research and is part of the National Institutes of Health. The PDQ clinical trials database contains a list of more than 2,000 cancer clinical trials worldwide. You can find details about how to search the database below.

The U.S. National Library of Medicine maintains a database called ClinicalTrials.gov that includes trials for many diseases and conditions, including cancer. The PDQ and ClinicalTrials.gov databases contain the same cancer treatment trial listings. The main difference

is in how information is searched and displayed. You may prefer one way over another.

Get a Copy of the Protocol Summary

Steps 4 and 5 describe where to look for cancer clinical trials. Whichever resource you use, be sure to get a copy of the protocol summary for each trial you are interested in. What is a protocol? It is the action plan for the trial. The protocol explains what will be done in the trial, how, and why. The protocol should also list the location(s) where the trial will enroll participants. Both PDQ and ClinicalTrials.gov (Step 4) provide detailed summaries of the official protocols for each trial listed on their Web sites. Other resources (Step 5) may or may not provide protocol summaries.

How to Search PDQ

You can search PDQ by telephone. Make a free telephone call—in English or Spanish—within the United States to the National Cancer Institute's Cancer Information Service (CIS) at 800-4-CANCER (800-422-6237). All calls to the CIS are strictly confidential. When you call the CIS, be ready with the details of your Diagnosis Checklist from Step 3.

The CIS is staffed with understanding and knowledgeable information specialists who will search PDQ for you. They can send you the search results and protocol summaries by e-mail, fax, or regular mail. The CIS can also provide you with reliable information about your type of cancer and the current standard therapy for treating it.

You can also look for trials yourself using the PDQ search form on the NCI website. You can find it online at www.cancer.gov/clinicaltrials. Remember to print out the protocol summaries for each trial you may be interested in.

If you would like help searching PDQ while you're online, consider using LiveHelp. Through LiveHelp, you can communicate confidentially and in real time with a CIS information specialist from the National Cancer Institute. The service is available Monday through Friday from 9:00 a.m. to 11:00 p.m. Eastern time.

Step 5: Search Other Resources

While PDQ and ClinicalTrials.gov have the most complete listing of cancer trials, you might want to check a few other resources, as well. Why? Because some may include a few trials not found in the federal databases or you may prefer their way of assisting you in your search.

TrialCheck®

TrialCheck (www.cancertrialshelp.org/trialcheck) is operated and maintained by the Coalition of Cancer Cooperative Groups (CCCG). The CCCG is made up of groups of doctors and other health professionals that carry out many of the large cancer clinical trials in the United States funded by the National Cancer Institute.

TrialCheck maintains comprehensive data on thousands of cancer clinical trials and contains a copyrighted cancer clinical trials screening questionnaire that will identify trials appropriate for a patient's individual medical condition. The TrialCheck Frequently Asked Questions (FAQs) page (at http://www.cancertrialshelp.org/trialcheck/default .aspx?intAppMode=11) provides helpful information about how to use TrialCheck.

Third-Party Clinical Trial Websites

There are a number of clinical trial websites that are not operated by funders, sponsors, or the organizations carrying out the trials. Some of these websites are operated by private companies—these may be funded through fees that industry sponsors pay to have their trials listed or according to how many participants the website refers to them. Keep the following points in mind:

- Most third-party clinical trials websites list or link to trials in PDQ or ClinicalTrials.gov.

- They may include a few more trials than you'll find in the federal databases, but they may also include fewer.

- Unlike the federal databases, these sites may not regularly update their content or links.

- Unlike the federal databases, these sites might require you to register to search for trials or to obtain contact information about the trials that interest you.

Industry-Sponsored Cancer Trials

Pharmaceutical and biotechnology companies sponsor many of the cancer clinical trials being carried out in the United States. Some of these trials are listed in the federal databases (PDQ and ClinicalTrials .gov), but many are not.

Federal law requires that U.S. researchers submit to ClinicalTrials.gov all phase II, III, and IV trials of therapies for serious or life-threatening

illnesses (including cancer) conducted as part of the approval process overseen by the U.S. Food and Drug Administration. However, this law is difficult to enforce and for business reasons, some drug companies have preferred to keep details about their clinical trials from the public.

If you are aware of an experimental cancer treatment and know the company that manufactures it, search the internet to find the website of the company. Find the company's customer service telephone number. When you call, ask to speak to the company's clinical trials department. Tell them you are looking for a trial that you might be eligible to join.

Cancer Advocacy Groups

Cancer advocacy groups work on behalf of people diagnosed with cancer and their loved ones. They provide education, support, financial assistance, and advocacy to help patients and families who are dealing with cancer. These organizations recognize that clinical trials are important to the cancer treatment process and, thus, work to educate and empower people to find information and access to treatment.

Because they work hard to know about the latest research advances in cancer treatment, these groups will sometimes have information about certain key government-sponsored trials, as well as some potentially significant trials sponsored by pharmaceutical companies or cancer care centers.

Contact the advocacy group for the type of cancer you are interested in and ask what they can tell you about ongoing clinical trials. The nonprofit Marti Nelson Cancer Foundation maintains a partial list of such groups on its CancerActionNow.org website.

Fee-Based Private Search Services

A number of private services will, for a fee, locate clinical trials for you. While having someone search for you may ease your stress, it is important to keep in mind that several of the resources mentioned earlier in this guide provide elements of this kind of service for free. Also, be sure to ask the following questions:

- What list or lists of clinical trials does the service search? Are those lists likely to provide you with an unbiased and largely complete source of options?

- Does the service receive any money for directing patients to certain trials or for including certain trials in their list?

Step 6: Make a List of Potential Trials

At this point you have created a Diagnosis Checklist, identified one or more trials you might be interested in, and obtained a protocol summary for each one. Now it's time to take a closer look at the protocol summaries you have obtained for the trials you're interested in. You should remove from your list those trials you aren't actually able to join and come up with one or more top possibilities.

What follows are some key questions to consider about each trial. However, don't worry if you cannot answer all of these questions just yet. The idea is to narrow the list if you can, but don't give up on one that you're not sure of.

Ideally, you should consult your doctor during this process, especially if you find the protocol summaries difficult to understand. But you can probably do Step 6 yourself if the protocol summary is relatively complete and easy to understand.

- **Trial objective:** What is the main purpose of the trial? Is it to improve your chances of a cure? To slow the rate at which your cancer may grow or return? To lessen the severity of treatment side effects? To establish whether a new treatment is safe and well tolerated? Read this information carefully to learn whether the trial's main objective matches your goals for treatment.

- **Eligibility criteria:** Do your diagnosis and current overall state of health match the eligibility criteria (sometimes referred to as enrollment or entry criteria)? This may tell you whether you could qualify for the trial. If you're not sure, keep the trial on your list for now.

- **Trial location:** Is the location of the clinical trial manageable for you? Some trials are available at more than one site. Look carefully at how often you will need to receive treatment during the course of the trial, and decide how far and how often you are willing to travel. You will also need to ask if the sponsoring organization will provide for some or all of your travel expenses.

- **Study duration:** How long will the study run? Not all protocol summaries list this information. If they do, consider the time commitment and whether it will work for you and your family.

If, after considering these questions, you are still interested in one or more of the clinical trials you have found, then you are ready for Step 7.

Step 7: Contact the Clinical Trial Team

There are several ways to contact the Clinical Trial Team.

You can contact the trial team directly. The protocol summary should include the name and telephone number of someone you can contact for more information. You do not need to talk to the lead researcher (called the "protocol chair" or "principal investigator") at this time, even if that is the name that is included with the telephone number. Instead, call the number and ask to speak with the "trial coordinator," the "referral coordinator," or the "protocol assistant." This person can answer questions from potential patients and their doctors. It is also this person's job to determine whether you are likely to be eligible to join the trial. (A final determination would be made only after you had gone in for a first appointment.)

You can ask your doctor or other health care team member to contact the trial team for you. Because the clinical trial coordinator will ask questions related to your diagnosis, you may want to ask your doctor or someone else on your health care team to contact the clinical trial team for you.

The trial team may contact you. If you have used some a third-party website and identified a trial that interests you, you may have provided your name, phone number, and e-mail address so that the clinical trial team can contact you.

You will need to refer to your Diagnosis Checklist (Step 3) during the conversation, so keep that handy.

Step 8: Ask Questions about the Trial

Whether you or someone from your health care team calls the clinical trial coordinator, this is the time to get answers to questions that will help you decide whether or not to join this particular clinical trial.

It will be helpful if you can talk about your diagnosis in a manner that is brief and to the point. Before you make the call, rehearse with a family member or friend how you will present the key details of your diagnosis. This will make you more comfortable when you are talking with the clinical trial coordinator and will enable you to answer his or her questions smoothly.

Here are some questions to ask the trial coordinator:

Is the trial still open?

On occasion, clinical trial listings will be out-of-date and will include trials that have actually closed to further enrollment.

Am I eligible for this trial?

The trial coordinator will ask you many, if not all, of the questions listed on your Diagnosis Checklist (Step 3). This is the time to confirm that you are indeed a candidate for this trial, although a final decision will likely await your first appointment with the clinical trial team (Step 10).

Why do researchers think the new treatment might be effective?

Results from earlier clinical trials will highlight the potential effectiveness of the treatment you may receive. The strength of the earlier evidence may influence your decision. You or someone who knows how to read the medical literature may also want to use a web-based service such as PubMed to explore any previously published evidence related to the trial you're interested in.

What are the risks and benefits associated with the treatments I may receive?

Every treatment has risks. Be sure you understand what risks and side-effects are associated with any of the treatments you might receive as a participant in this trial. Likewise, ask for a detailed description of how the treatments may benefit you.

Who will monitor my care and safety?

Primary responsibility for the care and safety of patients in a cancer clinical trial rests with the clinical trial health care team. In addition, clinical trials are governed by safety and ethical regulations set by the federal government and the institution or organization sponsoring and carrying out the trial, including a group called the Institutional Review Board (IRB). The trial coordinator will be able to give you more information.

May I get a copy of the protocol document?

In some cases, the trial coordinator may be allowed to release the full, detailed protocol document to you. However, the protocol summary and the informed consent document will probably answer most of your questions about the trial's design and intention.

May I get a copy of the informed consent document?

The U.S. Food and Drug Administration requires that potential participants receive complete information about the study. This process is

known as "informed consent" and must be in writing. It may be helpful to see a copy of this document before you decide whether or not to join the trial.

Is there a chance I will receive a placebo?

Placebos are rarely used in cancer treatment trials, but be sure you understand what possible treatments you may or may not receive for any trial you are thinking of joining.

Is the trial randomized?

In a randomized clinical trial, participants are assigned, by chance, to separate groups or "arms." Each arm receives a different treatment, and the results are compared. In a randomized trial, you may or may not receive the new treatment.

What is the treatment dose and schedule in each arm of the trial?

You will want to consider this when you are discussing your various treatment options with your health care team. Does the dose seem reasonable? Is the treatment schedule manageable for you?

What costs will I be responsible for?

In many cases, the research costs are paid by the group sponsoring the trial. Research costs include the treatments under study and any test performed purely for research purposes. However, you or your insurance plan would be responsible for paying "routine patient care costs." These are the costs of medical care (for example, doctor visits, hospital stays, x-rays) that you would receive whether or not you were in a clinical trial. Some insurance plans don't cover these costs once you join a trial. Consult your health plan, if you have one.

If I have to travel, who will pay for travel and lodging?

Some trials may pay for your travel and lodging expenses. Otherwise, you will be responsible for these costs.

Will participation in this trial require more time than if I had elected to receive standard care? Will participation require a hospital stay?

Understanding how much time is involved may influence your decision and help you make plans.

How will participating in the clinical trial affect my everyday life?

A cancer diagnosis can be very disrupting to the routine of everyday life. Many patients seek to keep those routines intact as they deal with their diagnosis and treatment. This information will be useful in evaluating any additional help you may need at home.

Step 9: Discuss Your Options with Your Doctor

To make a final decision, you will want to know the possible risks and benefits of all the various treatment options open to you. You may decide that joining a trial for which you are eligible is your best option, or you may decide not to join a trial. It is your choice.

Step 10: If You Want to Join a Trial, Schedule an Appointment

If you decide to participate in a clinical trial for which you are eligible, schedule an appointment with the trial coordinator you spoke to during Step 8.

You might also want your doctor to contact the study's principal investigator to further discuss your medical history and overall current state of your health. The principal investigator's name should be listed in the protocol summary.

Your doctor might disagree with your decision to participate in a clinical trial. If so, be sure you understand his or her concerns. You also may wish to seek a second opinion about your treatment options at this time. Ultimately, it is up to you to decide what treatment is in your best interest.

Diagnosis Checklist

The following questions should be included in your Diagnosis Checklist before you start looking for a clinical trial. The checklist will help you know which clinical trials you are eligible to join. See Step 3 for details about how to obtain the information you need for the checklist.

If you would like to download the PDF version of this guide and save it to your own computer, go to http://www.cancer.gov/clinicaltrials/finding/treatment-trial-guide-pdf. Then you can print it out and fill in the answers to these questions to keep for later use.

1. What kind of cancer do you have?

Write down the full medical name.

2. Where did the cancer first start?

Many cancers spread to the bones, liver, or elsewhere. However, the type of cancer you have is determined by where it first showed up. For example, breast cancer that spreads to the bone is still breast cancer.

3. What is the cancer's cell type?

This information will be in your pathology report.

4. If there's a solid tumor, what size is it?

5. If there is a solid tumor, where is it located?

If the tumor has spread, list all locations.

6. What stage is the cancer?

The stage describes the extent of cancer in the body and whether it has spread from the original site. There are different staging systems for different cancers.

7. Have you had cancer before, different from the one you have now?

If so, answer questions 1–6 for the other cancer, as well.

8. What is your current performance status?

An assessment from your doctor indicating how well you are able to perform ordinary tasks and carry out daily activities.

9. If you have not yet had any treatment for cancer, what treatment(s) have been recommended to you?

10. If you have had treatment(s) for cancer, what treatments have you had (for example: type of surgery, chemotherapy, immunotherapy, or radiation)?

11. Bone marrow function? (blood tests that check whether your blood count is normal)

- White blood cell count
- Platelet count
- Hemoglobin/hematocrit

12. Liver function? (blood tests that check whether your liver function is normal)

- Bilirubin
- Transaminases

13. Renal function? (blood test that checks whether your kidney function is normal)

- Serum creatinine

Part Six

Coping with the
Side Effects of Cancer and
Cancer Treatments

Chapter 38

Nausea and Vomiting

Overview

Nausea is an unpleasant wavelike feeling in the back of the throat and/or stomach that may or may not result in vomiting. Vomiting is the forceful elimination of the contents of the stomach through the mouth. Retching is the movement of the stomach and esophagus without vomiting and is also called dry heaves. Although treatments have improved, nausea and vomiting continue to be worrisome side effects of cancer therapy. Nausea may be even more distressing for patients than vomiting.

It is very important to prevent and control nausea and vomiting in patients with cancer. Uncontrolled nausea and vomiting can interfere with the patient's ability to receive cancer treatment and care for himself or herself by causing chemical changes in the body, loss of appetite, physical and mental difficulties, a torn esophagus, broken bones, and the reopening of surgical wounds.

Nausea and vomiting that are caused by cancer therapy are classified as acute, delayed, anticipatory, or chronic.

- **Acute nausea and vomiting:** Usually occurs within 24 hours after beginning chemotherapy.

- **Delayed nausea and vomiting:** Occurs more than 24 hours after chemotherapy. Also called late nausea and vomiting.

From PDQ® Cancer Information Summary. National Cancer Institute; Bethesda, MD. "Nausea and Vomiting (PDQ®): Patient Version." Updated 10/2009. Available at http://cancer.gov. Accessed April 27, 2010.

- **Anticipatory nausea and vomiting:** If a patient has had nausea and vomiting after the previous three or four chemotherapy treatments, he or she may experience anticipatory nausea and vomiting. The smells, sights, and sounds of the treatment room may remind the patient of previous episodes and may trigger nausea and vomiting before a new cycle of chemotherapy (or radiation therapy) has even begun.

- **Chronic nausea and vomiting:** May affect people who have advanced cancer. It is not well understood.

Studies strongly suggest that patients receiving chemotherapy experience more acute and delayed nausea and vomiting than is estimated by health care providers.

Causes

Nausea is controlled by a part of the central nervous system that controls involuntary bodily functions. Vomiting is a reflex controlled by a vomiting center in the brain. Vomiting can be stimulated by various triggers, such as smell, taste, anxiety, pain, motion, poor blood flow, irritation, or changes in the body caused by inflammation.

The most common causes of nausea and vomiting are chemotherapy drugs and radiation therapy directed at the gastrointestinal (GI) tract, liver, or brain. Nausea and vomiting are more likely to occur if the patient experienced severe episodes of nausea and vomiting after past chemotherapy sessions. Nausea and vomiting are also more likely to occur if the patient is female, younger than 50 years, has a fluid and/or electrolyte imbalance (hypercalcemia, dehydration, or an excess of fluid in the body's tissues), or has a tumor in the GI tract, liver, or brain. Other factors that make nausea and vomiting more likely are if the patient has constipation, is receiving certain drugs, has an infection or blood poisoning, has kidney disease, or experiences anxiety.

Anticipatory Nausea and Vomiting

Anticipatory nausea and vomiting occur after the patient has undergone several cancer treatments. It occurs in response to triggers, such as odors in the therapy room. For example, a person who begins chemotherapy and smells an alcohol swab at the same time, may later experience nausea and vomiting at the smell of alcohol alone. Patients usually do not experience nausea and/or vomiting before or during

chemotherapy until after they have received several courses of treatment. The following factors may help predict which patients are more likely to experience anticipatory nausea and vomiting:

- Being younger than 50 years
- Being female
- The severity of nausea and vomiting after the last chemotherapy session
- Feeling warm or hot after the last chemotherapy session
- A history of motion sickness
- Feeling dizzy or lightheaded after chemotherapy
- Sweating after the last chemotherapy session
- Experiencing weakness after the last chemotherapy session
- Having a high level of anxiety
- The type of chemotherapy (some are more likely to cause nausea and vomiting)
- Having morning sickness during pregnancy

Acute Nausea and Vomiting

Chemotherapy is the most common treatment-related cause of nausea and vomiting. The drug, dose, schedule of administration, route, and factors that are unique to the patient all determine how often nausea occurs and how severe it will be. Usually, these symptoms can be prevented or controlled. Acute nausea and vomiting are more likely to occur in patients who have experienced nausea and vomiting after previous chemotherapy sessions, are female, drink little or no alcohol, and are young.

Delayed Nausea and Vomiting

Delayed nausea and vomiting occurs more than 24 hours after chemotherapy. It is more likely to occur in patients who are receiving high-dose chemotherapy regimens, have experienced acute nausea and vomiting with chemotherapy, are female, drink little or no alcohol, and are young. Drugs to prevent nausea and vomiting may be given alone or in combinations to patients who are receiving chemotherapy.

Nausea and Vomiting in Advanced Cancer

Patients who have advanced cancer commonly experience chronic nausea and vomiting, which can significantly impair quality of life. Nausea and vomiting related to advanced cancer may be caused by the following:

- Use of opioids, antidepressants, and other pain medications

- Constipation (a common side effect of opioid use)

- Brain and colon tumors

- Abnormal levels of certain substances in the blood

- Dehydration

- Stomach ulcers

Radiation Therapy and Nausea and Vomiting

Radiation therapy may also cause nausea and vomiting, especially in patients who are undergoing radiation to the GI tract (particularly the small intestine and stomach) or brain. The risk for nausea and vomiting increases as the dose of radiation and area being irradiated increase. Nausea and vomiting associated with radiation therapy usually occurs one-half hour to several hours after treatment. Symptoms may improve on days the patient does not undergo radiation therapy.

Treatment

Anticipatory Nausea and Vomiting

Treatment of anticipatory nausea and vomiting is more likely to be successful when symptoms are recognized and treated early. Although anti-nausea drugs do not seem to be effective, the following may reduce symptoms:

- Guided imagery

- Hypnosis

- Relaxation

- Behavioral modification techniques

- Distraction (such as playing video games)

Acute/Delayed Nausea and Vomiting

Acute and delayed nausea and vomiting are most commonly treated with anti-nausea drugs. Some drugs last only a short time in the body, and need to be given more often; others last a long time and are given less frequently. Blood levels of the drug(s) must be kept constant to control nausea and vomiting effectively.

The following drugs are commonly given alone or in combinations to treat nausea and vomiting:

- Prochlorperazine

- Droperidol, haloperidol

- Metoclopramide

- Ondansetron, granisetron, dolasetron, palonosetron

- Aprepitant

- Dexamethasone, methylprednisolone

- Marijuana

- Dronabinol

- Lorazepam, midazolam, alprazolam

- Olanzapine

Nausea and Vomiting Related to Constipation and Bowel Obstruction in Advanced Cancer

In patients with advanced cancer, constipation is one of the most common causes of nausea. To prevent constipation and decrease the risk for nausea and vomiting, it is important that a regular bowel routine be followed, even if the patient isn't eating. High- fiber diets and bulk-forming laxatives with psyllium or cellulose require large amounts of fluid, however, and are not well tolerated by patients with advanced cancer. Laxatives that soften the stool or stimulate the bowel may be prescribed to prevent constipation, especially if the patient is being treated with opioids for cancer pain. The use of enemas and rectal suppositories is limited to short-term, severe episodes of constipation. Patients who have a loss of bowel function because of nerve damage (such as a tumor pressing on the spinal cord) may require suppositories for regular bowel emptying. Enemas and rectal suppositories should not be used in patients who have

damage to the bowel wall. Severe constipation may result in bowel obstruction.

Malignant Bowel Obstruction

Patients who have advanced cancer may develop a bowel obstruction that cannot be removed with surgery. The doctor may insert a nasogastric tube through the nose and esophagus into the stomach to temporarily relieve a partial obstruction. If the obstruction completely blocks the bowel, the doctor may insert a gastrostomy tube through the wall of the abdomen directly into the stomach to relieve fluid and air build-up. A gastrostomy tube also allows medications and liquids to be given directly into the stomach by pouring them down the tube. Sometimes, the doctor may create an ileostomy or colostomy by bringing part of the small intestine or colon through the abdominal wall to form an opening; or an expandable metal tube called a stent may be inserted into the bowel to open the blocked area. Injections or infusions of medications may be prescribed to relieve pain and/or nausea and vomiting.

Alternative Therapies for Nausea and Vomiting

Nausea and vomiting may be controlled without using drugs. The following may be helpful in relieving symptoms, especially for anticipatory nausea and vomiting, and may improve the effectiveness of anti-nausea drugs: Nutrition, hypnosis, acupuncture, acupressure, and guided imagery.

Chapter 39

Gastrointestinal Effects of Cancer Treatment

Overview

Constipation is the slow movement of feces (stool or body wastes) through the large intestine, resulting in infrequent bowel movements and the passage of dry, hard stools. The longer it takes for the stool to move through the large intestine, the more fluid is absorbed and the drier and harder the stool becomes.

Inactivity, immobility, or physical and social barriers (for example, bathrooms being unavailable or inconveniently located) can make constipation worse. Depression and anxiety caused by cancer treatment or cancer pain can also lead to constipation. The most common causes of constipation are not drinking enough fluids and taking pain medications.

Constipation is annoying and uncomfortable, but fecal impaction (a collection of dry, hard stool in the colon or rectum) can be life-threatening. Patients with a fecal impaction may not have gastrointestinal symptoms. Instead, they may have circulation, heart, or breathing problems. If fecal impaction is not recognized, the signs and symptoms will get worse and the patient could die.

A bowel obstruction is a partial or complete blockage of the small or large intestine by a process other than fecal impaction. Bowel obstructions are classified by the type of obstruction, how the obstruction

PDQ® Cancer Information Summary. National Cancer Institute; Bethesda, MD. "Gastrointestinal Complications (PDQ®): Patient Version." Updated 1/2009. Available at http://cancer.gov. Accessed August 14, 2009.

occurred, and where it is. Tumors growing inside or outside the bowel, and scar tissue that develops after surgery, can affect bowel function and cause a partial or complete obstruction. Patients who have colostomies are especially at risk of developing constipation, which can lead to bowel obstruction.

Diarrhea can occur at any time during cancer treatment. Although diarrhea occurs less often than constipation, it can be physically and emotionally devastating for patients who have cancer. Diarrhea can cause the following:

- Changes in eating patterns
- A loss of body fluids
- Chemical imbalances in the blood
- Impairments in physical function
- Excessive tiredness
- Skin problems
- A decrease in physical activity
- Problems that can be life threatening in some patients

Diarrhea is an abnormal increase in the amount of fluid in the stool that lasts more than four days but less than two weeks. It may also be described as an abnormal increase in the amount of fluid in the stool and the passage of more than three unformed stools during a 24-hour period. Diarrhea is considered a long-term problem when it lasts longer than two months.

Radiation enteritis is a condition in which the lining of the bowel becomes swollen and inflamed during or after radiation therapy to the abdomen, pelvis, or rectum. The large and small bowels are very sensitive to radiation. The larger the dose of radiation, the greater the damage to normal bowel tissue. Most tumors in the abdomen and pelvis need large doses, and almost all patients receiving radiation to the abdomen, pelvis, or rectum will show signs of acute enteritis.

Acute symptoms are those that appear during the first course of radiation therapy and up to eight weeks later. Chronic radiation enteritis may appear months to years after radiation therapy is completed, or it may begin as acute enteritis and continue after treatment stops. Only five percent to 15 percent of persons treated with radiation to the abdomen will develop chronic problems. Several factors affect how long the enteritis will last and how severe it will be:

- The dose of radiation given

- The tumor size and how much it has spread

- The amount of normal bowel treated

- Whether chemotherapy was given at the same time as the radiation therapy

- Whether radiation implants were used

- Whether the patient has high blood pressure, diabetes, pelvic inflammatory disease, or poor nutrition, or has had surgery to the abdomen or pelvis. These conditions can decrease blood flow to the bowel wall and affect bowel movement, increasing the chance of radiation injury.

Constipation

Description and Causes

Common factors that may cause constipation in healthy people are eating a low- fiber diet, postponing visits to the toilet, using laxatives and enemas excessively, not drinking enough fluids, and exercising too little. In persons with cancer, constipation may be a symptom of cancer, a result of a growing tumor, or a result of cancer treatment. Constipation may also be a side effect of medications for cancer or cancer pain and may be a result of other changes in the body (organ failure, decreased ability to move, and depression). Other causes of constipation include dehydration and not eating enough. Cancer, cancer treatment, aging, and declining health can contribute to causing constipation.

Changed Bowel Habits

- Repeatedly ignoring the urge to pass stool

- Using too many laxatives and enemas

Immobility and Lack of Exercise

- Spinal cord injury, spinal cord compression, bone fractures, fatigue, weakness, long periods of bedrest

- Inability to tolerate movement and exercise due to respiratory or cardiac problems

Medications

- Chemotherapy treatments

- Pain medications, including opioids
- Medications for anxiety and depression
- Stomach antacids
- Diuretics
- Vitamin supplements such as iron and calcium
- Sleep medications
- General anesthesia

Bowel Disorders

- Irritable colon
- Diverticulitis
- Tumor

Muscle and Nerve Disorders

Nerve damage can lead to loss of muscle tone in the bowel.

- Brain tumors
- Spinal cord compression from a tumor or other spinal cord injury
- Stroke or other disorders that cause muscle weakness or movement
- Weakness of the diaphragm or abdominal muscles making it difficult to take a deep breath and push to have a bowel movement

Body Metabolism Disorders

- Under-secretion of the thyroid gland
- Increased level of calcium in the blood
- Low levels of potassium or sodium in the blood
- Diabetes with nerve dysfunction

Environmental Factors

- Needing assistance to go to the bathroom
- Being in unfamiliar surroundings or a hurried atmosphere
- Living in extreme heat leading to dehydration

- Needing to use a bedpan or bedside commode
- Lack of privacy

Treatment

Treatment of constipation includes prevention (if possible), elimination of possible causes, and limited use of laxatives. Constipation caused by opioid pain medicine may be treated with a drug given by injection. Suggestions for the patient's treatment plan may include the following:

- Keep a record of all bowel movements.
- Increase the fluid intake by drinking eight-ounce glasses of fluid each day (patients who have kidney or heart disease may need to limit fluid intake).
- Exercise regularly, including abdominal exercises in bed or moving from the bed to chair if the patient cannot walk.
- Increase the amount of dietary fiber by eating more fruits (raisins, prunes, peaches, and apples), vegetables (squash, broccoli, carrots, and celery), and whole grain cereals, breads, and bran. Patients must drink more fluids when increasing dietary fiber or they may become constipated. Patients who have had a bowel obstruction or have undergone bowel surgery (for example, a colostomy) should not eat a high-fiber diet.
- Drink a warm or hot drink about one half-hour before the patient's usual time for a bowel movement.
- Provide privacy and quiet time when the patient needs to have a bowel movement.
- Help the patient to the toilet or provide a bedside commode instead of a bedpan.
- Take only medications prescribed by the doctor.
- Do not use suppositories or enemas unless ordered by the doctor. In some cancer patients, these treatments may lead to bleeding, infection, or other harmful side effects.

Impaction

Description and Causes

Five major factors can cause impaction: Opioid pain medications, inactivity over a long period, changes in diet, mental illness, and long-term

use of laxatives. Regular use of laxatives for constipation contributes most to the development of constipation and impaction. Repeated use of laxatives in higher and higher doses makes the colon less able to signal the need to have a bowel movement.

Patients with impaction may have symptoms similar to patients with constipation, or they may have back pain (the impaction presses on sacral nerves) or bladder problems (the impaction presses on the ureters, bladder, or urethra). The patient's abdomen may become enlarged causing difficulty breathing, rapid heartbeat, dizziness, and low blood pressure. Other symptoms can include explosive diarrhea (as stool moves around the impaction), leaking stool when coughing, nausea, vomiting, abdominal pain, and dehydration. Patients who have an impaction may become very confused and disoriented with rapid heartbeat, sweating, fever, and high or low blood pressure.

Treatment of Impaction

Impactions are usually treated by moistening and softening the stool with an enema. Enemas must be given very carefully as prescribed by the doctor since too many enemas can damage the bowel. Some patients may need to have stool manually removed from the rectum after it is softened. Glycerin suppositories may also be prescribed. Laxatives that stimulate the bowel and cause cramping must be avoided since they can damage the bowel even more.

Bowel Obstruction

Description and Causes

A bowel obstruction may be caused by a narrowing of the intestine from inflammation or damage to the bowel, tumors, scar tissue, hernias, twisting of the bowel, or pressure on the bowel from outside the intestinal tract. It can also be caused by factors that interfere with the function of muscles, nerves, and blood flow to the bowel. Most bowel obstructions occur in the small intestine and are usually caused by scar tissue or hernias. The rest occur in the colon (large intestine) and are usually caused by tumors, twisting of the bowel, or diverticulitis. Symptoms will vary depending on whether the small or large intestine is involved.

The most common cancers that cause bowel obstructions are cancers of the colon, stomach, and ovary. Other cancers, such as lung and breast

cancers and melanoma, can spread to the abdomen and cause bowel obstruction. Patients who have had abdominal surgery or radiation are at a higher risk of developing a bowel obstruction. Bowel obstructions are most common during the advanced stages of cancer.

Treatment of Acute Bowel Obstruction

Patients who have abdominal symptoms that continue to become worse must be monitored frequently to prevent or detect early signs and symptoms of shock and constricting obstruction of the bowel. Medical treatment is necessary to prevent fluid and blood chemistry imbalances and shock.

A nasogastric tube may be inserted through the nose and esophagus into the stomach, or a colorectal tube may be inserted through the rectum into the colon to relieve pressure from a partial bowel obstruction. The nasogastric tube or colorectal tube may decrease swelling, remove fluid and gas build-up, or decrease the need for multiple surgical procedures; however, surgery may be necessary if the obstruction completely obstructs the bowel.

Treatment of Chronic, Malignant Bowel Obstruction

Patients who have advanced cancer may have chronic, worsening bowel obstruction that cannot be removed with surgery. Sometimes, the doctor may be able to insert an expandable metal tube called a stent into the bowel to open the area that is blocked.

When neither surgery nor a stent placement is possible, the doctor may insert a gastrostomy tube through the wall of the abdomen directly into the stomach by a very simple procedure. The gastrostomy tube can relieve fluid and air build-up in the stomach and allow medications and liquids to be given directly into the stomach by pouring them down the tube. A drainage bag with a valve may also be attached to the gastrostomy tube. When the valve is open, the patient may be able to eat or drink by mouth without any discomfort because the food drains directly into the bag. This gives the patient the experience of tasting the food and keeping the mouth moist. Solid food should be avoided because it may block the tubing to the drainage bag.

If the patient's comfort is not improved with a stent or gastrostomy tube, and the patient cannot take anything by mouth, the doctor may prescribe injections or infusions of medications for pain and/or nausea and vomiting.

Diarrhea

Causes

In cancer patients, the most common cause of diarrhea is cancer treatment (chemotherapy, radiation therapy, bone marrow transplantation, or surgery). Other causes of diarrhea include antibiotic therapy, stress and anxiety related to being diagnosed with cancer and undergoing cancer treatment; and infection. Infection may be caused by viruses, bacteria, fungi, or other harmful microorganisms. Antibiotic therapy can cause inflammation of the lining of the bowel, resulting in diarrhea that often does not respond to treatment. Other causes of diarrhea in cancer patients include the cancer itself, physical reactions to diet, medical problems and diseases other than cancer, the laxative regimen, and bowel impaction with leakage of stool around the blockage.

Undergoing surgery to the stomach and/or intestines can affect normal bowel function and cause diarrhea. Some chemotherapy drugs cause diarrhea by affecting how nutrients are broken down and absorbed in the small bowel. Radiation therapy to the abdomen and pelvis can cause inflammation of the bowel. Patients may have problems digesting food, and experience gas, bloating, cramping, and diarrhea. These symptoms may last up to eight to 12 weeks after therapy or may not develop for months or years. Treatment may include diet changes, medications, or surgery. Patients who are undergoing radiation therapy while receiving chemotherapy often experience severe diarrhea. Hospitalization may not be required, since an outpatient clinic or special home care nursing may give the care and support needed. Each patient's symptoms should be evaluated to determine if intravenous fluids or special medication should be prescribed.

Patients who undergo donor bone marrow transplantation may develop graft-versus-host disease (GVHD). Stomach and intestinal symptoms of GVHD include nausea and vomiting, severe abdominal pain and cramping, and watery, green diarrhea. Symptoms may occur one week to three months after transplantation. Some patients may require long-term treatment and diet management.

Treatment

Diarrhea is treated by identifying and treating the problems causing diarrhea. For example, diarrhea may be caused by stool impaction and medications to prevent constipation. The doctor may make changes in medications, diet, and fluids. Diet changes that may help decrease

diarrhea include eating small frequent meals and avoiding some of the following foods:

- Milk and dairy products
- Spicy foods
- Alcohol
- Caffeine—containing foods and drinks
- Some fruit juices
- Gas-forming foods and drinks
- High- fiber foods
- High-fat foods

For mild diarrhea, a diet of bananas, rice, apples, and toast (the BRAT diet) may decrease the frequency of stools. Patients should be encouraged to drink up to three quarts of clear fluids per day including water, sports drinks, broth, weak decaffeinated tea, caffeine-free soft drinks, clear juices, and gelatin. For severe diarrhea, the patient may need intravenous fluids or other forms of intravenous nutrition.

To manage diarrhea caused by graft-versus-host disease (GVHD), the doctor may recommend a special 5-phase diet. During phase 1, the patient receives intravenous fluids and nothing by mouth to rest the bowel until the diarrhea slows down. In phase 2, the patient may begin drinking fluids. If the patient is able to drink fluids and the diarrhea improves, he or she may begin phase 3, eating solid foods that are low-fiber, low-fat, low-acid, and do not irritate the stomach. In phase 4, the patient is gradually allowed to eat regular foods. If the patient is able to eat regular foods without any episodes of diarrhea, he or she may begin phase 5, eating their regular diet. Many patients may continue to have problems digesting milk and dairy products.

Depending on the cause of the diarrhea, the doctor may change the laxative therapy regimen or may prescribe medications that slow down bowel activity, decrease bowel fluid secretions, and allow nutrients to be absorbed by the bowel.

Radiation Enteritis

Causes and Symptoms

Radiation therapy stops the growth of rapidly dividing cells, such as cancer cells. Since normal cells in the lining of the bowel also divide

rapidly, radiation treatment can stop those cells from growing, making it difficult for bowel tissue to repair itself. As bowel cells die and are not replaced, gastrointestinal problems develop over the next few days and weeks.

Acute Enteritis

Patients with acute enteritis may have the following symptoms:

- Nausea

- Vomiting

- Abdominal cramps

- Frequent urges to have a bowel movement

- Rectal pain, bleeding, or mucus -like discharge

- Watery diarrhea

With diarrhea, the gastrointestinal tract does not function normally, and nutrients such as fat, lactose, bile salts, and vitamin B12 are not well absorbed.

Symptoms of acute enteritis usually get better two to three weeks after treatment ends.

Chronic Enteritis

Patients with chronic enteritis may have the following symptoms:

- Wave-like abdominal pain

- Bloody diarrhea

- Frequent urges to have a bowel movement

- Greasy and fatty stools

- Weight loss

- Nausea

- Vomiting

Less common symptoms of chronic enteritis are bowel obstruction, holes in the bowel, and heavy rectal bleeding.

Symptoms usually appear six to 18 months after radiation therapy ends. Before determining that chronic radiation enteritis is

causing these symptoms, recurrent tumors need to be ruled out. The radiation history of the patient is important in making the correct diagnosis.

Treatment of Acute Radiation Enteritis

Treatment of acute enteritis includes treating the diarrhea, loss of fluids, poor absorption, and stomach or rectal pain. These symptoms usually get better with medications, changes in diet, and rest. If symptoms become worse even with this treatment, then cancer treatment may have to be stopped, at least temporarily.

Medications that may be prescribed include antidiarrheals to stop diarrhea, opioids to relieve pain, and steroid foams to relieve rectal inflammation and irritation. If patients with pancreatic cancer have diarrhea during radiation therapy, they may need pancreatic enzyme replacement, because not having enough of these enzymes can cause diarrhea.

Nutrition

Nutrition also plays a role in acute enteritis. Intestines damaged by radiation therapy may not make enough or any of certain enzymes needed for digestion, especially lactase. Lactase is needed for the digestion of milk and milk products. A lactose-free, low-fat, and low-fiber diet may help to control symptoms of acute enteritis.

Foods to avoid include the following:

- Milk and milk products, except buttermilk and yogurt. Processed cheese may not cause problems because the lactose is removed during processing. Lactose-free milkshake supplements, such as Ensure, may also be used.

- Whole-bran bread and cereal

- Nuts, seeds, and coconut

- Fried, greasy, or fatty foods

- Fresh and dried fruit and some fruit juices (such as prune juice)

- Raw vegetables

- Rich pastries

- Popcorn, potato chips, and pretzels

- Strong spices and herbs

- Chocolate, coffee, tea, and soft drinks with caffeine
- Alcohol and tobacco

Foods to choose include the following:

- Fish, poultry, and meat that are cooked, broiled, or roasted
- Bananas, applesauce, peeled apples, and apple and grape juices
- White bread and toast
- Macaroni and noodles
- Baked, boiled, or mashed potatoes
- Cooked vegetables that are mild, such as asparagus tips, green and waxed beans, carrots, spinach, and squash
- Mild processed cheese, eggs, smooth peanut butter, buttermilk, and yogurt

Helpful Hints

- Eat food at room temperature.
- Drink three liters (about 12 eight-ounce glasses) of fluid a day.
- Allow carbonated beverages to lose their fizz before drinking them.
- Add nutmeg to food to help decrease movement of the gastrointestinal tract.
- Start a low-fiber diet on the first day of radiation therapy.

Treatment of Chronic Radiation Enteritis

Treatment of the symptoms of chronic radiation enteritis is the same as treatment of acute radiation enteritis. Surgery is used to treat severe damage. Fewer than two percent of affected patients will need surgery to control their symptoms. Two types of surgery may be used:

- Intestinal bypass, a procedure in which the doctor creates a new pathway for the flow of bowel contents.
- Complete removal of the diseased intestines.

The patient's general health and the amount of damaged tissue are considered before surgery is attempted, however, because wound

healing is often slow and long-term tube feeding may be needed. Even after surgery, many patients still have symptoms.

To lower the risk that chronic radiation enteritis will occur, different treatment methods are used to reduce the area that is exposed to radiation. Patients may be positioned to protect as much of the small bowel as possible from the radiation treatment, or may be asked to have a full bladder during treatment to help push the small bowel out of the way. The amount of radiation may be adjusted to deliver lower amounts more evenly or higher amounts to specific areas. If a patient has surgery, clips may be placed at the tumor site to help show the area to be irradiated.

Chapter 40

Controlling Cancer-Related Pain

Introduction

Having cancer doesn't mean that you'll have pain. But if you do, you can manage most of your pain with medicine and other treatments. You don't have to accept pain.

People who have cancer don't always have pain. Everyone is different. But if you do have cancer pain, you should know that you don't have to accept it. Cancer pain can almost always be relieved.

Pain Specialists Can Help

Cancer pain can be reduced so that you can enjoy your normal routines and sleep better. It may help to talk with a pain specialist. These may be oncologists, anesthesiologists, neurologists, surgeons, other doctors, nurses, or pharmacists. If you have a pain control team, it may also include psychologists and social workers.

Pain and palliative care specialists are experts in pain control. Palliative care specialists treat the symptoms, side effects, and emotional problems of both cancer and its treatment. They will work with you to find the best way to manage your pain. Ask your doctor or nurse to suggest someone. Or contact one of the following for help finding a pain specialist in your area:

- Cancer center

Excerpted from "Pain Control: Support for People with Cancer," National Cancer Institute (www.cancer.gov), January 24, 2008.

- Your local hospital or medical center

- Your primary care provider

- People who belong to pain support groups in your area

- The Center to Advance Palliative Care, http://www.getpalliativecare .org/ (for lists of providers in each state)

When cancer pain is not treated properly, you may be tired, depressed, angry, worried, lonely, or stressed. When cancer pain is managed properly, you can enjoy being active, sleep better, enjoy family and friends, improve your appetite, enjoy sexual intimacy, and prevent depression.

Types and Causes of Cancer Pain

Cancer pain can range from mild to very severe. Some days it can be worse than others. It can be caused by the cancer itself, the treatment, or both.

You may also have pain that has nothing to do with your cancer. Some people have other health issues or headaches and muscle strains. But always check with your doctor before taking any over-the-counter medicine to relieve everyday aches and pains.

Different Types of Pain

Here are the common terms used to describe different types of pain:

- Acute pain ranges from mild to severe. It comes on quickly and lasts a short time.

- Chronic pain ranges from mild to severe. It either won't go away or comes back often.

- Breakthrough pain is an intense rise in pain that occurs suddenly or is felt for a short time. It can occur by itself or in relation to a certain activity. It may happen several times a day, even when you're taking the right dose of medicine. For example, it may happen as the current dose of your medicine is wearing off.

Causes of Cancer Pain

Cancer and its treatment cause most cancer pain. Major causes of pain include the following:

Pain from medical tests: Some methods used to diagnose cancer or see how well treatment is working are painful. Examples may be a biopsy, spinal tap, or bone marrow test. If you are told you need the procedure, don't let concerns about pain stop you from having it done. Talk with your doctor ahead of time about what will be done to lessen any pain you may have.

- **Pain from a tumor:** If the cancer grows bigger or spreads, it can cause pain by pressing on the tissues around it. For example, a tumor can cause pain if it presses on bones, nerves, the spinal cord, or body organs.

- **Spinal cord compression:** When a tumor spreads to the spine, it can press on the spinal cord and cause spinal cord compression. The first sign of this is often back or neck pain, or both. Coughing, sneezing, or other motions may make it worse.

- **Pain from treatment:** Chemotherapy, radiation therapy, surgery, and other treatments may cause pain for some people.

- **Neuropathic pain:** This is pain that may occur if treatment damages the nerves. The pain is often burning, sharp, or shooting. The cancer itself can also cause this kind of pain.

- **Phantom pain:** You may still feel pain or other discomfort coming from a body part that has been removed by surgery. Doctors aren't sure why this happens, but it's real.

How much pain you feel depends on different things. These include where the cancer is in your body, what kind of damage it is causing, and how you experience the pain in your body. Everyone is different.

Listen to Your Body

If you notice that everyday actions, such as coughing, sneezing, or moving, cause new pain or your pain to get worse, tell your doctors right away. Also let them know if you have unusual rashes or bowel or bladder changes.

Pain Control Is Part of Treatment

Controlling pain is a key part of your overall cancer treatment. The most important member of the team is you. You're the only one who knows what your pain feels like. Talking about pain is important. It gives your health care team the feedback they need to make you feel better.

Some people with cancer don't want to talk about their pain. They think that they'll distract their doctors from working on ways to help treat their cancer. Or they worry that they won't be seen as "good" patients. They also worry that they won't be able to afford pain medicine. As a result, people sometimes get so used to living with their pain that they forget what it's like to live without it.

But your health care team needs to know details about your pain and whether it's getting worse. This helps them understand how the cancer and its treatment are affecting your body. And it helps them figure out how to best control the pain.

Try to talk openly about any other medical problems and fears you have. And if money worries are stopping you, be sure to read the Financial Issues section. There may be ways to help you get the medicine you need.

Tell your health care team if you are taking any medicine to treat other health problems, taking more or less of the pain medicine than prescribed, allergic to certain drugs, or using any over-the-counter medicines, home remedies, or herbal or alternative therapies.

This information could affect the pain control plan your doctor suggests for you. If you feel uneasy talking about your pain, bring a family member or friend to speak for you. Or let your loved one take notes and ask questions. Remember, open communication between you, your loved ones, and your health care team will lead to better pain control.

Talking about Pain

The first step in getting your pain under control is talking honestly about it. Try to talk with your health care team and your loved ones about what you are feeling. This means telling them facts such as the following:

- Where you have pain
- What it feels like (sharp, dull, throbbing, constant, burning, or shooting)
- How strong your pain is
- How long it lasts
- What lessens your pain or makes it worse
- When it happens (what time of day, what you're doing, and what's going on)
- If it gets in the way of daily activities

You will be asked to describe and rate your pain. This provides a way to assess your pain threshold and measure how well your pain control plan is working.

Your doctor may ask you to describe your pain in a number of ways. A pain scale is the most common way. The scale uses the numbers 0 to 10, where 0 is no pain, and 10 is the worst. You can also use words to describe pain, like pinching, stinging, or aching. Some doctors show their patients a series of faces and ask them to point to the face that best describes how they feel.

No matter how you or your doctor keep track of your pain, make sure that you do it the same way each time. You also need to talk about any new pain you feel.

It may help to keep a record of your pain. Some people use a pain diary or journal. Others create a list or a computer spreadsheet. Choose the way that works best for you.

Your Pain Control Plan

Your pain control plan will be designed for you and your body. Everyone has a different pain control plan. Even if you have the same type of cancer as someone else, your plan may be different.

Take your pain medicine dose on schedule to keep the pain from starting or getting worse. This is one of the best ways to stay on top of your pain. Don't skip doses. Once you feel pain, it's harder to control and may take longer to get better.

Here are some other things you can do:

- Bring your list of medicines to each visit.

- If you are seeing more than one doctor, make sure each one sees your list of medicines, especially if he or she is going to change or prescribe medicine.

- Never take someone else's medicine. What helped a friend or relative may not help you. Do not get medicine from other countries or the Internet without telling your doctor.

- Don't wait for the pain to get worse.

- Ask your doctor to change your pain control plan if it isn't working.

- The best way to control pain is to stop it before it starts or prevent it from getting worse.

Don't wait until the pain gets bad or unbearable before taking your medicine. Pain is easier to control when it's mild. And you need to take

pain medicine often enough to stay ahead of your pain. Follow the dose schedule your doctor gives you. Don't try to "hold off" between doses. If you wait your pain could get worse, it may take longer for the pain to get better or go away, or you may need larger doses to bring the pain under control.

Keep a List of All Your Medicines

Make a list of all the medicines you are taking. If you need to, ask a member of your family or health care team to help you. Bring this list of medicines to each visit. You can take most pain medicines with other prescription drugs. But your health care team needs to know what you take and when. Tell them each drug you are taking, no matter how harmless you think it might be. Even over-the-counter medicines, herbs, and supplements can interfere with cancer treatment.

When You Need a New Plan

Here are a few things to watch out for and tell your health care team about:

- Your pain isn't getting better or going away.
- Your pain medicine doesn't work as fast as your doctor said it would.
- Your pain medicine doesn't work as long as your doctor said it would.
- You have breakthrough pain.
- You have side effects that don't go away.
- Pain interferes with things like eating, sleeping, or working.
- The schedule or the way you take the medicine doesn't work for you.

If you have trouble breathing, dizziness, or rashes, call your doctor right away. You may be having an allergic reaction to the pain medicine.

Don't Give Up

If you are still having pain that is hard to control, you may want to talk with your health care team about seeing a pain or palliative care specialist. Whatever you do, don't give up. If one medicine doesn't work, there is almost always another one to try. Also, new medicines

are created all the time. And unlike other medicines, there is no "right" dose for many pain medicines. Your dose may be more or less than someone else's. The right dose is the one that relieves your pain and makes you feel better.

Medicines to Treat Cancer Pain

Your doctor prescribes medicine based on the kind of pain you have and how severe it is. In studies, these medicines have been shown to help control cancer pain. Doctors use three main groups of drugs for pain: nonopioids, opioids, and other types. You may also hear the term analgesics used for these pain relievers. Some are stronger than others. It helps to know the different kinds of medicines, why and how they're used, how you take them, and what side effects you might expect.

Nonopioids

Nonopioids are drugs used to treat mild to moderate pain, fever, and swelling. On a scale of 0 to 10, a nonopioid may be used if you rate your pain from 1 to 4. These medicines are stronger than most people realize. In many cases, they are all you'll need to relieve your pain. You just need to be sure to take them regularly.

You can buy most nonopioids without a prescription. But you still need to talk with your doctor before taking them. Some of them may have things added to them that you need to know about. And they do have side effects. Common ones, such as nausea, itching, or drowsiness, usually go away after a few days. Do not take more than the label says unless your doctor tells you to do so.

Nonopioids include acetaminophen, which you may know as Tylenol®. Acetaminophen reduces pain. It is not helpful with inflammation. Most of the time, people don't have side effects from a normal dose of acetaminophen. But taking large doses of this medicine every day for a long time can damage your liver. Drinking alcohol with the typical dose can also damage the liver.

Make sure you tell the doctor that you're taking acetaminophen. Sometimes it is used in other pain medicines, so you may not realize that you're taking more than you should. Also, your doctor may not want you to take acetaminophen too often if you're getting chemotherapy. The medicine can cover up a fever, hiding the fact that you might have an infection.

Nonopioids also include nonsteroidal anti-inflammatory drugs (NSAIDs), such as ibuprofen (which you may know as Advil® or Motrin®) and aspirin. NSAIDs help control pain and inflammation. With NSAIDs,

the most common side effect is stomach upset or indigestion, especially in older people. Eating food or drinking milk when you take these drugs may stop this from happening.

NSAIDs may also keep blood from clotting the way it should. This means that it's harder to stop bleeding after you've hurt yourself. NSAIDs can also sometimes cause bleeding in the stomach.

Opioids

If you're having moderate to severe pain, your doctor may recommend that you take stronger drugs called opioids. Opioids are also known as narcotics. You must have a doctor's prescription to take them. They are often taken with aspirin, ibuprofen, and acetaminophen. Common opioids include the following:

- Codeine
- Fentanyl
- Hydromorphone
- Levorphanol
- Meperidine
- Methadone
- Morphine
- Oxycodone
- Oxymorphone

Over time, people who take opioids for pain sometimes find that they need to take larger doses to get relief. This is caused by more pain, the cancer getting worse, or medicine tolerance. When a medicine doesn't give you enough pain relief, your doctor may increase the dose and how often you take it. He or she can also prescribe a stronger drug. Both methods are safe and effective under your doctor's care. Do not increase the dose of medicine on your own.

Some pain medicines may cause constipation, drowsiness, nausea, or vomiting (throwing up). Other less common side effects include dizziness, confusion, breathing problems, itching, or trouble urinating. Usually these side effects last only a few days. But if they last longer, your doctors can change the medicine or dose you're taking. Or they may also add another medicine to your pain control plan to control the side effects.

Almost everyone taking opioids has some constipation. This happens because opioids cause the stool to move more slowly through your system, so your body takes more time to absorb water from the stool. The stool then becomes hard. Keep in mind that constipation will only go away if it's treated. Your health care team can talk with you about other ways to relieve side effects. Don't let side effects stop you from getting your pain under control.

You may be able to take less medicine when the pain gets better. You may even be able to stop taking opioids. But it's important to stop taking opioids slowly, with your doctor's advice. When pain medicines are taken for long periods of time, your body gets used to them. If the medicines are stopped or suddenly reduced, a condition called withdrawal may occur. This is why the doses should be lowered slowly. This has no relation to being addicted.

Stopping your pain medicines slowly makes withdrawal symptoms mild. But if you stop taking opioids suddenly, you may start feeling like you have the flu. You may sweat and have diarrhea or other symptoms. If this happens, tell your doctor or nurse. He or she can treat these symptoms. Any symptoms from withdrawal may take a few days to a few weeks to go away.

Medicine Tolerance and Addiction

When treating cancer pain, addiction is rarely a problem. Addiction is when people can't control their seeking or craving for something. They continue to do something even when it causes them harm. People with cancer often need strong medicine to help control their pain. Yet some people are so afraid of becoming addicted to pain medicine that they won't take it. Family members may also worry that their loved ones will get addicted to pain medicine. Therefore, they sometimes encourage loved ones to "hold off" between doses. But even though they may mean well, it's best to take your medicine as prescribed.

People in pain get the most relief when they take their medicines on schedule. And don't be afraid to ask for larger doses if you need them. Developing a tolerance to pain medicine is common. But taking cancer pain medicine is not likely to cause addiction. If you're not a drug addict, you won't become one. Even if you have had an addiction problem before, you still deserve good pain management. Talk with your doctor or nurse about your concerns.

Some people think that they have to save stronger medicines for later. They're afraid that their bodies will get used to the medicine and that it won't work anymore. But medicine doesn't stop working—it just doesn't work as well as it once did. As you keep taking a medicine over time, you may need a change in your pain control plan to get the same amount of pain relief. This is called tolerance. Tolerance is a common issue in cancer pain treatment.

Medicine tolerance is not the same as addiction. As mentioned, medicine tolerance happens when your body gets used to the medicine you're taking. The result is that the dose no longer works as well. Each person's body is different. Many people don't develop a tolerance to opioids. But

if tolerance happens to you, don't worry. Under your doctor's care, you can increase your dose in small amounts, add a new kind of medicine, or change the kind of medicine that you're taking for pain.

The goal is to relieve your pain. Increasing the dose to overcome tolerance does not lead to addiction. Taking pain medicine will not cause you to "get high."

Most people do not "get high" or lose control when they take cancer pain medicines as prescribed by the doctor. Some pain medicines can cause you to feel sleepy when you first take them This feeling usually goes away within a few days. On occasion, people get dizzy or feel confused when they take pain medicines. Tell your doctor or nurse if this happens to you. Changing your dose or type of medicine can usually solve this problem.

Other Types of Pain Medicine

Doctors also prescribe other types of medicine to relieve cancer pain. They can be used along with nonopioids and opioids. Some include antidepressants, anticonvulsants, and steroids:

- **Antidepressants:** Some drugs can be used for more than one purpose. For example, antidepressants are used to treat depression, but they may also help relieve tingling and burning pain. Nerve damage from radiation, surgery, or chemotherapy can cause this type of pain.

- **Antiseizure medicines (anticonvulsants):** Like antidepressants, anticonvulsants or antiseizure drugs can also be used to help control tingling or burning from nerve injury.

- **Steroids:** Steroids are mainly used to treat pain caused by swelling.

Be sure to ask your health care team about the common side effects of these medicines.

How Pain Medicine Is Given

To relieve cancer pain, doctors often prescribe pills or liquids. But there are also other ways to take medicines:

- **Mouth:** Some pain medicine can be put inside the cheek or under the tongue.

- **Injections (shots):** There are two different kinds of shots. Under the skin: Medicine is placed just under the skin using a small needle. These are called subcutaneous injections. In the vein: Medicine

goes directly into the vein through a needle. These are called intravenous (IV) injections. Patient-controlled analgesia (PCA) pumps are often used with these kinds of injections. PCA pumps let you push a button to give yourself a dose of pain medicine.

- **Skin patches:** These bandage-like patches go on the skin. They slowly but steadily, release medicine for 2 to 3 days.

- **Rectal suppositories:** These are capsules or pills that you put inside your rectum. The medicine dissolves and is absorbed by the body.

- **Around the spinal cord:** Medicine is placed between the wall of the spinal canal and the covering of the spinal cord (called an epidural).

Other Ways to Relieve Pain

Along with your pain medicine, your health care team may suggest you try other methods to control your pain. However, unlike pain medicine, some of these methods have not been tested in cancer pain studies. But they may help improve your quality of life by helping you with your pain, as well as stress, anxiety, and coping with cancer. Some of these methods are called complementary or integrative.

These treatments include everything from cold packs, massage, acupuncture, hypnosis, and imagery to biofeedback, meditation, and therapeutic touch. Once you learn how, you can do some of them by yourself. For others, you may have to see a specialist to receive these treatments. If you do, ask if they are licensed experts.

Medicine doesn't always relieve pain in some people. In these cases, doctors use other treatments to reduce pain:

- **Radiation therapy:** Different forms of radiation energy are used to shrink the tumor and reduce pain. Often one treatment is enough to help with the pain. But sometimes several treatments are needed.

- **Neurosurgery:** A surgeon cuts the nerves that carry pain messages to your brain.

- **Nerve blocks:** Anesthesiologists inject pain medicine into or around the nerve or into the spine to relieve pain.

- **Surgery:** A surgeon removes all or part of a tumor to relieve pain. This is especially helpful when a tumor presses on nerves or other parts of the body.

- **Chemotherapy:** Anticancer drugs are used to reduce the size of a tumor, which may help with the pain.

- **Transcutaneous electric nerve stimulation (TENS):** TENS uses a gentle electric current to relieve pain. The current comes from a small power pack that you can hold or attach to yourself.

Your Feelings and Pain

Having pain and cancer affects every part of your life. Research shows that people in pain may feel sad or anxious and may get depressed more often. At other times they may feel angry and frustrated. And they can feel lonely, even if they have others around them.

A common result of having cancer and being in pain is fear. For many, pain and fear together feel like suffering. People get upset worrying about the future. They focus their thoughts on things that may or may not happen. You may feel fear about many things, such as fear of the cancer getting worse, the pain being too much to handle, your job or daily tasks becoming too hard to do, not being able to attend special trips or events, or loss of control.

This roller coaster of feelings often makes people look for the meaning that cancer and pain have in their life. Some question why this could happen to them. They wonder what they did to deserve it. Others may turn to religion or explore their spirituality more, asking for guidance and strength. Don't lose hope.

If you have feelings like these, know that you're not alone. Many people with cancer pain have had these kinds of feelings. Having negative thoughts is normal. And some people have positive thoughts, too, finding benefits in facing cancer. But if your negative thoughts overwhelm you, don't ignore your feelings. Help is there for you if you're distressed or unsure about your future.

Financial Issues

When you're in pain, the last thing you want to think about is paying for your medicine. Yet money worries have stopped many people from getting the pain treatment they need. Talk with your oncology social worker if you have questions. He or she should be able to direct you to resources in your area. Here are some general tips:

Insurance

- Call your insurance company and find out what treatments are covered. Sometimes insurance companies pay for only certain

types of medicines. If the medicine you need isn't covered, your doctor may need to write a special appeal letter. Or your doctor may need to prescribe a different treatment.

- Ask if your insurance company can give you a case manager to help you with your coverage.

- Check to make sure that your plan will cover any specialists your doctor refers you to. If it does not, check with your insurance company to see which doctors are included in your plan. Ask your doctor to refer you to someone on your plan's list.

- Find out whether you have to pay copayments up front and how much they cost.

- Find out how you should pay your balance. For example, do you file a claim? Does the insurance company pay first? Or do you pay and get reimbursed?

- Tell the insurance company if you believe you've received an incorrect bill. You should also tell your doctor or the hospital or clinic that sent the bill. Don't be afraid to ask questions.

Government Health Insurance

Medicare is health insurance for people age 65 or older. However, people under 65 who are on kidney dialysis or have certain disabilities may also qualify.

Medicare Part B only pays for outpatient medicine given by a pump or by vein. It doesn't pay for pills, patches, or liquids.

Medicare Part D is a benefit that covers outpatient prescription medicines. It comes from private insurance plans that have a contract with Medicare. These plans vary in what they cost and the medicines they cover. Find out which medicines a plan covers before you join to make sure that it meets your needs. You should also know how much your copays and deductible will be.

Medicaid gives health benefits to low income people and their families. Some may have no health insurance or not enough, and therefore need this help.

If you have Medicaid, you should know that it pays for medicine given by mouth (orally) or by vein (intravenous). Each state has its own rules about who is eligible for Medicaid.

To learn more about Medicare and Medicaid talk with your oncology social worker. You can also go to the Medicare and Medicaid Web site, http://www.cms.gov, or call the helpline at 800-MEDICARE (800-

633-4227). Specialists can answer your questions or direct you to free counseling in your area.

Tips for Saving Money on Pain Medicine

Don't be embarrassed to tell your health care team if you're having trouble paying for your medicine. They may be able to prescribe other medicine that better fits your budget.

If you feel that you're overwhelmed, the stress may seem like too much to handle. You might try getting help with financial planning. Talk with the business office where you get treatment. There are many free consumer credit counseling agencies and groups. Talk with your oncology social worker about your choices.

If the cost of pain medicine is an issue for you, consider the following tips:

- Ask your doctor if there are generic brands of your medicine available. These usually cost less than brand name medicines.

- Ask your doctor for medicine samples before paying for a prescription. You can't get samples of opioids. But you can ask your doctor to write only part of the prescription. This way you can make sure that the medicine works for you before buying the rest of it. This will only help if you pay by the amount you buy. For some insurance plans, you pay the same amount for part of or the whole prescription. Find out what will work best for you.

- Ask about drug companies that have special programs to give free drugs to patients in financial need. Your doctor should know about these programs.

- Remember that pills may cost less than other forms of medicine.

- Use a bulk-order mail pharmacy. But first make sure that the medicine works for you. Also, be aware that you can't order opioids in bulk or through the mail. Ask your oncology social worker or pharmacist about bulk-order mail pharmacies.

- Contact NeedyMeds. They are a nonprofit organization that helps people who cannot afford medicine or health care costs. Go to http://www.needymeds.com, or ask someone to do it for you.

Chapter 41

Lymphedema

About Lymphedema

Lymphedema is the build-up of fluid in soft body tissues when the lymph system is damaged or blocked.

Lymphedema occurs when the lymph system is damaged or blocked. Fluid builds up in soft body tissues and causes swelling. It is a common problem that may be caused by cancer and cancer treatment. Lymphedema usually affects an arm or leg, but it can also affect other parts of the body. Lymphedema can cause long-term physical, psychological, and social problems for patients.

The lymph system is a network of lymph vessels, tissues, and organs that carry lymph throughout the body.

The parts of the lymph system that play a direct part in lymphedema include the following:

- **Lymph:** A clear fluid that contains lymphocytes (white blood cells) that fight infection and the growth of tumors. Lymph also contains plasma, the watery part of the blood that carries the blood cells.

- **Lymph vessels:** A network of thin tubes that helps lymph flow through the body and returns it to the bloodstream.

PDQ® Cancer Information Summary. National Cancer Institute; Bethesda, MD. "Lymphedema (PDQ®): Patient Version." Updated 01/2010. Available at http:// cancer.gov. Accessed April 27, 2010.

- **Lymph nodes:** Small, bean-shaped structures that filter lymph and store white blood cells that help fight infection and disease. Lymph nodes are located along the network of lymph vessels found throughout the body. Clusters of lymph nodes are found in the underarm, pelvis, neck, abdomen, and groin.

The spleen, thymus, tonsils, and bone marrow are also part of the lymph system but do not play a direct part in lymphedema.

When Lymphedema Occurs

When the lymph system is working as it should, lymph flows through the body and is returned to the bloodstream.

- Fluid and plasma leak out of the capillaries (smallest blood vessels) and flow around body tissues so the cells can take up nutrients and oxygen.

- Some of this fluid goes back into the bloodstream. The rest of the fluid enters the lymph system through tiny lymph vessels. These lymph vessels pick up the lymph and move it toward the heart. The lymph is slowly moved through larger and larger lymph vessels and passes through lymph nodes where waste is filtered from the lymph.

- The lymph keeps moving through the lymph system and collects near the neck, then flows into one of two large ducts:

- The right lymph duct collects lymph from the right arm and the right side of the head and chest.

- The left lymph duct collects lymph from both legs, the left arm, and the left side of the head and chest.

- These large ducts empty into veins under the collarbones, which carry the lymph to the heart, where it is returned to the bloodstream.

When part of the lymph system is damaged or blocked, fluid cannot drain from nearby body tissues. Fluid builds up in the tissues and causes swelling.

Two Types of Lymphedema

Lymphedema may be either primary or secondary:

- Primary lymphedema is caused by the abnormal development of the lymph system. Symptoms may occur at birth or later in life.

- Secondary lymphedema is caused by damage to the lymph system. The lymph system may be damaged or blocked by infection, injury, cancer, removal of lymph nodes, radiation to the affected area, or scar tissue from radiation therapy or surgery.

This chapter is about secondary lymphedema that is caused by cancer or cancer treatment.

Cancer-Related Risks Factors for Lymphedema

Lymphedema can occur after any cancer or treatment that affects the flow of lymph through the lymph nodes, such as removal of lymph nodes. It may develop within days or many years after treatment. Most lymphedema develops within three years of surgery. Risk factors for lymphedema include the following:

- Removal and/or radiation of lymph nodes in the underarm, groin, pelvis, or neck. The risk of lymphedema increases with the number of lymph nodes affected. There is less risk with the removal of only the sentinel lymph node (the first lymph node to receive lymphatic drainage from a tumor).

- Being overweight or obese.

- Slow healing of the skin after surgery.

- A tumor that affects or blocks the left lymph duct or lymph nodes or vessels in the neck, chest, underarm, pelvis, or abdomen.

- Scar tissue in the lymph ducts under the collarbones, caused by surgery or radiation therapy.

Lymphedema often occurs in breast cancer patients who had all or part of their breast removed and axillary (underarm) lymph nodes removed. Lymphedema in the legs may occur after surgery for uterine cancer, prostate cancer, lymphoma, or melanoma. It may also occur with vulvar cancer or ovarian cancer.

Signs of Lymphedema

- Swelling of an arm or leg, which may include fingers and toes

- A full or heavy feeling in an arm or leg

- A tight feeling in the skin

- Trouble moving a joint in the arm or leg

- Thickening of the skin, with or without skin changes such as blisters or warts

- A feeling of tightness when wearing clothing, shoes, bracelets, watches, or rings

- Itching of the legs or toes

- A burning feeling in the legs

- Trouble sleeping

- Loss of hair

A doctor should be consulted if any of these problems occur. Other conditions may cause the same symptoms. These symptoms may occur very slowly over time or more quickly if there is an infection or injury to the arm or leg.

Diagnosing Lymphedema

It is important to make sure there are no other causes of swelling, such as infection or blood clots. The following tests and procedures may be used to diagnose lymphedema:

- **Physical exam and history:** An exam of the body to check general signs of health, including checking for signs of disease, such as lumps or anything else that seems unusual. A history of the patient's health habits and past illnesses and treatments will also be taken.

- **Lymphoscintigraphy:** A procedure used to make pictures (called scintigrams) of the lymph system to check for blockages or anything else that seems unusual. A radioactive substance is injected under the skin, between the first and second fingers or toes of each hand or foot. The substance is taken up by the lymph vessels and detected by a scanner. The scanner makes images of the flow of the substance through the lymph system on a computer screen.

- **MRI (magnetic resonance imaging):** A procedure that uses a magnet, radio waves, and a computer to make a series of detailed

pictures of areas inside the body. This procedure is also called nuclear magnetic resonance imaging (NMRI).

The swollen arm or leg is usually measured and compared to the other arm or leg. Measurements are taken over time to see how well treatment is working.

Stages to Describe Lymphedema

- **Stage I:** The limb (arm or leg) is swollen and feels heavy. Pressing on the swollen area leaves a pit (dent). This stage of lymphedema may go away without treatment.

- **Stage II:** The limb is swollen and feels spongy. A condition called tissue fibrosis may develop and cause the limb to feel hard. Pressing on the swollen area does not leave a pit.

- **Stage III:** This is the most advanced stage. The swollen limb may be very large. Stage III lymphedema rarely occurs in breast cancer patients. Stage III is also called lymphostatic elephantiasis.

Managing Lymphedema

Taking preventive steps may keep lymphedema from developing. Health care providers can teach patients how to prevent and take care of lymphedema at home. If lymphedema has developed, these steps may keep it from getting worse.

Preventive steps include the following:

Be Alert

Tell your health care provider right away if you notice symptoms of lymphedema. The chance of improving the condition is better if treatment begins early. Untreated lymphedema can lead to problems that cannot be reversed.

Prevent Infection

Keep skin and nails clean and cared for. Bacteria can enter the body through a cut, scratch, insect bite, or other skin injury. Fluid that is trapped in body tissues by lymphedema makes it easy for bacteria to grow and cause infection. Look for signs of infection, such as redness, pain, swelling, heat, fever, or red streaks below the surface of the skin.

Call your doctor right away if any of these signs appear. Careful skin and nail care helps prevent infection:

- Use cream or lotion to keep the skin moist.

- Treat small cuts or breaks in the skin with an antibacterial ointment.

- Avoid needle sticks of any type into the limb (arm or leg) with lymphedema. This includes shots or blood tests.

- Use a thimble for sewing.

- Avoid testing bath or cooking water using the limb with lymphedema. There may be less feeling (touch, temperature, pain) in the affected arm or leg, and skin might burn in water that is too hot.

- Wear gloves when gardening and cooking.

- Wear sunscreen and shoes when outdoors.

- Cut toenails straight across. See a podiatrist (foot doctor) as needed to prevent ingrown nails and infections.

- Keep feet clean and dry and wear cotton socks.

Avoid Blocking the Flow of Fluids

It is important to keep body fluids moving, especially through an affected limb or in areas where lymphedema may develop.

- Do not cross legs while sitting.

- Change sitting position at least every 30 minutes.

- Wear loose jewelry and clothes without tight bands or elastic.

- Do not carry handbags on the arm with lymphedema.

- Do not use a blood pressure cuff on the arm with lymphedema.

- Do not use elastic bandages or stockings with tight bands.

Also, keep blood from pooling in the affected limb:

- Keep the limb with lymphedema raised higher than the heart when possible.

- Do not swing the limb quickly in circles or let the limb hang down. This makes blood and fluid collect in the lower part of the arm or leg.

- Do not apply heat to the limb.

Exercise

It is not known how exercise affects lymphedema related to breast cancer. In the past, women with lymphedema related to breast cancer were warned against certain types of exercise. Recently, studies have been done to learn how exercise affects this type of lymphedema. In these studies, exercise did not seem to make the lymphedema worse. More studies are needed.

Treatment of Lymphedema

Damage to the lymph system cannot be repaired. The goal of treatment is to control the swelling and other problems caused by lymphedema and keep other problems from developing or getting worse.

Physical (non-drug) therapies and combinations of several methods are the standard treatment. The goal of these treatments is to help patients continue with activities of daily living, to decrease pain, and to improve the ability to move and use the limb (arm or leg) with lymphedema. Drugs are not usually used for long-term treatment of lymphedema. Treatment of lymphedema may include the following:

Exercise

Both light exercise and aerobic exercise (physical activity that causes the heart and lungs to work harder) may help the lymph vessels move lymph out of the affected limb and decrease swelling.

Pressure Garments

Pressure garments are made of fabric that puts a controlled amount of pressure on different parts of the arm or leg to help move fluid and keep it from building up. Some patients may need to have these garments custom-made for a correct fit. Wearing a compression sleeve during exercise may help prevent more swelling in an affected limb. It is important to use pressure garments during air travel, because lymphedema can become worse at high altitudes. Pressure garments are also called compression sleeves and lymphedema sleeves or stockings.

Bandages

Once the lymph fluid is moved out of a swollen limb, bandaging (wrapping) can help prevent the area from refilling with fluid. Bandages

also increase the ability of the lymph vessels to move lymph along. Lymphedema that has not improved with other treatments is sometimes helped with bandaging.

Massage Therapy

Massage therapy (manual therapy) for lymphedema is a treatment in which the soft tissues of the body are lightly kneaded, rubbed, tapped, and stroked. Massage may help move lymph out of the swollen area into an area with working lymph vessels.

Massage therapy is usually not used in patients who had radiation therapy to the area with lymphedema or who have any of the following conditions:

- Cellulitis (infection of the deep tissues of the skin and muscle) or other inflammation of the swollen limb

- Cancer remaining in the area with lymphedema

- Deep vein thrombosis (blood clot in a vein)

- Congestive heart failure (weakness of the heart muscle, which leads to a build-up of fluid in body tissues)

Skin Care

The goal of skin care is to prevent infection and to keep skin from drying and cracking.

Combined Therapy

Combined physical therapy is a program of massage, bandaging, exercises, and skin care managed by a trained therapist. At the beginning of the program, the therapist gives many treatments over a short time to decrease most of the swelling in the limb with lymphedema. Then the patient continues the program at home to keep the swelling down. Combined therapy is also called complex decongestive therapy.

Compression Device

Compression devices are pumps connected to a sleeve that wraps around the arm or leg and applies pressure on and off. The sleeve is inflated and deflated on a timed cycle. This pumping action may help move fluid through lymph vessels and veins and keep fluid from building up in the arm or leg. Compression devices may be helpful

when added to combined therapy. The use of these devices should be supervised by a trained professional because too much pressure can damage lymph vessels near the surface of the skin.

Weight Loss

In patients who are overweight, lymphedema may improve with weight loss.

Laser Therapy

Laser therapy may help decrease lymphedema swelling and skin hardness after a mastectomy. A hand-held, battery-powered device is used to aim low-level laser beams at the area with lymphedema.

Drug Therapy

Lymphedema is not usually treated with drugs. Antibiotics may be used to treat and prevent infections. Other types of drugs, such as diuretics or anticoagulants (blood thinners), are usually not helpful and may make the lymphedema worse.

Surgery

Lymphedema caused by cancer is rarely treated with surgery.

Lymphangiosarcoma

When lymphedema is severe and does not get better with treatment, other problems may be the cause.

Sometimes severe lymphedema does not get better with treatment or it develops several years after surgery. If there is no known reason, doctors will try to find out if the problem is something other than the original cancer or cancer treatment, such as another tumor.

Lymphangiosarcoma is a rare, fast-growing cancer of the lymph vessels. It is a problem that occurs in some breast cancer patients and appears an average of 10 years after a mastectomy. Lymphangiosarcoma begins as purple lesions on the skin, which may be flat or raised. A computed tomography (CT) scan or magnetic resonance imaging (MRI) is used to check for lymphangiosarcoma. Lymphangiosarcoma usually cannot be cured.

Chapter 42

The Effects of Cancer Treatments on Blood Cells

Chapter Contents

Section 42.1

Anemia

Anemia is a decrease in the number of red blood cells (RBCs). Since most cancer therapies destroy cells that grow at a fast rate, and red blood cells have relatively rapid growth rates, they are often affected. An important part of the RBC is hemoglobin, the protein that carries oxygen throughout your body. Therefore, when your hemoglobin is low, oxygen levels are decreased, and your body has to work harder in order to compensate. The end result is that your body becomes tired.

Normal hemoglobin levels for women are usually in the range of 11.8 to 15.5 gm/dL; for men, the normal level is from 13.5 gm/dL to 17.5 gm/dL. While receiving cancer therapy, your hemoglobin level may drop to lower than these normal levels, so your hemoglobin level will be checked periodically throughout the course of treatments. Any time that your hemoglobin level drops below 10.0 gm/dL you are considered to be anemic.

The signs and symptoms of anemia include:

- Weakness or fatigue

- Dizziness

- Headache

- Shortness of breath or difficulty breathing

- Palpitations or rapid heartbeat

- Pale skin

- Feeling cold, particularly in the hands and feet

What can I do to prevent anemia?

Since red blood cells are destroyed as a side effect of cancer therapy, there is nothing specifically that you can do to prevent anemia from

occurring. Anemia may cause you to feel weak and tired. Some ways to help yourself include:

- Saving energy

- Get plenty of sleep

- Avoid prolonged or strenuous activity

- Pace yourself; take rest periods during activities that make you feel tired. Take short naps when needed

- Prioritize your activities so you will have enough energy for important activities or the activities that you enjoy most

- Ask friends and family to help you prepare meals or do chores when you're tired

- Avoiding injury

- Change positions slowly, especially when going from lying to standing to prevent dizziness

- When getting out of bed, sit on the side of the bed for a few minutes before standing

- Eat a well-balanced diet

- Eat foods high in iron, including green leafy vegetables, liver and cooked red meats

- Drink plenty of fluids

- Avoid caffeine and big meals late in the day if you're having trouble sleeping at night

- Take iron supplements only if you have been told to by your oncologist or nurse

When should I call my doctor?

Call your doctor immediately if you have any one or more of the following:

- Dizziness

- Shortness of breath or difficulty breathing

- Excessive weakness or fatigue

- Palpitations or chest pain

How is anemia treated?

Depending on the cause and severity of the anemia, there are several ways that anemia can be treated. Your doctor may instruct you to take over-the-counter iron pills on a daily basis or may order blood transfusions.

Your doctor may also choose to order injections of a "growth factor," which can be used to stimulate the growth of red blood cells, in certain patients. By increasing your body's production of red blood cells, this growth factor may decrease your risk of becoming anemic, and may also decrease the number of blood transfusions that may be required during your treatment.

Growth factors are administered by injection. You may receive the injections from the oncology nurse, or you and/or a family member may be taught how to give the injections at home. Once your red blood cell count has returned to a normal level, the injections will be stopped.

If necessary, your oncologist may decide to delay further treatments until your red blood cell count has returned to normal levels.

Section 42.2

Neutropenia

"Low White Blood Cell Count (Neutropenia)," reprinted
with permission from www.oncolink.org. Copyright 2001 by the
Trustees of the University of Pennsylvania. All rights reserved.

Neutropenia is a low level of white blood cells. Because radiation therapy and chemotherapy destroy cells that grow at a fast rate, white blood cells are often affected. Patients receiving a combination of radiation therapy and chemotherapy are at greater risk for neutropenia.

Since white blood cells play an important role in preventing infection, any time your white blood cell count drops, you are at higher risk of getting an infection. Since these cells also help to fight off infections once in the body, it may be harder to get over an infection when your white blood cell counts are low. Therefore, you need to take precautions to decrease the chance that you will become infected while receiving treatment.

Normal white blood cells counts are usually in the range of 4,000–11,000 per mm3 of blood. While receiving radiation therapy, your white count may drop to lower levels. Your white blood cell count will be checked periodically throughout the course of your treatments to monitor your white count.

Any time that your white blood cell count drops below 1,000 per mm3, you will be considered to be neutropenic. Should this happen, a nurse will review with you special steps that you must take in order to decrease the chance that you will get an infection. These neutropenic precautions are discussed below.

What can I do to prevent neutropenia?

Since white blood cells are destroyed as a side effect of chemotherapy, there is nothing specifically that you can do to prevent neutropenia from occurring. Nonetheless, there are several things that you can do to reduce your risk of getting an infection when your white blood cells are low.

Taking action at the first signs of infection can help prevent it from spreading and getting worse. There are several signs and symptoms of infection that you should look for, including:

- Oral temperature above 100.5° degrees, chills or sweats

- Cough, excess mucous, shortness of breath or painful breathing

- Soreness or swelling in your mouth, ulcers or white patches in your mouth, or a change in the color of your gums

- Pain or burning with urination or an odor to your urine

- Change in the odor, character or frequency of your stool, especially diarrhea

- Redness, pain or swelling of any area of your skin

- Redness, pain, swelling or drainage from any tube you may have (e.g., Hickman catheter, feeding tube, urinary catheter)

- Pus or drainage from any open cut or sore

- An overall feeling of being sick, even if you don't have a temperature or any other sign of an infection

Perform excellent daily personal hygiene:

- Wash your hands frequently, especially before eating and after using the bathroom.

- Use alcohol-free, antiseptic mouthwashes daily.

- Do not cut or pick at cuticles. Use a cuticle cream instead. Even if you have a manicure, only cuticle cream should be used.

- Use a deodorant rather than an antiperspirant. Antiperspirants block sweat glands and, therefore, may promote infection.

- When menstruating, use sanitary napkins rather than tampons, which may promote infection in a neutropenic patient.

- Avoid situations that will increase your chance of getting an infection.

- Stay away from people with colds or other infections.

- Avoid contact with anyone who has recently been vaccinated, including infants and children.

- Avoid crowds as much as possible. When going to places where there are often a lot of people (i.e., church, shopping), try going at off-peak times, when they're not as crowded.

- If possible, don't use public transportation. If you must, travel during off-peak times.

Use extra precautions to decrease the chance of injury and infection:

- Always wear shoes to prevent cuts on your feet.

- Protect your hands from cuts and burns. When doing dishes, wear rubber gloves, always use pot holders or some other protective covering when cooking or baking; wear gloves when gardening.

- Wear sunscreen with a sun protection factor (SPF) of at least 15 and avoid getting sunburned.

- When shaving under your arms or your legs, use an electric razor to avoid breaks in the skin.

- Do not receive any vaccination, including the flu vaccine, unless it has been approved by your oncologist.

- Avoid activities that are prone to falling and/or injury, including but not necessarily limited to bicycling, roller-blading, skating, and skiing.

- If you cut or scrape the skin, clean the area immediately with soap and water and bandage as necessary.

What are neutropenic precautions?

If your white blood cell count drops to 1,000 per mm3 or below, you are considered to be neutropenic. Until your count rises, it will be necessary for you to take additional measures to further decrease your risk for infection.

These are referred to as "neutropenic precautions" and include:

- Take your temperature by mouth four times each day. Call your oncologist immediately if your oral temperature is above 100.5° Fahrenheit.

- Eliminate uncooked foods, which may contain germs, from your diet, including:

  - cold soups made from fresh fruits or vegetables

  - salads of raw vegetables or fruits

  - raw meats or fish salads

  - natural cheeses

  - uncooked eggs

  - fresh, frozen and dried fruits

  - uncooked herbs, spices and black pepper

  - instant iced tea, coffee or punch

  - sushi and sashimi

- Avoid fresh flowers and plants which may have germs in the soil.

- Avoid enemas, rectal suppositories and rectal temperatures.

Unless an emergency, do not have any dental work performed. If you have an emergency that requires dental work, inform your dentist when you schedule your appointment that you are receiving chemotherapy and what your most recent white blood cell count is. You may want to suggest that your dentist contact your oncologist prior to your scheduled dental work.

When should I call my doctor?

Even if you have taken great care to prevent an infection, you may still become infected. If any of the following signs or symptoms of infection occur, call your doctor or nurse immediately. Do not take any

medications, even aspirin or other products to lower your temperature, before talking to your doctor.

Call your doctor if you have any one or more of the following:

- Oral temperature above 100.5° degrees, chills or sweats

- Cough, excess mucous, shortness of breath or painful breathing

- Soreness or swelling in your mouth or throat, ulcers or white patches in your mouth, or a change in the color of your gums

- Pain or burning with urination or an odor to your urine

- Change in the odor, character or frequency of your stool, especially diarrhea

- Redness, pain or swelling of any area of your skin

- Redness, pain, swelling in the area surrounding any tube you may have (e.g., Hickman catheter, feeding tube, urinary catheter)

- Pus or drainage from any open cut or sore

- An overall feeling of being sick, even if you don't have a temperature or any other sign of an infection

How is neutropenia treated?

One of the most significant advances in the past decades has been the development of "growth factors," which stimulate the body's production of specific substances. One growth factor stimulates the growth of white blood cells and is used frequently with cancer patients, especially those receiving chemotherapy and radiation therapy. By increasing your body's production of white blood cells, this growth factor can decrease your risk of developing an infection.

Growth factors are administered by injection. You may receive the injections from the radiation oncology nurse or you and/or a family member may be taught how to give the injections at home. Once your white blood cell count has returned to a normal level, the injections will be stopped.

If you develop an infection, your doctor will order medications to treat it. Depending on the cause and severity of the infection, the medications may be given either by mouth or through a vein using an intravenous (IV) catheter. If you require IV medications, you may be able to remain at home and have the medications administered by specially trained nurses. Some patients require admission to the hospital in order to effectively treat their infection.

If necessary, your oncologist may decide to delay further treatments until your white blood cell count has returned to normal levels and/or you are free of infection.

Section 42.3

Thrombocytopenia

Thrombocytopenia is a low level of platelets. Radiation therapy and certain chemotherapy medications can damage platelets and lead to thrombocytopenia. Patients receiving a combination of radiation therapy and chemotherapy are at greater risk for thrombocytopenia.

Platelets play an important role in blood clotting, so thrombocytopenia puts you at higher risk of bleeding. Therefore, while you are receiving therapy, use caution to avoid any activities that could result in bleeding. Even the most minor of injuries, such as a small cut or bump, can result in excessive bleeding when your platelets are low.

A normal platelet counts ranges from 150,000–400,000 per mm3 of blood. While receiving chemotherapy or radiation therapy, your platelet count may drop. Your platelet count will be checked throughout the course of your treatments. Any time your platelet count drops below 50,000 per mm3 you are considered to be at increased risk for bleeding. If your platelet count drops below 10,000 per mm3, you may require a transfusion of platelets.

Keep track of your blood counts.

What can I do to prevent bleeding?

Since platelets are destroyed as a side effect of radiation therapy and chemotherapy, there is nothing specifically that you can do to prevent thrombocytopenia from occurring. Nonetheless, there are several things that you can do to reduce your risk of injury when your platelets are low.

Taking prompt action at the first signs of a low platelet count is essential as it may help to prevent a bleeding episode. The signs and symptoms of a low platelet count include:

- Excessive bruising of your skin

- Tiny, pinpoint red spots on your skin (called petechiae)

- Bleeding gums

- Nosebleeds that will not stop

- Excessive bleeding from a small cut, or bleeding that won't stop even after pressure has been applied

- Dark colored urine or blood in your urine

- Blood from your rectum, blood in your stool or black colored stool

- Menstrual bleeding that is heavier than usual, lasts longer than usual or occurs between periods

Perform daily personal hygiene in ways that minimize the risk of bleeding.

- Keep your mouth clean and moist.

- Brush your teeth gently with a soft bristle toothbrush. If you cannot use a toothbrush, use a sponge toothette to clean your teeth and gums.

- Rinse your mouth after each meal with a baking soda solution (2 tsp. baking soda to 8 oz. water).

- Do not use dental floss.

- Avoid any commercial mouthwashes that contain alcohol. Alcohol can dry out your mouth, which may lead to bleeding.

- Use petroleum jelly or other lip balms to keep your lips moist and to prevent cracking.

- Take sips of water or juice frequently if your tongue or mouth feel dry.

- Modify feminine hygiene practices.

- Use sanitary napkins rather than tampons during menstruation.

- Avoid vaginal douching.

Take these other general precautions:

- Do not cough forcefully or harshly. If you have a persistent cough, notify your doctor or nurse who may recommend a cough syrup.

- Do not blow your nose too hard.

- Avoid straining too much with bowel movements. If you have a problem with constipation, ask your doctor for a stool softener or laxative.

- Do not use rectal thermometers, suppositories or enemas.

- Use an electric razor for shaving.

- Do not take any medications that affect blood clotting.

- Do not take aspirin or any product that contains aspirin. Check the labels of all drugs you are taking for salicylic acid, the chemical name for aspirin. If you are not sure about a drug or cannot tell by reading the label, check with your oncologist, nurse or a pharmacist.

- Do not take any non-steroidal, anti-inflammatory medications (NSAIDs) such as Motrin®, Aleve®, Advil®, etc.

- For headaches or other pain, use acetaminophen (Tylenol®).

Adjust your lifestyle to minimize the risk of bleeding.

- Avoid strenuous activity, lifting heavy objects, and bending over from the waist.

- Avoid sports and activities that could result in falling and/or injury including but not necessarily limited to bicycling, roller-blading, skating and skiing.

- Adjust your diet.

- Drink eight to ten, 8-ounce glasses of non-alcoholic fluid a day to keep your mouth moist, avoid constipation and keep the intestinal lining in good condition.

- Avoid raw and course vegetables that are hard to digest and may cause damage to the intestinal lining.

- Eat protein-rich foods and beverages such as chicken, turkey, cheese, cooked eggs, milk.

- Avoid drinking alcoholic beverages, including beer and wine.

- Wear shoes or slippers at all times to protect your feet.

- Do not wear tight-fitting clothing.

- Use a water-based lubricant and avoid vigorous thrusting during sexual intercourse.

What if I start to bleed?

Even if you have taken special precautions to decrease the chance of injury and bleeding, it is still possible that bleeding will occur. If bleeding occurs, apply firm pressure for five minutes to the area. If bleeding does not stop after five minutes, continue to apply pressure until it has stopped completely.

If you have a nosebleed, apply pressure with your fingers below the bridge of your nose until the bleeding stops. Keep your head raised.

When should I call my doctor?

Call your doctor immediately if you have any one or more of the following:

- Bleeding that does not stop after you have applied pressure for 10 to 15 minutes.

- Blood in your urine or your urine appears dark in color.

- Blood from your rectum, blood in your stool or your stool is black.

- A change in your vision.

- A persistent headache, blurred vision or a change in your level of consciousness such as a decreased attention span, excessive sleeping, confusion, and/or difficulty being awakened.

If you have a major injury or start spontaneously bleeding, go immediately to the nearest hospital emergency room. Make sure you inform the doctor that you are receiving cancer therapy and that your platelet count may be low.

How is thrombocytopenia treated?

If your platelet count drops to a point that your oncologist is concerned about significant risk of bleeding, they may order transfusions of platelets. These transfusions are most often done in an outpatient treatment center. Unless other problems exist, patients rarely are admitted to the hospital just to receive platelet transfusions.

If necessary, your oncologist may decide to delay further treatments until your platelet count has returned to normal levels.

Chapter 43

Fever, Sweats, and Hot Flashes

Introduction

Fever is a rise in body temperature above the normal temperature. In a person who has cancer, fever may be caused by infection, a tumor, drug reactions, or blood transfusion reactions. Sweating is the body's way of decreasing body temperature by causing heat loss through the skin and, in a person who has cancer, may be associated with fever, a tumor, or cancer treatment. Hot flashes can also cause excessive sweating and may occur in natural menopause or in patients who have been treated for breast cancer or prostate cancer. This chapter briefly summarized the causes and treatment for fever, sweats, and hot flashes.

Fever

Normal human body temperature changes during each 24-hour period according to a definite pattern. It is lowest in the morning before dawn and highest in the afternoon. Normal body temperature is maintained by temperature control activities in the body that keep a balance between heat loss and heat production.

An abnormal increase in body temperature is caused by either hyperthermia (an unusual increase in body temperature above normal)

PDQ® Cancer Information Summary. National Cancer Institute; Bethesda, MD. "Fever, Sweats, and Hot Flashes (PDQ®): Patient Version." Updated 01/2010. Available at: http://cancer.gov. Accessed April 27, 2010.

or fever. Hyperthermia is caused by a breakdown in the body's temperature control activities. In fever, the temperature controls in the body are working correctly, but body temperature increases as the body responds to chemicals produced by microorganisms that cause infection or works to kill harmful microorganisms such as bacteria or viruses. There are three phases to fever. In the first phase, the body raises its temperature to a new level by causing the blood vessels in the skin to constrict and move blood from the skin surface to the interior of the body, which helps to retain heat. The skin becomes cool, the muscles contract causing shivering or chills, and the body produces more heat. The body's efforts to retain and produce heat continue until a new higher temperature is reached. In the second phase, heat production and heat loss are equal, shivering stops, and the body maintains the new higher temperature. In the third phase, body temperature is lowered to normal as the body gets rid of the excess heat by causing the blood vessels in the skin to open and move blood from the interior of the body to the skin surface. Sweating occurs and helps to cool the body.

Fever is most likely to cause harmful effects in older persons or the very young. In older persons, the hypothalamus' temperature regulating centers do not work as well and the body temperature may rise above normal causing irregular heartbeat, lack of blood flow, changes in the ability to think clearly, or heart failure. Children between six months and six years old may have seizures due to a fever.

Causes

The main causes of fever in cancer patients are infections, tumors, reactions to drugs or blood transfusions, and graft-versus-host-disease. Graft-versus-host-disease occurs when transplanted bone marrow or peripheral stem cells attack the patient's tissue. Infection is a common cause of fever in cancer patients and can cause death. Tumor cells can produce various substances that can cause fever. A wide variety of medications can cause fever including chemotherapy drugs, biological response modifiers, and antibiotics, such as vancomycin and amphotericin.

Other causes of fever in cancer patients include drug withdrawal; neuroleptic malignant syndrome; blockages of the bladder, bowel, or kidney, and blockage of an artery by tumor fragments. Other medical conditions occurring at the same time as the cancer such as blood clots, connective tissue disorders, and central nervous system hemorrhage or stroke, may also cause fever.

Assessment

The doctor will ask questions about past medical problems, review all medications the patient is taking, and perform a thorough physical examination to determine the cause of fever. Patients who are suspected of having an infection, especially those who have neutropenia (a very low white blood cell count) and fever, will undergo very careful inspection of the skin, body openings (mouth, ears, nose, throat, urethra, vagina, rectum), needle stick sites, biopsy sites, and skin folds (for example, the breasts, armpits, or groin). The teeth, gums, tongue, nose, throat, and sinuses will be carefully examined. Any tubes that are inserted into veins or arteries or other tubes placed in the body, such as stomach tubes, are common sources of infection. Urine, sputum, and blood specimens will be examined for signs of infection. Patients with neutropenia may not show the usual symptoms of infection, so they should be examined frequently.

Treatment of Underlying Causes

The symptoms of fever in very weakened cancer patients may include fatigue, muscle pain, sweating, and chills. Possible treatments to manage fever include those that treat the underlying cause, giving intravenous fluids, nutritional support, and other measures to make the patient more comfortable. The specific treatments are determined by the stage of cancer and the patient's goals for care. For example, some patients who are nearing the end of life may decide not to be treated for the underlying cause such as pneumonia or other infections, but may still request general comfort measures and fluids to maintain their quality of life. Other patients may choose antibiotics to relieve symptoms such as cough, fever, or shortness of breath that occur because of the infection.

Antibiotics may be used to treat fever caused by infection. Antibiotic therapy regimens and drugs to treat fungal infections are prescribed by the doctor. Fever caused by a tumor is usually treated by prescribing standard therapies for the specific type of cancer. If the therapy is not successful, the therapy takes awhile to work, or there is no therapy available, the doctor may prescribe nonsteroidal anti-inflammatory drugs (NSAIDs).

Sometimes fever may be caused by a reaction to drugs given to treat the cancer or prevent infection. Drugs that are known to cause fever include biological response modifiers, amphotericin B, and bleomycin. Suspected drug-related fever may be treated by stopping the drug

that is causing the fever. When a biological response modifier, certain chemotherapy drugs, or antibiotics cause the fever, the doctor may control the fever by adjusting the type of drug, how the drug is given, the amount of drug given, or how often the drug is given. Acetaminophen, NSAIDs, and steroids may also be given before the patient receives the drug that causes the fever. Meperidine may be given to stop chills associated with a drug-related fever.

Neuroleptic malignant syndrome (NMS) is a rare but sometimes fatal reaction to drugs that a patient is given for psychotic conditions, delirium, or nausea and vomiting. The symptoms of NMS are fever, muscle stiffness, confusion, loss of control of body functions, and an increase in white blood cell count. A delirious patient who does not improve when treated with medication should be examined for NMS. Treatment for NMS includes stopping the drug, treating the symptoms, and sometimes using other drugs.

Cancer patients may develop a fever as a reaction to blood products (for example, receiving a blood transfusion). Removing white blood cells from the blood or treating the blood product with radiation before transfusing it into the patient can lessen the reaction. The possibility of fever due to receiving blood products can also be lessened by giving patients acetaminophen or antihistamines before the transfusion.

General Treatments to Relieve Fever

Along with treatment of the underlying cause of fever, comfort measures may also be helpful in relieving the discomfort that goes along with fever, chills, and sweats. During periods of fever, giving the patient plenty of liquids, removing excess clothing and linens, and bathing or sponging the patient with lukewarm water may give relief. During periods of chills, replace wet blankets with warm, dry blankets, keep the patient away from drafts, and adjust the room temperature to improve patient comfort.

Nonsteroidal anti-inflammatory drugs (NSAIDs) or acetaminophen may also be prescribed to relieve symptoms. Aspirin may be effective in decreasing fever, but should be used with caution in patients with Hodgkin lymphoma and cancer patients who are at risk for developing a decrease in the number of platelets in the blood. Aspirin is not recommended in children with fever because of the risk of developing Reye syndrome.

Sweats

Sweat is made by sweat glands in the skin. Sweating helps to keep the body cool and can occur with disease or fever, when in a warm environment, exercising, or as part of hot flashes experienced with menopause.

Most breast cancer and prostate cancer patients report having moderate-to-severe hot flashes. Distressing hot flashes seem to be less frequent and gradually decrease with time in most postmenopausal women who do not have breast cancer. Hot flashes occur in most men with prostate cancer who have had surgery to remove the testicles or who receive drugs to stop the testicles from making testosterone.

Causes

Sweats in the cancer patient may be associated with the tumor, cancer treatment, or other medical conditions that are not related to the cancer. Sweats are a typical symptom of certain types of tumors such as Hodgkin lymphoma, pheochromocytoma, or tumors involving the nervous system and endocrine system. Sweats may also be caused by the following conditions:

- Fever
- Female menopause (natural menopause, surgical removal of the ovaries, or damage to ovaries from chemotherapy, radiation, or hormone therapy)
- Male menopause (surgical removal of the testicles or hormone therapy)
- Drugs such as tamoxifen, aromatase inhibitors, opioids, antidepressants, and steroids
- Problems in the hypothalamus in the brain
- Sweating disorders

Treatment

Treatment of sweats caused by fever is directed at the underlying cause of the fever. (Refer to the fever treatment section above for more information.) Sweats caused by a tumor are usually controlled by treatment of the tumor.

A variety of medications are being used for general treatment of cancer-related sweats. The use of loose-fitting cotton clothing, fans, and behavioral techniques such as relaxation training is also recommended.

Hot Flashes

Hot flashes associated with natural or treatment-related menopause can be effectively controlled with estrogen replacement. Many women are not able to take estrogen replacement (for example, women

with breast cancer). Hormone replacement therapy that combines estrogen with progestin may increase the risk of breast cancer or breast cancer recurrence.

Studies of non-estrogen drugs to treat hot flashes have reported that many of them are not as effective as estrogen replacement or have unwanted side effects. The most effective of these include megestrol (a drug similar to progesterone) and certain antidepressants, including venlafaxine. It is important to know that some antidepressants may change how other drugs, such as tamoxifen, work in the body. Soy and black cohosh have not proven to be helpful in relieving hot flashes. Soy contains estrogen-like substances; the effect of soy on the risk of breast cancer growth or recurrence is not clear.

Relaxation training has been found to decrease hot flash discomfort in postmenopausal women who are in general good health.

Treatment of hot flashes in men may include estrogens, progesterone, antidepressants, and anticonvulsants. Certain hormones (such as estrogen) can make some cancers grow. The effect of hormone use on the growth of prostate cancer is being studied.

Chapter 44

Treatment-Related Neuropathy

Peripheral neuropathy (also called neuropathy) is a term used to describe damage to nerves that are outside of the brain and spinal cord (peripheral nerves).

Peripheral neuropathy is not one specific disease. Many different conditions that can damage the peripheral nerves can cause it. This information is about cancer related causes of peripheral neuropathy and mainly on neuropathy caused by anti-cancer drugs.

The nervous system is made up of the brain, the spinal cord and a network of nerves that thread throughout the body. It has two main parts:

- **The central nervous system (CNS)**, which is made up of the brain and spinal cord

- **The peripheral nervous system (PNS)**, which is made up of nerves that carry messages between the brain, the spinal cord and the rest of the body

Nerves carry nerve impulses back and forth between the body and the brain.

They are made up of nerve cells called neurons. Some neurons are very small, but others can be up to three feet long. When a nerve ending is stimulated—for example by heat, touch, or sound vibrations—it creates a tiny electrical pulse. This sends a signal along the nerve cell.

When it reaches the end of the cell, the signal triggers the release of chemicals. These carry the signal to the next nerve cell. In this way, messages can be sent from nerves anywhere in the body to the spinal cord and then up to the brain.

The Nervous System

When a nerve ending is stimulated, for example by heat, touch, or sound vibrations, it creates a tiny electrical pulse. This sends a signal along the nerve cell. When it reaches the end of the cell, the signal triggers the release of chemicals.

These carry the signal to the next nerve cell. In this way, messages can be sent from nerves anywhere in the body to the spinal cord and then up to the brain.

There are different types of nerves:

- **Motor nerves** carry messages from the brain to the muscles. When a muscle receives a message, it reacts with a movement. Messages can be sent from the brain to any part of the body.

- **Sensory nerves** carry messages from the body to the brain. These nerves have endings (receptors) that are sensitive to sensations such as pain, temperature, touch and vibration. They enable us to feel different sensations.

- **Autonomic nerves** carry messages back and forth between internal organs and the brain. They control the actions of muscles that aren't under our voluntary control. They are responsible for maintaining our blood pressure, and for the workings of our bowel and bladder.

Although we are not aware of it, our brain is constantly receiving messages from sensory nerves throughout our body. These messages tell our brain where each part of our body is and are important for balance, coordination and walking.

Causes of Peripheral Neuropathy

There are several ways in which cancer and treatments for cancer may cause peripheral neuropathy:

- Some anti-cancer drugs can cause nerve damage. This is the most common cause of peripheral neuropathy in people with cancer.

- Cancer can cause peripheral neuropathy in one area of the body if the tumour is growing close to a nerve and presses on it.

- Surgery may damage nerves and cause symptoms in the affected area; for example, numbness or tingling and pain in the arm after breast cancer surgery.

- Rarely, radiotherapy may damage nerves within the treated area, causing symptoms such as numbness and weakness. These may develop months or years after treatment.

Occasionally, in some types of cancer, the body makes substances that damage peripheral nerves. This is called paraneoplastic peripheral neuropathy. It most commonly occurs in people with cancers of the lung, breast or ovaries, and in people with myeloma or Hodgkin lymphoma.

Symptoms

The symptoms of peripheral neuropathy vary depending on which nerves are affected. Anti-cancer drugs that cause nerve damage are most likely to affect sensory nerves but some can also affect the motor nerves and the autonomic nerves.

Peripheral neuropathy often affects the hands, feet and lower legs. This is because the longer a nerve is, the more vulnerable it is to injury. Nerves going to the hands, feet and lower legs are some of the longest in the body.

Symptoms of peripheral neuropathy are usually mild to begin with and gradually get worse.

Symptoms may include:

- **A change in sensation:** A feeling of heaviness, burning or pins and needles in the affected area. Alternatively, you may notice unusual sensations such as a feeling of warmth or burning when touching something cold.

- **Increased sensitivity:** You may find that even the lightest touch or pressure in the affected area feels uncomfortable or painful.

- **Pain:** This can be mild or more severe. The pain may be felt as sharp and stabbing or as a burning sensation, or it may feel like minor electric shocks. There are treatments to help to relieve pain.

- **Numbness:** There may be a loss of sensitivity or feeling in the affected area. Often the feet and fingertips are the first places to be affected.

- **Muscle weakness:** A muscle may lose strength if it isn't being stimulated by a nerve. Depending on which muscles are affected, this may make it difficult to walk, climb stairs or do other tasks. You may be given physiotherapy or special exercises to help with this.

- **Difficulty buttoning clothes or picking up small objects:** If the nerve endings in the fingers are affected, you may not be able to do "fiddly" tasks such as fastening small buttons or tying shoelaces.

- **Difficulty with balance, walking and coordination:** You may find that you stumble or trip when walking. Walking on uneven surfaces may be particularly difficult. You may feel clumsy at times, or that your body is not doing what you want it to do. Your sense of where things are around you may become less certain.

- **Constipation and feeling bloated:** Drinking at least two liters (three and a half pints) of fluid a day, and increasing the fibre in your diet may help to prevent constipation. If it does develop, you can contact your doctor or nurse for advice. You may need to take laxatives or other treatment prescribed by your doctor.

- **Feeling lightheaded or dizzy when you stand up:** Standing up more slowly may help as it gives your body more time to adjust to the change in position.

Anti-Cancer Drugs and Peripheral Neuropathy

There are many different chemotherapy drugs. The types that most frequently cause peripheral neuropathy are:

- **Vinca alkaloids:** These include vinblastine (Velbe®), vincristine (Oncovin®), vinorelbine (Navelbine®) and vindesine. Vincristine is the most likely one of these drugs to cause peripheral neuropathy.

- **The platinum based drugs** cisplatin, oxaliplatin (Eloxatin®) and carboplatin (Paraplatin®).

- **Taxanes** docetaxel (Taxotere®) and paclitaxel (Taxol®).

- **Other anti-cancer drugs** that may cause peripheral neuropathy include thalidomide, bortezomib (Velcade®) and alpha interferon.

Are some people more at risk of peripheral neuropathy when having these drugs?

You may be at higher risk if you:

- Are having more than one type of drug or treatment that can cause nerve damage.

- Have had previous anti-cancer drugs that can cause peripheral neuropathy.

- Have diabetes.

- Have low levels of certain minerals and vitamins (such as vitamin E, and B-vitamins). This may be because of diet, how much alcohol you drink, or for another reason.

What can I do to reduce my risk?

Let your doctor know if you think you drink quite a lot of alcohol. Taking vitamin B1 tablets can help to prevent nerve damage in this situation. Your doctor can prescribe these for you.

If you think your diet may be low in vitamins or minerals, talk to your doctor about whether you should take vitamin supplements. It's important not to take high doses of vitamins or minerals without your doctor's knowledge, in case this interferes with how well your treatment works.

If you already have peripheral neuropathy and need to have chemotherapy, there are a large number of chemotherapy drugs that do not cause or aggravate peripheral neuropathy. Your doctor can discuss the possible options with you.

Assessment

If you are being given a drug that can cause peripheral neuropathy, your doctor will monitor you for signs of nerve damage before each treatment. Symptoms are often mild to begin with and gradually become more troublesome and severe. The earlier that nerve damage is detected, the better. It is therefore important to tell your doctor if you notice any new symptoms that may be caused by the treatment or if your symptoms are getting worse.

If an anti-cancer drug is causing peripheral neuropathy, your doctor will assess how much your nerves are affected. This information helps them to decide whether to continue your treatment, reduce the

dose or stop the drug. There are various ways your doctor may assess your symptoms:

- Finding out how your symptoms are affecting your daily activities. Establishing your ability to sense where parts of your body are when your eyes are closed.

- Checking whether the reflexes in your ankles, knees and wrists are working. Everyone has points on our body which, if hit gently with a rubber hammer, will normally respond with an automatic (reflex) movement.

- Testing for numbness or loss of sensation (pinprick test). This test measures whether you have lost some or any feeling in particular areas of the body such as the feet, lower legs and hands. You will be asked to say if you can feel a pin gently touching your skin in the areas of your body that may be affected by nerve damage.

- Assessing your balance and coordination. for example, by asking you to walk in a straight line.

Other, more specialized, tests are also sometimes done:

- Nerve conduction studies assess the number of nerve cells that are working, and test the speed at which your nerves conduct an impulse.

- Electromyography (EMG) records the response of the nerve or muscle to an electrical impulse.

- Nerve conduction studies. These assess the number of nerve cells that are working, and test the speed at which your nerves conduct an impulse.

- Electromyography (EMG). This records the response of the nerve or muscle to an electrical impulse.

- Management of peripheral neuropathy. There isn't a treatment to prevent or reverse nerve damage caused by anti-cancer drugs. Studies are looking at various drug treatments, such as amifostine and xaliproden to see if they can help to protect against nerve damage during anti-cancer treatment. There are also studies looking into whether any treatments can reverse nerve damage that has occurred. But, at the moment, there isn't enough evidence that any of these drugs work.

The most effective treatment for peripheral neuropathy is to prevent further damage to the nerves. Sometimes it can help to lower the dose of the drug that is causing the problem. If your symptoms continue to get worse, your doctors may have to stop the drug.

In most people symptoms gradually improve once the drug is stopped, but they can sometimes continue to get worse for a few weeks. This is known as coasting.

Stopping treatment because of symptoms can be very difficult for some people to accept, especially if the treatment is working well. Your doctors will usually discuss with you whether another type of anti-cancer drug can be given instead.

Alternatively, some other kind of treatment such as radiotherapy may be suggested. It is extremely important not to stop treatment without first talking to your cancer specialist.

Most people find that their symptoms gradually improve with time as the nerves slowly recover. This may take several months or more. For some people nerve damage will be permanent. In this situation, however, many people find that their symptoms become less troublesome over time, as they adapt and find ways of coping with the changes.

Treating Pain

If you have nerve pain, sometimes called neuropathic pain, this can be managed in a number of ways.

Drugs: Some types of drugs can alter nerve impulses and so help to relieve nerve pain. Drugs that act in this way include antidepressants, anticonvulsants (drugs that are used to treat epilepsy) and some heart drugs. If your doctor suggests an antidepressant drug, this is because of the way it acts on nerves, and not because they think that the pain is in your mind. Drugs such as morphine can also sometimes be helpful.

Injections: A local anaesthetic may be injected around the damaged nerve. The anaesthetic works by blocking pain impulses for several days or weeks.

Transcutaneous electrical nerve stimulation (TENS): This may help to reduce pain. TENS uses pads, put onto the skin, that give off small electrical pulses. This causes a tingling sensation, which aims to stimulate nerves close to the area where the pain is. It is thought that this may work by blocking pain messages from being carried along

the nerves to the brain. TENS is unlikely to cause any side-effects, so can be worth trying.

Acupuncture: Acupuncture uses very fine needles that are placed through the skin at particular points. It isn't clear exactly how this works but it may help to block pain messages from being sent to the brain.

Psychological support: This may help to reduce the anxiety, tension and fear caused by the pain and can make it more bearable. This kind of support can be offered by psychotherapists and counsellors.

Other Types of Help

If your symptoms are mild, you may not need any additional help in managing them. If you have more troublesome symptoms, support is available to help you cope with them.

A physiotherapist will be able to offer treatment and advice if you are having problems with coordination, muscle weakness, balance, or walking.

If you are having difficulty in carrying out daily tasks because of peripheral neuropathy, you can ask to be referred to an occupational therapist. They will be able to assess your needs and recommend appropriate aids and equipment to help you. There are organizations which provide equipment for people who need help with daily tasks.

If symptoms continue for more than six months and cause you difficulty in walking or in carrying out daily activities you may be entitled to financial help.

Things You Can Do

- If your hands or feet are affected, it is important to protect them as much as possible.

- Keep them warm (wear gloves and warm socks in cold weather).

- Wear gloves when working with your hands—for example when gardening or washing-up.

- Use pot holders and take care to avoid burning your hands when cooking.

- Wear well-fitting shoes or boots.

- Avoid walking around barefoot and check your feet regularly for any problems.

- Test the temperature of water with your elbow to make sure it isn't too hot before baths, showers or doing the washing-up. Turn the temperature control to a lower setting for hot water or have a temperature control (thermostat) fitted.

- If your balance, coordination or walking is affected, you may be at more risk of accidents and falls.

- Make sure rooms are well lit, and always put on a light if you get up during the night.

- Keep areas that you walk through, such as halls, free of clutter and make sure there aren't things such as loose rugs you could trip over.

- Get advice from a physiotherapist about walking aids if your balance is affected.

Your Feelings

How peripheral neuropathy affects each person and how much practical and emotional support is needed to cope with it varies from person to person. You may find that your life is not affected very much, or, you may have many more challenges and difficulties to cope with.

If the peripheral neuropathy is severe and causing changes to your lifestyle, it is natural to feel isolated and frustrated. You may have different emotions, including anger, resentment, guilt, anxiety and fear.

These are all normal reactions and are part of the process many people go through in trying to come to terms with side effects caused by their treatment.

Chapter 45

Cancer Treatment and Physical Appearance

Chapter Contents

Section 45.1

Hair Loss (Alopecia)

A common side effect of chemotherapy is hair loss. This information answers questions about hair loss and offers alternatives for coping with this condition.

Why does chemotherapy cause hair loss?

Chemotherapy attacks cells in our body that are rapidly growing, such as cancer cells. Some normal cells that also grow rapidly, like hair cells, are also affected.

Does all chemotherapy cause hair loss?

Many chemotherapy drugs have no affect on your hair. Others cause mild hair thinning or complete hair loss. Your doctor or nurse can tell you if hair loss is expected with your treatment.

Scalp hair is the most frequently affected, but loss of eyelashes, eyebrows, facial hair, pubic hair and body hair can also occur.

The degree of hair loss will depend on several factors, including the chemotherapy drug(s) and dose received, how it is given and other treatments.

When will the hair loss occur?

Hair loss usually begins two weeks after your first treatment. Some people notice achiness or tingling of the scalp as the hair loss begins. If complete hair loss is expected, the hair may come out in large amounts and is usually completed within three to seven days.

Is the hair loss permanent?

Hair loss caused by chemotherapy is usually temporary. Your hair will start to re-grow after your treatment is completed. Some people

experience a small amount of re-growth during treatment. Most people experience significant hair re-growth three to five months after treatment is completed. It is common for hair to grow back curlier and a slightly different color.

Can I apply ice packs to my scalp to decrease hair loss?

No. It generally does not work. It may actually decrease the ability of the chemotherapy to kill cancer cells in this area.

How should I care for my hair while receiving chemotherapy?

Even if your chemotherapy treatment is not expected to cause significant hair changes, some precautions are still recommended. If hair thinning is expected, these precautions may decrease damage to your hair:

- Use a soft bristle brush and a gentle, pH balanced shampoo
- Avoid using hair dryers, hot rollers or curling irons too much
- Avoid bleaching or coloring your hair
- Avoid permanent waves
- Avoid braiding or placing hair in a pony tail
- Sleep on a satin pillowcase to decrease friction.
- Wear a hat when in the sun

If your hair is long, cutting it shorter may help decrease the impact of your hair loss when it occurs.

Should I get a wig?

Each person responds differently when learning that they may experience partial or total hair loss. There is no right or wrong response. Do what's comfortable for you.

If you plan to purchase a wig, make an appointment with a wig stylist before the hair loss is expected so that the color, style and texture of your hair can be matched to a wig. If hair loss begins before your appointment with the wig stylist, save some pieces of your hair and take them with you.

Types of wigs:

- **Natural hair:** More expensive Requires more care
- **Synthetic:** Less expensive

Some insurance companies provide coverage for the purchase of wigs. Consider scarves, turbans and hats to conceal hair loss. They are cooler, can be more comfortable and overall require less care than wigs. There are many attractive, stylish, and creative head covers available.

Why am I so upset about my hair loss?

It is normal to be upset about hair loss from cancer treatment. It may effect how you feel about yourself. It is also a visible reminder of your cancer. Share your feelings with your doctor, nurse, family and friends. There are many educational and supportive programs available.

Section 45.2

Nail and Skin Care

"Nail and Skin Care Tip Sheet," by Carolyn Vachani, RN, MSN, AOCN, reprinted with permission from www.oncolink.org. Copyright © 2006 by the Trustees of the University of Pennsylvania. All rights reserved.

During cancer therapy, you may notice changes in your skin and/or nails. These changes vary based on the type and dose of therapy you are receiving. Some common changes with radiation therapy include redness, peeling, thin or fragile skin and/or increased sensitivity to sunlight. If you are receiving chemotherapy, you may notice changes in skin tone or pigmentation, very dry skin, rashes, redness, peeling, and/or increased sensitivity to sunlight. If you develop any of these problems, be sure to show them to your oncology healthcare team, as they can be signs of reactions to some medications or can require adjustments to the doses of chemotherapy or radiation. Your fingernails may become weak, break or lift off, or develop ridges (which will grow out over time).

General tips for caring for your skin:

• Wash with warm water and a mild, unscented soap.

- You can use your normal deodorant. If a product appears to cause irritation, stop using it and try another brand. You may benefit from a "non-allergenic" product.

- Use an electric razor for shaving to avoid cuts.

- Avoid tight clothing or irritating fabrics, such as wool, that may rub your skin.

- Protect your skin from sunlight. Use SPF 30 or higher, even on overcast days. Wear a hat and long sleeved clothing to cover exposed skin and/or carry an umbrella when out during peak sun hours.

- Protect your skin from extreme cold or heat.

Dry skin is a common side effect. Tips for dealing with dry skin include:

- Use an emollient, which are creams that soften skin and moisturize. Creams tend to be more effective than lotions. Some examples are Eucerin®, Aquaphor®, Nivea®, and Cetaphil®.

- Avoid perfumed or scented lotions, as these can be irritating.

- Apply your moisturizer or cream after your shower or bath when skin is still damp.

- Don't forget to moisturize your lips! Try an eye or face cream to moisten the sensitive skin on your face.

- Drink 8–10 glasses of non-alcoholic fluid a day.

Nails can be affected by cancer therapy too. Here are some tips to dealing with nail changes:

- Avoid cutting cuticles; this can be a source of infection. Use a cuticle cream instead. If you need to cut your cuticle, be sure to clean the clipper before using it.

- Artificial fingernails can harbor bacteria and lead to infections, so you should not use them.

- Nails absorb water and expand, then contract as they dry out. The more they expand and contract, the weaker they become, so wear gloves to protect your nails when doing housework or gardening.

- Keep your hands moisturized and your nails cut short.

- You may want to use nail polish to give your nails extra strength and cover imperfections.

- Soaking your nails in or massaging the nail with oil, such as vegetable or olive, helps replace moisture lost from water exposure. These natural oils lack the alcohol containing fragrance often found in commercial nail products.

If your nails break or lift off, try to keep them clean and protected. Covering the nail with a band-aid can protect it from trauma. Clean with soap and warm water and apply an antibiotic ointment twice a day.

If the nail or nail bed appears infected (redness, swelling, warm to the touch), inform your healthcare team.

Chapter 46

Cognitive-Related Effects of Cancer Treatment

Overview

Cognitive disorders and delirium are conditions in which the patient experiences a confused mental state and changes in behavior. People who have cognitive disorders or delirium may fall in and out of consciousness and may have problems with the following:

- Attention
- Thinking
- Awareness
- Emotion
- Memory
- Muscle control
- Sleeping and waking

Delirium occurs frequently in patients with cancer, especially in patients with advanced cancer.

Delirium usually occurs suddenly and the patient's symptoms may come and go during the day. This condition can be treated and is often temporary, even in people with advanced illness. In the last 24 to 48

PDQ® Cancer Information Summary. National Cancer Institute; Bethesda, MD. "Cognitive Disorders and Delirium (PDQ®): Patient Version." Updated 09/2008. Available at: http://cancer.gov. Accessed August 14, 2009.

hours of life, however, delirium may be permanent due to problems such as organ failure.

Causes of Cognitive Disorders and Delirium

Cognitive disorders and delirium may be complications of cancer and cancer treatment, especially in people with advanced cancer. In patients with cancer, cognitive disorders and delirium may be due to the direct effects that cancer has on the brain, such as the pressure of a growing tumor. Cognitive disorders and delirium may also be caused by indirect effects of cancer or its treatment, including the following:

- Organ failure

- Electrolytc imbalances

- Infection

- Symptoms caused by the cancer but that occur apart from the local or distant spread of the tumor (paraneoplastic syndromes), such as inflammation of the brain

- Medication side effects

- Withdrawal from drugs that depress (slow down) the central nervous system

Patients with cancer usually take many medications. Some drugs have side effects that include delirium and confusion. The effects of these drugs usually go away after the drug is stopped.

Risk factors for delirium include having a serious disease and having more than one disease. Other conditions besides having cancer may place a patient at risk for developing delirium. Risk factors include the following:

- Advanced cancer or other serious illness

- Having more than one disease

- Older age

- Previous mental disorder, such as dementia

- Low levels of albumin (protein) in the blood

- Infection

- Taking medications that affect the mind or behavior

- Taking high doses of pain medication

Early identification of risk factors may help prevent the onset of delirium or may reduce the length of time it takes to correct it.

Effects on the Patient, Family, and Healthcare Providers

Cognitive disorders and delirium can be upsetting to the family and caregivers, and may be dangerous to the patient if judgment is affected. These conditions can cause the patient to act unpredictably and sometimes violently. Even a quiet or calm patient can suddenly experience a change in mood or become agitated, requiring increased care. The safety of the patient, family, and caregivers is most important.

Cognitive disorders and delirium may affect physical health and communication.

Patients with cognitive disorders or delirium are more likely to fall, be incontinent (unable to control bladder and/or bowels), and become dehydrated (drink too little water to maintain health). They often require a longer hospital stay than patients without cognitive disorders or delirium.

The confused mental state of these patients may hinder their communication with family members and the healthcare providers. Assessment of the patient's symptoms becomes difficult and the patient may be unable to make decisions regarding care. Agitation in these patients may be mistaken as an expression of pain. Conflict can arise among the patient, family, and staff concerning the level of pain medication needed.

Diagnosis of Cognitive Disorders and Delirium

Possible signs of cognitive disorders and delirium include sudden personality changes, impaired thinking, or unusual anxiety or depression.

A patient who suddenly becomes agitated or uncooperative, experiences personality or behavior changes, has impaired thinking, decreased attention span, or intense, unusual anxiety or depression, may be experiencing cognitive disorders or delirium. Patients who develop these symptoms need to be assessed completely.

The symptoms of delirium are similar to symptoms of depression and dementia.

Early symptoms of delirium are similar to symptoms of anxiety, anger, depression, and dementia. Delirium that causes the patient to be very inactive may appear to be depression. Delirium and dementia

are difficult to tell apart, since both may cause disorientation and impair memory, thinking, and judgment. Dementia may be caused by a number of medical conditions, including Alzheimer disease. Some differences in the symptoms of delirium and dementia include the following:

- Patients with delirium often go in and out of consciousness. Patients who have dementia usually remain alert

- Delirium may occur suddenly. Dementia appears gradually and gets worse over time

- Sleeping and waking problems are more common with delirium than with dementia

In elderly patients who have cancer, dementia is often present along with delirium, making diagnosis difficult. The diagnosis is more likely dementia if symptoms continue after treatment for delirium is given.

In patients aged 65 or older who have survived cancer for more than five years, the risk for cognitive disorders and dementia is increased, apart from the risk for delirium.

Regular screening of the patient and monitoring of the patient's symptoms can help in the diagnosis of delirium.

Treatment of Delirium

Patient and family concerns are addressed when deciding the treatment of delirium. Deciding if, when, and how to treat a person with delirium depends on the setting, how advanced the cancer is, the wishes of the patient and family, and how the delirium symptoms are affecting the patient.

Monitoring alone may be all that is necessary for patients who are not dangerous to themselves. In other cases, symptoms may be treated or causes of the delirium may be identified and treated.

Changing the Patient's Surroundings

Controlling the patient's surroundings may help reduce mild symptoms of delirium. The following changes may be effective:

- Putting the patient in a quiet, well-lit room with familiar objects

- Placing a clock or calendar where the patient can see it

- Reducing noise

- Having family present

- Limiting changes in caregivers

To prevent a patient from harming himself or herself or others, physical restraints also may be necessary.

Treatment of the Causes of Delirium

The standard approach to managing delirium is to find and treat the causes. Symptoms may be treated at the same time. Identifying the causes of delirium will include a physical examination to check general signs of health, including checking for signs of disease. A medical history of the patient's past illnesses and treatments will also be taken. In a terminally ill delirious patient being cared for at home, the doctor may do a limited assessment to determine the cause or may treat just the symptoms.

Treatment may include the following:

- Stopping or reducing medications that cause delirium

- Giving fluids into the bloodstream to correct dehydration

- Giving drugs to correct hypercalcemia (too much calcium in the blood)

- Giving antibiotics for infections

Treatment with Medication

Drugs called antipsychotics may be used to treat the symptoms of delirium. Drugs that sedate (calm) the patient may also be used, especially if the patient is near death. All of these drugs have side effects and the patient will be monitored closely by a doctor. The decision to use drugs that sedate the patient will be made in cooperation with family members after efforts have been made to reverse the delirium.

Delirium and Sedation

The decision to use drugs to sedate the patient who is near death and has symptoms of delirium, pain, and difficult breathing presents ethical and legal issues for both the doctor and the family. When the symptoms of delirium are not relieved with standard treatment approaches and the patient is experiencing severe distress and suffering,

the doctor may discuss the option to give drugs that will sedate the patient. This decision is guided by the following principles:

- Healthcare professionals who have experience in palliative care make repeated assessments of the patient's response to treatments. The family is always included.

- The need to use drugs that sedate the patient is evaluated by a multidisciplinary team of healthcare professionals.

- Temporary sedation should be considered.

- A multidisciplinary team of healthcare professionals will work with the family to ensure that the family's views are assessed and understood.

Chapter 47

Fighting Cancer Fatigue

Treating the Symptoms of Fatigue

Treating the causes of cancer fatigue can sometimes help to reduce tiredness. Help is also available for the symptoms of fatigue. There are some suggestions below. You may find that some of our suggestions don't work for you. It may take some trial and error to learn how to manage fatigue and know what works for you. This may take some time. But the first step is to tell your doctors and nurses about your fatigue. More than half of cancer patients with fatigue never tell their doctor about it. But if you tell your doctor, they can find ways of helping you.

Treating Anemia

Most people with cancer will have anemia at some point during their illness. Although it's not usually life threatening, fatigue caused by anemia can have a big effect on your daily life. You may need a blood transfusion to bring your red cell count up again and make you feel more energetic. Up to a third of chemotherapy patients may need a blood transfusion for anemia. There are many different types of anemia and you may have anemia for a number of reasons. In some situations it may not be helpful to have a blood transfusion. Your doctor or specialist nurse can assess you to see if it would be helpful for you.

"Treating Cancer Fatigue," reprinted with permission from CancerHelp UK, www.cancerhelp.org.uk, the patient information website of Cancer Research UK, © 2009.

Another treatment for anemia is a drug called erythropoietin or EPO. EPO is a hormone made by your kidneys that encourages the body to make more red blood cells. A number of studies have shown that EPO can raise hemoglobin levels in the body and improve people's quality of life. But some research has found that EPO may also increase the chance of some types of cancer coming back after treatment. The benefits of EPO may outweigh the risks for some people, but it should be prescribed carefully.

EPO is available on the NHS for people with cancer, in some circumstances. In May 2008, NICE (National Institute for Health and Clinical Excellence) decided that EPO (with iron injections) should only be given to:

- People with anemia related to their cancer treatment if they cannot have blood transfusions;

- Women with ovarian cancer who have had platinum-based chemotherapy, such as carboplatin or cisplatin.

Exercising

Exercise may be the last thing you feel like doing. You may feel so tired that doing any exercise seems ridiculous. But sometimes, the less you do, the less you feel like doing. We know that light to moderate exercise every day helps people with cancer to feel better and can give them more energy. Many people with cancer get out of condition while they are going through treatment and recovering afterwards. If you feel run down and unfit, one of the best ways to feel more energetic is to build up the amount of exercise you do.

Just a short walk each day helps. Try and increase the distance you go each day. You can walk with a friend to support you along the way. A pedometer is a great way of keeping track of how active you are. Pedometers are about the size of a matchbox and they clip to your waistband or belt. The pedometer counts every step you take so you can easily keep track of how your exercise is building up each day.

You can buy a pedometer from a sports shop. As a guide, health experts advise that a healthy adult should walk about 10,000 steps a day. Obviously if you are having treatment or have advanced cancer, that might be too much for you. Talk to your doctor or a physiotherapist about where to start so that you can find a realistic goal.

Try doing your exercise at different times in the day to find out when suits you best. Some people find the early morning a good time. Doing a bit of exercise every day will make you feel less tired and your appetite is

likely to improve too. Overall, you may be more able to cope with things and be happier in yourself. But don't overdo it. If you are really aching the next day, you are doing too much. Drink plenty of water whenever you exercise to prevent dehydration. And remember to get advice from your doctor before starting any heavy exercise program.

Exercise can also help people in the advanced stages of cancer. You may not be able to go for a long walk but even gentle exercises in bed or standing up can help. Your hospital physiotherapist can help you plan an exercise program that suits your needs and how much you can do.

Getting Support from Other People

This can mean:

- Finding out more about your cancer;
- Talking to other people at the outpatient department;
- Going to a support group;
- Having some counseling.

Just about everyone needs support from someone else when they have cancer. You can get some support from family and friends, or doctors and nurses. But support from other people who've been through the same thing can make all the difference. Talking to other people in a support group can show you that you are not alone. It can confirm that fatigue is something many people with cancer have and that fatigue will lessen with time after a cancer has been successfully treated.

Resting

If you have advanced cancer and are very tired, it is important to set yourself a few rest times throughout the day. This can be difficult to stick to and you may try to push yourself to keep going. But that won't help. You'll be more tired and less able to cope. You don't have to sleep during these rest times. If you are having trouble sleeping at night it may be better not to actually sleep. Just sit or lie down somewhere quiet. Pace yourself, have some ëyou' time and recharge those batteries! Just sitting or lying down to rest will help. And remember you don't have to do everything, only the things that are important to you right now. Everything else can wait. There is more information on saving your energy below.

If you have short term fatigue, caused by treatment you may be better off taking a little exercise than resting.

Sleeping

Sleepless nights can make you feel tired, cranky and a bit dazed. If you often have trouble sleeping at night, it may help to change a few things about when and where you sleep. If you have cancer related fatigue, sometimes getting a lot of sleep may not help much because lots of other things are causing your fatigue. But to make sure you sleep as well as possible.

- Try to sleep in a quiet, calm room.

- Go to bed and get up at the same time each day.

- Make sure the room that you sleep in is a comfortable and soothing place—an untidy room may be distracting and make you feel anxious.

- Make sure the temperature is right.

- Sleep with the window open if you prefer, as long as there isn't too much noise outside.

- Spend time relaxing before you go to bed—have a bath, read or listen to music

- Do some light exercise each day to help tire yourself out.

- Don't drink too much alcohol before bed—you may fall asleep to start with but you'll have a disturbed night.

- Avoid caffeine (coffee, tea, chocolate and cola drinks) after early afternoon.

- Limit daytime naps to 45 minutes so it doesn't stop you sleeping at night.

- Have a light snack before you go to bed to stop hunger waking you up.

- Practice relaxation before sleeping—you could imagine somewhere beautiful you'd like to be.

- Listen to a relaxation tape.

When you really can't sleep, get up and watch TV, read, or listen to music until you feel sleepy. Or try the simple things your Mum may have suggested, like taking a warm bath and a warm milky drink. The amino acids in milk are thought to encourage sleep. Then go back to bed and try again. Do let your doctor know if you often have trouble sleeping.

Improving Your Diet

Eating enough to keep up your energy levels can be hard if side effects from your treatment are making you sick or have diarrhea. But it is important to try and eat what you can, as your diet plays an important role in controlling fatigue. There are some good tips on how to control diarrhea and sickness in the main chemotherapy section of CancerHelp UK (online at www.cancerhelp.org.uk).

Changing Your Medicines

Although some medicines can cause fatigue, some can help to control the side effects of cancer treatment that cause fatigue, including:

- Drugs that stimulate your appetite—steroids or progesterone;
- Painkillers;
- Drugs that treat anemia;
- Sleeping tablets;
- Antidepressants.

Doctors have to find a balance between the positive and negative effects of these drugs.

Learning to Manage Fatigue

You can do many things in your everyday life that will help to save your energy. Taking short cuts on some things or getting help from other people may both help you feel less tired. You could:

- Try not to rush—plan ahead where possible and give yourself plenty of time to get to places, preferably not in the rush hour.
- Put chairs around the house so that you can easily stop and rest if you need to.
- Sit down to dry off after your bath, or simply put on a toweling dressing gown and let that do the work.
- Have some handrails fitted in your bathroom to hold on to when you get in and out of the shower or bath (the hospital can help to arrange this for you).
- Prepare your clothes and lay them out in one place before you dress.

- Get dressed sitting down, as far as you can. Try not to bend too much—rest your foot on your knee to put socks and shoes on.

- Fasten your bra at the front first and then turn it to the back.

- Wear loose-fitting clothes, and things with few buttons to do up.

- Where possible do household tasks sitting down—peeling vegetables, ironing (or better still, buy clothes that don't need ironing).

- Use a duster on a long stick and sit to do your dusting.

- Write a shopping list and go when the shops are quiet.

- If you have children, play games that you can do sitting or lying down—reading, puzzles, board games or drawing.

- Ask family and friends for help with shopping, housework or collecting the children from school.

- Have plenty of nutritious snacks and drinks in, so you can have something quickly and easily whenever you feel like eating.

- Don't forget to do things that you enjoy—it will take your mind off your cancer and make you feel more relaxed.

Keeping a Fatigue Diary

Keep a record of how you are feeling, and how your energy levels change. This will help you to tell if you are more or less tired than before, and help you to identify which activities make you feel better or worse.

If you are tired and don't feel like cooking, buy ready made meals at your local shop or supermarket. Or buy ready prepared vegetables or pre-grated cheese. Every bit of work done for you will save your energy.

Causes of Long-Term Fatigue

Remember that fatigue for people having treatment for cancer is different from the fatigue some people feel long after finishing their treatment. Things that can cause long-term fatigue include:

- Bone marrow transplants—in some cases, these can cause fatigue for many years after the transplant;

- Cancer treatment in childhood, especially for brain tumors;

- Taking tamoxifen for several years.

Many people with cancer find it helpful to talk to other people who have the same symptoms as them. If you think this may help, look for an organization that can put you in touch with a local support group. (You can find suggestions through a link at the www.cancerhelp.org. uk website.) Sharing your feelings with someone in the same situation may make you feel less anxious about your fatigue, and you can often get tips on how to cope better from talking about your own situation.

Part Seven

Women's Issues in Cancer Survivorship

Chapter 48

Living with Cancer

Chapter Contents

Section 48.1

Cancer Changes Everything

From "Coping with Cancer: Tools to Help You Live,"
by Rosalie Canosa, LCSW-R, MPA. © 2008 Cancer Care, Inc.
All rights reserved. Reprinted with permission.

What do I tell my children? How is my husband going to react? Am I going to be able to continue working? How do I pay for treatment? What happens after my treatment is finished?

The answers to these questions are different for everyone because no two people experience cancer in the same way. The diagnosis may make you feel worried, sad, confused, or even angry. Your new world is filled with information and medical terms you never wanted to learn. And in addition to the physical difficulties, there are emotional and financial issues that you must learn to manage. Without a doubt, cancer turns your world upside down.

This information will help you understand the challenges that are a part of living with cancer and provide you with the tools you need to cope better with this experience. Importantly, you will learn that you are not alone—there are sources of support available to you, and many people have made this journey before you.

For more than 60 years, CancerCare®—a national non-profit organization—has helped people with cancer and their loved ones with exactly these kinds of challenges (visit www.cancercare.org). CancerCare provides professional counseling, educational programs, financial guidance, and referrals to helpful resources—all completely free of charge. CancerCare oncology social workers know that when someone is first diagnosed, it seems overwhelming. From the moment of diagnosis, life will never be the same. But the tips and advice outlined here will give you tools you need to truly live with cancer.

Treating the Whole Person

When someone is diagnosed with cancer, it seems everyone is focused—and rightly so—on the person's physical well being: treatments, side effects, doctor visits, tests. But we know there are other parts of

life affected by cancer: your self-image, work, family, and your approach to living. These are the psychosocial aspects of cancer.

People diagnosed with cancer face a whole range of concerns about finances, medical worries, and emotional issues. For example, you may feel that you are "complaining" if you express sadness at losing your hair because of treatment. You may think you should "just be glad to be alive" and that worrying about a "little thing" like hair loss shouldn't concern you. Or, if you're a caregiver having a particularly difficult day, you may feel like you don't have "the right" to be upset because of what your partner is experiencing. But it is not wrong to be as concerned about psychosocial effects as your physical state. In fact, in October 2007, the National Institute of Medicine (IOM) released a report called "Cancer Care for the Whole Patient: Meeting Psychosocial Health Needs." In the report, the IOM recommends that the standard of care for all cancer patients must include addressing the emotional and practical effects of cancer.

The report names CancerCare® as one of the leaders in providing such psychosocial services. That's because at CancerCare, we understand the complex issues raised by cancer. More importantly, we know that finding ways to cope with these concerns brings an enormous sense of relief to both the person with cancer and his or her loved ones.

Coping: What It Really Means

At CancerCare we often use the word "coping" to describe how people deal with their cancer situation. People sometimes mistakenly think that coping means just living with a problem, whether you like it or not. But coping actually means managing a problem, and finding ways to take control of it. You can't control the fact that you or a loved one has cancer. But you can control how you react to and live with cancer.

Coping Is...

- Managing and understanding what you need to live with your problems
- Making efforts to bring your problems under control
- Maintaining a healthy balance of realism and cautious optimism

Coping Is Not...

- Hopeless acceptance of a problem

- Being happy about your whole life all the time in spite of cancer

- A hands-off attitude that says you don't have to make an effort to overcome problems

Learning about Medicine

One of the biggest challenges for people with cancer is learning all the complex medical aspects of the disease. As the science of treating cancer has advanced, researchers have developed better, more effective treatments, which means patients have more choices than they did a few decades ago. At CancerCare, we often hear patients say they are not sure how to choose the "right" treatment. The "wrong" choice, they worry, could make their condition worse.

One of the reasons why making choices is often overwhelming and confusing is the vast amount of information available on the internet, some of it unreliable. Advertisements on television and health stories in newspapers and magazines add to this outpouring of information. It's difficult to sift through everything. Throw into that mix the different doctors involved in your care, along with well-meaning friends and family offering opinions, and it all adds up to what people with cancer describe as "too many voices."

People with cancer know they are expected to take part in care and treatment decisions. Because treatment nowadays often takes place in an outpatient setting, it allows for greater freedom. But it also means that patients and their loved ones will spend less time with doctors and nurses and more time taking greater responsibility for their own care.

So how do you cope with this situation? Here are some tips:

- As a health care consumer, it is your right to have a good health care team that listens to your questions and concerns. Get to know all the members of your team and learn how each one helps you.

- Identify one person on the medical team who is in charge of your care and "funnel" all information through that person.

- As you visit different websites or hear about new treatments, write down questions as they arise. At your next doctor's visit, bring these questions with you so you can keep track of what you need to know.

- During your doctor's visits, take notes or ask a family member to take notes. Also ask your doctor if you can tape-record your visits.

This will allow you to go back later and listen carefully to all the information presented by your doctor.

- Ask your doctor to recommend books, brochures, and websites. For tips on evaluating websites, see the information below.

- Find trustworthy educational programs about your cancer. CancerCare® offers more than 50 free Telephone Education Workshops every year that provide people with reliable information from experts on a range of cancer diagnoses and topics.

Can I Trust This Website?

Questions You Should Ask

What is the purpose of the website—educational or commercial? For example, a website sponsored by a pharmaceutical company isn't likely to give you unbiased information about a competing drug. But because that site must meet the standards of the U.S. Food and Drug Administration, it will be an excellent source on a particular product.

What is the source of the information? Generally, nationally known cancer centers, medical schools, large non-profit organizations, and government agencies provide the highest quality information.

Are you able to find contact information for the people behind the website? If you can't communicate with them, find another source.

Are the links relevant and appropriate for the site?

Websites that refer you to unreliable or frankly commercial sources of information should be rejected.

Remember: The internet is not a substitute for individual medical care. Use credible information you find on these sites to help you communicate more effectively with your doctor.

Finding Financial Help

Cancer is an expensive illness. Half of the people who contact CancerCare® each year cite financial need as a major source of difficulty. Some have no health insurance, some are insured but don't have coverage for parts of their treatment such as prescription drugs, and many do not have extra income to meet new costs such as child care or transportation to treatment. People with cancer and their caregivers often have to cut back on time spent at work, which means their income goes down at the same time their bills pile up.

Financial stress often causes emotional stress. When a family is under new financial pressures, it can create feelings of resentment

and sadness. Because cancer treatment often means years of medical care, financial concerns can influence major life decisions about work, housing, and school.

There is assistance available, and CancerCare can help you navigate the maze of different forms, government and non-profit programs, and other sources of financial relief.

Here are some of the things you can do:

- Talk to your insurance company. Many companies will assign a case manager to help you work through insurance concerns, clarify benefits, and suggest ways to get other health services.

- Talk to your medical care providers about your needs. Many treatment centers have social workers who help you sort through financial concerns. CancerCare social workers can also help you.

- Find out which government programs (entitlements) you are eligible for and apply promptly. You can order a free fact sheet from CancerCare called "Getting to Know Your Entitlements" that outlines all the different sources of help available.

- Learn how private organizations can help you. Many pharmaceutical companies have programs to help low-income patients pay for prescription drugs.

- Talk directly to your creditors if you expect to—or have already—run out of money and cannot meet your daily living expenses. Many utility and mortgage companies will work out a payment plan with you before a crisis develops.

Dealing with the Emotional Impact

The words "you have cancer" are frightening and overwhelming. Some people experience feelings of helplessness and hopelessness and question whether they know how to deal with these feelings. At times, people may be reluctant to tell their doctor about their concerns because they don't want to distract him or her from the primary goal of treatment.

Emotional needs vary from person to person, depending on age, closeness of family and friends, access to medical care, and other factors. For example, a 25-year-old person with a cancer diagnosis has different pressures and responsibilities than a person who is 75. Younger people may feel more confusion about having cancer at an age when they usually feel invincible, and none of their friends is ill. On the other hand, an older person may have fewer family members to rely on; perhaps

children have moved away and started their own families, or there is no spouse at home who can care for his or her medical needs.

But no matter what our stage in life, cancer takes an emotional toll on the person diagnosed, as well as everyone close to that person. At CancerCare®, we work to individualize support for each person, offering help that fits your needs now.

Strengthening the Spirit

When you or a loved one is diagnosed with cancer, you might find yourself turning to your spiritual side more often to help you cope. Or, you may begin to question your faith. Both of these reactions are normal.

Whether you are in the process of strengthening or reevaluating your spiritual beliefs, you might want to try the following:

- Take time to meditate or pray regularly. This can bring a sense of calm and stability during difficult times.

- Read spiritual writings such as the Bible, the Koran, the Book of Psalms, Bhagavad Gita, or other faith-based texts. Delving into sacred texts can put you in touch with ancient traditions of wisdom and give you a sense of connection with a more divine reality.

- Seek the help of others. You might begin an ongoing dialogue with your clergy or counselor, or join a group for meditation, prayer, and support.

- Retreat to spiritual spaces, natural settings, or concerts and museums to cultivate a spiritual sense of peace.

- Keep a journal to express your feelings, thoughts, and memories. It can contribute to your process of self-discovery and spiritual development.

A diagnosis of cancer can start a process of looking inward for a stronger connection to what is most meaningful and sacred. Out of the turmoil of this crisis, you may find strength and deeper meaning in your life.

It's important to remember that everyone experiences some kind of sadness or helplessness when confronted with cancer—and that many people have come through these experiences.

Life will never be the same after cancer, but it doesn't mean you stop living. There are many things you can do to handle the emotional impact of cancer.

To cope better emotionally, you can:

- Keep track of your feelings. Many people find it helpful to keep a journal or record their emotions through photography, drawing, painting, music, or other expressions.

- Share your feelings with people close to you. Sometimes, caregivers and people with cancer feel as if they are a "burden" to their loved ones by "complaining" about their problems. Remember that you are entitled to every emotion you have. Don't be afraid to share these emotions with the people close to you.

- Seek individual counseling with a professional. Oncology social workers, psychologists, and psychiatrists help you sort through your many complex emotions. CancerCare provides free individual counseling to people with cancer and caregivers across the country.

- Join a support group or "buddy" program. Talk with someone who has had a similar experience. Support groups help you feel less isolated. They provide reassurance, suggestions, and insight, allowing you to share similar concerns with your peers in a safe and supportive environment. CancerCare® provides free, professionally run support groups on the telephone, online, and face to face.

- Tell your doctor and nurse about your feelings. Doctors understand, better than ever before, that patients are concerned about good quality of life as they go through treatment. Sometimes, people benefit from a referral for counseling or a medicine for anxiety or depression.

Your Inner Power

Life changes in many ways when you or a loved one is diagnosed with cancer. The educational, financial, and emotional challenges are great. But there is one thing that even cancer does not have the power to change: the fact that you are the expert on your own life. You can manage many aspects of cancer that will help you cope better with the disease.

Section 48.2

Tips for Cancer Patients

Living with a serious disease is not easy, and we hope these tips will help you throughout your treatment.

- Adopt a fighting spirit.

- It's okay to discourage false cheerfulness and to share how you're feeling.

- Seek support from your family and friends.

- As a member of your health care team, learn about your disease and ask questions.

- Be an active participant in your treatment and recovery efforts.

- Make positive changes in your lifestyle that will improve your outcomes, such as quitting smoking, incorporating exercise and getting good nutrition.

- Find something to laugh about each day. Good humor is healthy for the body and soul.

- For safety's sake, when not feeling your best, ask for transportation assistance to your medical appointments.

- Participation in a support group can help you learn from others.

- Pay attention to how you are feeling and get plenty of rest, good nutrition, and take time for personal care.

- Find ways to express your feelings by speaking with a mental health provider or the Cancer Center Social Worker (visit http://cancer.ucsd.edu).

- Consider complementary therapies, such as massage, aromatherapy, acupuncture, yoga to help relieve stress and other symptoms.

- Just be yourself and continue to do the things that you already enjoy doing.

- Continue your current sports activities as much as physically possible.

- Allow yourself private time apart from your family and friends to do nothing, or something important to you.

- If you are currently employed, continue to work if physically possible.

- Practice guided visualization and/or meditation.

- Nourish yourself spiritually through prayer or guidance from a religious leader.

- Listen to relaxing music that can bring about serenity.

- Read uplifting books.

- If you have a significant person in your life, keep the romance going by selecting romantic movies to watch.

- Take time for simple pleasures, such as a warm bath, a manicure or pedicure.

- Keep in mind that your memory function and energy level will fluctuate according to your treatment and medications. Let your caregiver know when you need help.

- Consider writing down your feelings in a journal.

- Keep a calendar and or log of activities and appointments to help stay organized.

Chapter 49

Eating Well When You Have Cancer

Good nutrition is vital at every stage of your cancer treatment and recovery. Eating well gives you energy, helps you feel better and keeps your body strong so that you can cope with side effects from treatment. It will also help you heal and recover after treatment.

People's responses to food during their cancer experience vary widely. Some continue to enjoy eating and their appetite stays strong. Others find that just when they need to eat well, they feel unable to do so. Side effects or emotions like fear and anxiety can make eating more challenging. To help you eat well during difficult times, you might:

- Try to present your food in an attractive way on the plate to make it more appealing.

- Make mealtimes relaxed and pleasant. (Try music or soft lighting if this helps.)

- Experiment with different foods—some that didn't taste good before might taste good now.

This chapter begins with "Eating Well When You Have Cancer," and also includes "Special Nutrition Needs," "Food Safety Issues," and "Eating Well after Treatment," © 2009 Canadian Cancer Society. All rights reserved. Reprinted with permission. Accessed August 13, 2009. To view these documents along with additional information, visit http://www.cancer.ca/Canadawide.aspx?sc_lang=en.

- Remind yourself that eating difficulties are temporary. Try to be patient and know that you will be able to eat with pleasure again—perhaps as soon as tomorrow.

Try to make your food choices as balanced and varied as possible so that your body gets all the nutrients it needs. Weight loss is common in cancer patients, but weight gain is also possible. Many people with cancer, especially those who are losing weight or who have side effects that affect their ability to eat well, need to make changes to what they eat—perhaps by "building up" their diet with extra protein and calories.

Special Nutrition Needs

Snacking Is Okay

Many people with cancer find it hard to eat full meals. If this is a challenge for you, try eating smaller amounts more often throughout the day. Snacking is a good way to get the calories and nutrients your body needs. Healthy snacks—like vegetables or fruit with dip, yogurt, cottage cheese, nuts, and grain products—can also give you an energy boost between meals. So feel free to "graze," or reach for nutritious snacks, as often as you like.

Keeping Your Strength Up

Whether eating snacks or full meals, many people with cancer need to consume plenty of calories and protein. This may be different than what you've heard in the past about healthy eating—but when you're fighting cancer, taking in more calories and protein than usual can help you maintain your strength. Extra calories and extra protein can also help prevent weight loss and provide the energy you need to get through the day.

Food Safety Issues

People with cancer need to be especially careful about food safety. This is because cancer and treatments like chemotherapy can weaken your immune system. Your body may be less able to fight infection from bacteria or other organisms that could be in foods.

Your healthcare team or a registered dietitian can help you make food choices that are safest for you. They will know your treatment schedule and will be watching you closely for signs of a weakened immune system.

They can help with any particular concerns you have about food safety steps that you should take or foods that you should avoid. The suggestions below are just a starting point.

Prepare, Cook, and Store Your Foods with Care

- Wash your hands with warm soapy water before and after preparing food and before eating.

- Wash vegetables and fruit thoroughly under running water before peeling or cutting.

- Avoid vegetables and fruit that can't be washed well (for example, raspberries).

- Scrub vegetables and fruit that have firm surfaces such as potatoes, carrots, oranges, and melons.

- Cut away any damaged or bruised areas on produce. Bacteria can thrive in these places.

- Wash the top lids of canned foods with soap and water before opening.

- Rinse packaged salads under running water even when marked "pre-washed".

- Refrigerate foods at or below 4° C (40° F).

- Thaw meat, fish or poultry in the microwave or refrigerator (not on the counter).

- Put food in the refrigerator within two hours of serving. Foods containing eggs, cream or mayonnaise should be refrigerated after no more than one hour.

- Use defrosted foods right away and do not refreeze them.

- Cook meats until well done, with no traces of pink in the center. Red meats should be cooked to an internal temperature of 77° C (170° F) or 71° C (160° F) if the meat is ground. Poultry should be cooked to an internal temperature of 85° C (185° F) or 74° C (165° F) if ground or in pieces (breast, legs, thighs). A meat thermometer is your only way to be sure of the internal temperature.

- Use different spoons to taste and stir your food while you're cooking it.

591

- Cool hot foods, uncovered, in the refrigerator. Place in storage containers after cooling. Freeze what you do not plan to use within the next two to three days. Throw out all prepared foods after three days in the refrigerator.

- Throw out entire food packages or containers with any mold, including yogurt, cheese, cottage cheese, fruit, vegetables, jelly, and bread and pastry products.

Keep Work Surfaces and Kitchen Equipment Clean

- Use separate cutting boards for raw foods and cooked foods. Use one cutting board for fresh produce and a different one for raw meat, poultry and seafood.

- Wash cutting boards after each use in hot, soapy water or in the dishwasher.

- Get rid of worn cutting boards.

- Keep appliances, counter tops and kitchen surfaces free of food crumbs.

- Consider using paper towels to wipe kitchen surfaces or change dishcloths daily to avoid the possibility of cross-contamination and the spread of bacteria.

- Wash dishcloths in the hot cycle of the washing machine.

- Avoid using sponges because they are harder to keep bacteria-free.

- Clean and sanitize counter tops, cutting boards and utensils each week with a disinfectant cleaner or a mild bleach solution of 5 mL (1 teaspoon) of bleach per 750 mL (3 cups) of water.

Shop for Food with Care

- Read food labels to make sure food isn't past its "sell by" date.

- Keep raw meat, poultry, seafood and eggs separate from other foods in your grocery cart.

- Buy only pasteurized, refrigerated milk and dairy products.

- Pick up perishable foods last, and plan to go directly home from the grocery store.

- Avoid foods from bulk bins, salad bars, delicatessens, buffets, potlucks, and sidewalk vendors.

Try to Avoid

- Raw or undercooked eggs (like in Caesar salad dressing)

- Raw and undercooked meat, fish, shellfish, poultry and tofu

- Unwashed raw vegetables and fruit, and those with visible mold

- Home-canned vegetables, fruit, meats, and fish

- Well water, unless tested yearly and found safe

Your dietitian may suggest other foods to stay away from, depending on your situation.

Eating Well after Treatment

Once you have completed treatment, your interest in food often returns as the side effects from treatment improve. This is a gradual process and is an opportunity to slowly start eating a wider variety of foods.

Changes will not happen overnight, so be patient with yourself. Your interest in food might not come back as quickly as you would like it to. Your body needs plenty of time to recover. If side effects persist, talk to your healthcare team about how to manage them as you gradually return to your usual activities.

As you recover from treatment, eating well will help your body regain strength and rebuild healthy cells. It will also make you feel better. You may still need extra calories and extra protein in your diet until you reach a weight that is healthy for you. As you become more active, make sure you are eating enough to maintain your healthy weight.

As food regains its appeal, you can slowly return to regular eating habits. Here are a few suggestions to help:

- Pull out some simple recipes you used to like making—and eating.

- Remember what made meal times enjoyable—candles, music, your best dishes or tablecloth—and try these things again.

- Eat a nice meal with close friends or family. You can even ask them to supply the food!

- Make your meal a picnic—inside or out.

- Keep trying to eat foods you previously enjoyed. What doesn't taste good today might taste good tomorrow.

- Visit a gourmet or specialty food shop and indulge in a special treat.

Diet and Cancer Recurrence

Many people wonder if a healthy diet can prevent cancer from returning. Research has shown that eating a healthy diet can help prevent some cancers from developing in the first place. As far as cancer coming back, some research does suggest that eating a healthy diet may prevent cancer from returning. Research has also shown that obesity increases the risk of some cancers returning, so maintaining a healthy body weight is important.

Living with Advanced Cancer

If you are living with advanced cancer, you will have different challenges in trying to eat well and maintain your body weight. Talk to your healthcare team about ways to meet your nutritional needs. Eating as healthy a diet as possible will help you feel better, keep up your strength, and cope with side effects such as fatigue and loss of appetite.

Chapter 50

Exercise During Cancer Treatment and Beyond

Exercising during Cancer Treatment

If you have been recently diagnosed with cancer or are undergoing treatment, it's important to take special care of yourself. Studies show that one of the best ways to do this is to stay physically active.

That doesn't, of course, mean you should run a marathon or scale a mountain. But it's wise to add some form of regular exercise to your daily life—even during cancer therapy. Moderate aerobic exercise, such as riding a stationary bicycle or taking a daily walk, coupled with the use of light weights for strength training, can enhance physical well-being and spur recovery.

Exercise Reduces Fatigue

Research has found no harmful effects on patients with cancer from moderate exercise and, in fact, has demonstrated that those who exercised regularly had 40% to 50% less fatigue, the primary complaint during treatment.

Engaging in regular exercise increases muscle strength, joint flexibility and general conditioning, all of which may be impaired by surgery and some therapies. Exercise is known to improve cardiovascular

Adapted with permission from the NCCN Living with Cancer Articles posted on www.nccn.com. © 2009 National Comprehensive Cancer Network. Available at: http://www.nccn.com. Accessed August 1, 2009. To view the most recent and complete version of these articles, go online to www.nccn.com.

function and to protect bones. It also elevates mood, offering drug-free relief for the feelings of depression that may accompany a cancer diagnosis.

Finally, exercise helps control weight—a crucial factor, as studies have shown that gaining weight during and after treatment raises the risk of a cancer recurrence, particularly breast, colon, and prostate cancers.

When to Begin

The sooner you start exercising, the better you'll feel, the fewer medications you're likely to need, and the lower your risk will be for complications, says Andréa Leiserowitz, physical therapy supervisor at the Seattle Cancer Care Alliance, an affiliate of the Fred Hutchinson Cancer Research Center. She recommends implementing an exercise routine before treatment gets underway—especially if you have been inactive.

Leiserowitz advises asking your doctor for a referral to a physical therapist who works with cancer patients and can design an individualized exercise program. For example, exercises can be prescribed to improve range of motion and prevent lymphedema, a chronic arm swelling that affects some breast cancer patients after lymph node removal.

Exercise with Impact

An effective exercise program has three components:

- An aerobic workout that pumps up your heart rate. Examples include brisk walking (outdoors or on a treadmill), jogging, swimming, or bicycling.

- Strength training to tone and build muscles. This includes lifting weights or working with a machine circuit or resistance bands. (Be sure to get instruction if you're new to this type of exercise; light weights are sufficient to maintain strength.)

- Stretching to keep muscles and joints limber.

Proceed with Care

It is important to discuss with your doctor or physical therapist the type of exercise you are considering to ensure it will be safe.

The National Comprehensive Cancer Network (NCCN) Cancer-Related Fatigue Guidelines [available through the NCCN website at

www.nccn.org] advise starting slowly and progressing incrementally. Depending on fitness and comfort level, some people may want to start with a 10-minute walk around the block; others may find they can exercise for 20 minutes (or longer) right away.

Your goal should be at least 30 minutes of aerobic exercise five days a week or more. But be cautious: if you try to do too much, you may become discouraged and stop exercising altogether. On the other hand, if you were a regular at the gym before cancer, you may have to lower the intensity of workouts for awhile.

Here are some additional suggestions:

- If you don't have the energy to exercise a full half hour, break it up; try three 10-minute walks during the day.

- Make exercise enjoyable; recruit a walking partner or listen to music with headphones while on a recumbent bike or treadmill.

- Dress comfortably and drink plenty of water.

- Warm up by swinging your arms or marching in place and cool down with gentle stretches.

- Do some gardening or house cleaning—both provide physical workouts.

- Consider yoga and tai chi; though not aerobic, they integrate movement and meditation and enhance wellness.

- Look for programs designed for cancer patients. Some health clubs and hospitals offer exercise classes that address the challenges and needs of people with cancer.

- If on radiation therapy, avoid swimming pools; they can expose you to bacteria that may cause infections and the chlorine may irritate radiated skin.

- Listen to your body; don't exercise if you're not feeling well or running a fever.

Exercise for Life

Just as physical activity has been shown to reduce the risk of ever getting cancer, research indicates that exercise decreases the risk of a cancer recurrence and improves survival. Oncologists agree that one of the best things cancer survivors can do to remain healthy is to get regular exercise.

The Benefits

Studies have found that breast cancer patients who exercised moderately (three to five hours of normal-pace walking a week) had improved emotional well-being and better survival rates and than their more sedentary peers.

Being overweight increases the chance that some cancers, such as prostate, colon, and breast cancers, will return, and exercise helps control weight gain. In breast cancer, physical activity reduces excess fat cells that produce the high levels of estrogen associated with cancer. Exercise also may inhibit other hormones and growth factors believed to play a role in breast tumor development.

While long-term data aren't yet available, exercise may turn out to have more influence on breast cancer than diet, says Alexandra Heerdt, MD, an attending surgeon in the breast service at Memorial Sloan-Kettering Cancer Center in New York City. She is leading a pilot study in which breast cancer patients are taught a home-based regimen that combines aerobic exercise and strength training; the latter is aimed at preventing lymphedema, a painful arm swelling that troubles some women after lymph node removal. The goal is for women to learn the program at the center while waiting for treatment, and to be motivated enough to continue it on their own.

In studies of colon cancer patients, scientists at the Dana-Farber Cancer Institute in Boston found that patients who routinely exercised lowered their risk for a cancer recurrence and increased by 50 percent their overall chance for survival compared to inactive patients.

In addition to possibly preventing another bout of cancer, physical activity helps protect against heart disease, diabetes, and the bone-thinning disease osteoporosis. It also builds strength and stamina, boosts the immune system, and enhances quality of life by lessening fatigue and depression and raising self-esteem.

Getting the Right Amount

The Centers for Disease Control and Prevention (CDC) recommend that adults get a minimum of 30 minutes of "moderate-intensity physical activity" on five days or more, or at least 20 minutes of "vigorous-intensity activity" on three days or more. In addition to the aerobic component, adults need muscle-strengthening activities at least two days a week.

Don't worry if you've never been an athlete; there are many ways to be active. Moderate aerobic activity can encompass anything from brisk

walking to square dancing to playing with your grandkids; vigorous activity can be jogging, playing singles tennis, or downhill skiing.

Muscle strengthening—such as lifting weights, using resistance bands, or practicing yoga—should target the body's major muscle groups, with each movement done until you find it too taxing to do another repetition.

Making It a Habit

Solidifying exercise as a lifetime habit is a challenge. However, the period following treatment is an opportune time, since many cancer survivors are looking for new, empowering "tools" to keep them healthy, says Harriet Berman, PhD, executive vice president of clinical programs at the Wellness Community-Greater Boston.

The key is finding something you enjoy and will stick with. If you lack motivation to exercise alone, find a buddy or join a class.

That's what Randi Fox Tabb did. Never much of an exerciser, the Penfield, New York, preschool principal was overweight when she was diagnosed with breast cancer in 2001 and gained another 20 pounds during treatment. After two hip replacements, Tabb bought a cross trainer and joined a Zumba class, an energetic dance workout done to salsa music. She dropped 70 pounds and is now a Zumba enthusiast: "I just love it... I miss it when I don't do it."

Nancy Passavant, a breast cancer survivor from Newton, Massachusetts, and retired marketing specialist, found something even more novel—dragon boat racing. Dating back to ancient China, the sport is gaining popularity among cancer survivors, who find it builds physical strength, support, and camaraderie. The colorfully decorated boats seat up to 20 paddlers who keep pace to a drummer's beat.

Now captain of the Wellness Community's dragon boat team, which is comprised of male and female cancer survivors who practice on Boston's Charles River, Passavant, 61, says nothing compares to the rush she gets when paddling with her teammates. "I feel so alive when I'm out on the water," she says. "I don't think about my cancer at all."

Chapter 51

Coping with the Emotions of Cancer

Psyche

Cancer is one of those life crises that can provide new meaning and purpose in life. But that comes later. Awaiting the diagnosis and hearing the news can be the most emotionally difficult period of the entire cancer experience. Here are some suggestions and resources that can help you gather information and make decisions with presence of mind.

Know Yourself

There's no "right" way to cope with cancer. Each person handles the emotional challenges differently. Think about how you usually function in an emergency and expect to react the same way. It may help to understand the strengths that brought you through adversity before. Ask yourself whose support you usually count on in trying times, including family, friends, spiritual advisors and mental health professionals. Do what works for you. But if your reactions to crises generally interfere with your ability to function at home or at work, and you are unable to make treatment, family or workplace decisions, reach out to traditional or new support systems now.

This chapter includes "Psyche" and "Stress," reprinted with permission. © Cosmetic Executive Women Foundation's Cancer and Careers. For additional information visit www.cancerandcareers.org. All rights reserved.

What Does Cancer Mean to You?

Cancer triggers a terror different from most other diseases, even though they may have worse consequences. Any sense of doom you may have probably comes more from this historic dread than from the current realities concerning your type of cancer and its treatment. Cancer is not a death sentence for most people. It does not necessarily lead to helplessness, pain, disfigurement, disability or the end of your career. Accept that these exaggerated fears are normal, but do not let them prevent you from having a worrisome lump or symptom checked out or from deciding to undergo recommended treatment. And do not conclude that you will not have the energy or focus to pursue life goals. Most people find that their anxiety diminishes greatly once treatment begins and they are taking active steps to combat the disease.

Let It Out

Express your feelings, no matter how awful or embarrassing they may seem to you. Keeping them bottled up may prevent you from moving beyond the distress. However, at work or at home, you may need to promote the image that you are in greater control than you may feel. In that case, you need to find a person you can trust or a safe place— at a support group, in a therapy session with someone who has had cancer—where you can vent your anger, fear, sadness and even those alternating hopeful and hopeless feelings. It may also help to find a quiet place to become aware of the full range of your emotions—by meditating or writing in a journal, for example—and to appreciate that you can get through this.

It's a Control Problem

Uncertainty and lack of control over your body and your future often underlie the anxiety that people experience at the time of diagnosis. People who have always felt in control of their futures, their careers and their families may have particular difficulty, as will those who find it difficult to deal with change. Becoming a medical patient and enduring the passive waiting that tests and treatments entail can provoke a feeling of loss of autonomy. Distinguishing between what you can and cannot control will help restore confidence and competence. For example, although you can't control the outcome of tests or treatments, you can collect information to understand the illness, choose doctors whom you trust, and participate in all decisions. On a smaller, day-to-day scale, although you can't always control waiting time, you

can make it more comfortable by bringing a CD player and listening to your favorite music. Delegating essential daily chores to people you trust will also help you understand that you remain in charge of your life. At work, delegating tasks to trusted colleagues will help you—and them—to appreciate that you are managing your responsibilities during this personal crisis.

It's Not Your Fault

Resist blaming your personality, attitude, coping style, emotions, lifestyle or personal habits for your cancer. Cancer experts repeatedly emphasize that there is absolutely no scientific basis for these conclusions. The more you blame yourself, the less empowered you will feel to combat the disease.

Find Your Inner Warrior

Thinking of cancer as a battle to be won can help restore your self-confidence and self-esteem. People with a fighting spirit demand the best possible care for themselves. When confronted with a rigid bureaucracy, they insist on their rights. They don't take no for an answer. They are not necessarily "good" or "nice" patients. But if that's not your style, deputize someone to fight on your behalf.

Be Positive, But Be Real

Hopefulness and a positive outlook can be very motivating, but don't fake it or feel guilty when your spirits sink. Setting short-term goals can help to shore up your confidence. You have every right to feel lousy or dispirited even if other people pressure you to be more positive; there is no scientific research that links a positive attitude to recovery from cancer. But quality of life is directly affected by how you feel, and although it is normal to feel grief , loss, sadness and fear from time to time, persistent anxiety and depression are not part-and-parcel of having cancer. Tell your doctor. Ask for help. You need your emotional energy to tackle the disease, not to mention all the other responsibilities that are important to your life.

Reach Out

Research shows that people who have strong ties to others deal with crisis best. Reach out to loved ones and close friends. Although some people may disappoint you—because of their own fear of cancer—be

open to others who may unexpectedly offer concern and assistance. At home and at work, ask those you trust to help out with essential responsibilities and chores. During the period of uncertainty before treatment begins, cancer education programs and support groups can be sources of information as well as safe havens for emotional expression and understanding. Hospitals, the American Cancer Society, your church or synagogue, and Cancer Care can provide information about cancer support groups. Cancer support chat rooms on the internet can also help. Groups vary; if you don't feel comfortable in one, look for another.

Meeting one-on-one with someone with your type of cancer can help to validate your concerns. The American Cancer Society (www. cancer.org), for example, pairs breast cancer patients with long-term survivors. Cancer Care (www.cancercare.org; click on "Helping Hand Resource Guide") has a patient-to-patient network.

Psychologists, social workers, nurses and psychiatrists trained in psychosocial oncology can be a godsend to people who are trying to manage the distresses associated with a cancer diagnosis. A previous history of depression or emotional problems may trigger a recurrence during this crisis. Your oncologist's office or any cancer treatment center can provide information.

Distract Yourself

Hard as it may be in the beginning of this journey, schedule some time off from thinking about your illness. Keep doing things you enjoy, including exercise, if you are up to it, and remember that there's life plenty of it—beyond cancer. For some people, the workplace is where they best concentrate on their continuing competence and enjoy time away from the sick role.

Stress

When it comes to life stresses, cancer is certainly one of the most traumatic. Over time, the strain of coping with your diagnosis and the realities of treatment will probably be compounded by other stresses, such as keeping up with work and dealing with the worries of family and friends. If left unchecked, your body's reaction to these stresses— through increased blood pressure, a more rapid heart rate, decreased digestion, increased muscle tension, and higher levels of stress hormones like adrenaline—can lead to impaired immune function and an assortment of troubling stress symptoms. Preventing these effects

requires planning, an awareness of your needs and limitations, and a mastery of stress-reduction techniques that can stop your body's "stress response" before it gets out of hand.

Avoiding Stress

Obviously, the best way to prevent the negative effects of stress is to avoid getting stressed in the first place. While some sources of stress are unavoidable, others are surprisingly predictable and can be prevented with a few evasive maneuvers.

At Home

Let People Know What You Need

When family and friends say they want to help, believe them. Delegate chores that you don't feel up to doing, whether it's doing the laundry, cleaning the bathroom, or making dinner.

Cut Yourself Some Slack

No one expects you to be Martha Stewart and maintain a picture-perfect home while dealing with cancer.

Don't Be Afraid to Say No

It's OK to opt out of activities if you're feeling fatigued, ill, or just want to be alone.

Schedule Lots of Leisure Time

Now, more than ever, you need lots of downtime to relax, recover from treatment side effects, or just process your feelings about your illness. Make it a priority by scheduling time for stress-reducing activities such as attending a support group, meditation, gardening, exercise or just taking a long hot bath.

Listen to Your Body

As your treatment progresses, you'll be able to predict when you are likely to feel unwell. Pay attention to the patterns and adjust your schedule accordingly. Let friends and family know when you are most likely to need help around the house, and plan "must do" chores for the days when you tend to be feeling your best.

Be Honest about Your Feelings

Although you may not want to burden others with your fears, keeping them bottled up will only increase your stress level. If you are feeling scared, or depressed, or anxious, let others know. Be sure you have a place to discuss these feelings openly—whether it's with a therapist, a member of your treatment team or a support group.

At Work

Delegate

If you're someone who likes to do everything yourself, it's time to get over it! Look over your workload for the next several months to determine what requires your personal attention and what can be distributed to others. Keep in mind that you can provide guidance and direction without being on-site.

Keep the Lines of Communication Open

If you decide to tell your colleagues, be as open as possible with them about your needs—and possible limitations—as your treatment progresses.

Get a Massage

Everyone feels great after a massage. But the benefits of a good rubdown go beyond that immediate feeling of relaxation. In addition to relaxing tense muscles, massage also stimulates the nerves, increases lymph circulation, and enhances blood flow to tissues that have been deprived of oxygen by unrelenting stress. In fact, research has shown that the amount of oxygen reaching the body's cells increases by 15 percent after a massage. If your treatment team can't suggest a massage therapist, you can find one through the American Massage Therapy Association (http://www.amtamassage.org).

Relaxation Strategies

Effective Breathing

1. Sit up straight in a comfortable chair, feet flat on the floor, neck and shoulders relaxed.

2. Take a deep breath through your nose, with your mouth closed. Use your diaphragm when inhaling—consciously pushing your

belly outward as you inhale. Put one hand on your abdomen, if you like, to feel how it rises and falls.

3. Exhale slowly through your mouth, with your lips pursed as if you were whistling (or about to give someone a peck on the cheek). Make your exhalation twice as long as your inhalation, pulling your diaphragm in as you empty the air from your lungs.

4. Repeat three or more times, until you feel yourself relax.

Progressive Relaxation

1. Remove your shoes and any uncomfortable or restrictive clothing, including eyeglasses.

2. Remove any possible distractions. Turn off the television, radio and phone, and dim the lights to a comfortable level.

3. Sit in a comfortable chair, head and neck relaxed, with your hands at rest in your lap, palms up. (You can lie down if you prefer, just don't fall asleep!)

4. Close your eyes and breathe deeply.

5. Keeping your eyes closed, focus your mind on your feet and toes. Slowly tighten the muscles in your feet, hold for a beat, and slowly relax.

6. Repeat this tightening and relaxing pattern with each of the muscle groups in your body, gradually working upward. Move your focus from the calves to the thighs to the glutes, through your back, chest and head, including your face. Don't forget your hands and arms.

7. Continue to breathe deeply until you feel relaxed and calm. You can test your level of relaxation by putting your hands against your face or neck. Warm hands mean a relaxed body. If they're still cool, continue the exercise until they warm up.

Visualization

1. Remove your shoes and any uncomfortable or restrictive clothing, including eyeglasses.

2. Remove any possible distractions. Turn off the television, radio and phone, and dim the lights to a comfortable level.

3. Sit in a comfortable chair, head and neck relaxed, with feet flat on the floor and your hands resting in your lap, palms up. (You can lie down or sit on a mat if you prefer—just be sure you are comfortable enough to stay in this position for ten to 20 minutes.)

4. Close your eyes and picture yourself in a pleasant, restful place—a green meadow by a cool lake, the soft sand of a Caribbean beach, a warm rock by a clear mountain stream.

5. Fill in every detail as you breathe in deeply through your nose and exhale slowly through your mouth.

6. With each breath, slowly let the tension ease out of your body's muscles. Allow the muscles in your feet, your legs, your back, shoulders, arms, hands and feet to relax as you sink further into the restful world of your inner picture.

Chapter 52

Talking to Your Children about Cancer

Telling Your Children

As a clinical psychologist, Carolyn Ingram is an expert at helping people cope with life's challenges. But after she was diagnosed with breast cancer in 1994, she had to handle a problem that was new territory for her: Deciding how she and her husband should best tell their daughter Leslie Ann, then 8, about the cancer.

More than 200,000 women will learn they have breast cancer this year, and more than 400,000 others will learn they have other forms of cancer, according to American Cancer Society projections. Many will still have young children at home.

So it's crucial to deal not only with the cancer, but with communicating information to your children. Here, tips from Ingram, who practices in Marin County, California, and others on how to do your best when you may be feeling your worst.

First, Pull Yourself Together

Being emotional and distressed after a cancer diagnosis is normal. But before you call the kids in for a meeting, pull yourself together, experts advise. "We're not saying a mother should never show irritability

or tears," says Patti Brandt, Ph.D., a nurse practitioner at the University of Washington, Seattle, who has researched the topic. "But if she finds herself constantly sobbing or preoccupied with her own health, that's saying she needs to take some time out, to do some care taking of herself."

Call a Meeting

"Set a time when the phone doesn't ring," says Leslie Gebhart, a life coach in Palm Springs, California, and the sister of Carolyn Ingram. Or turn off the phone and other distractions. The sisters are both breast cancer survivors and together wrote *The Not-So-Scary Breast Cancer Book* (see their site, http://www.childvoice.com/ for more information) to help women cope, including tips on how to talk about their cancer with their kids.

"Include everyone who lives under your roof," Gebhart says. Decide on an age-appropriate length of time, Gebhart says, and set a timer in the kitchen to keep yourself on track.

Starting the conversation isn't easy; just remember to keep it simple. What works: "Mom's going to be taking special medicine to help the cancer go away." Let the children know it will of course affect the family and how the kids can help.

Keep the Goals in Mind

One point of the meeting, says Gebhart, is to ease tension. For you as the mother, it's also a way to practice asking for what you need. If you are like most mothers, you are not good at this.

You can be specific, telling the kids, "I might need you to make the beds." "I might need you to make sure the dog has fresh water."

If you will need outside help, pick and choose which chores you want to relinquish, Brant suggests. "Keep your personal connection with the kids," she says. So, hire someone to do laundry but not to pick up the kids from soccer practice.

Talk positively to set the tone. "Say, 'We are going to get through this'," Brandt suggests. Be brief and to the point. "You don't want to overload them with details about how often you will see the doctor, how many treatments you will have."

Picking a Good Setting

Use whatever environment you have used in the past to deliver news, good or bad, Brandt suggests. "Sometimes it works [to talk] after

a favorite TV show," she says. Maybe you want to order in a favorite dinner, and talk when you are done.

Don't schedule a meeting when kids have something important coming up on their agenda, such as a big school function or a test.

One Meeting Isn't Enough

One meeting won't do it all. Ongoing communication and discussion are crucial. How often you decide to meet to talk about your cancer depends on a lot of factors: the age of your children, the stage of your cancer, the personalities in your family.

Some experts suggest weekly meetings, but only you can decide how often is enough. Know that when children get no explanation for the changes swirling around them, experts say they are likely to make up their own explanation. And that could mean blaming themselves, especially in the case of young children, even if it makes no sense to you as a parent.

Between meetings, give your kids an opportunity to get their questions answered. Gebhart suggests keeping a sheet of paper on the refrigerator. Kids can jot down questions or concerns to be brought up at the next family meetings. Such as: "Sam's mother had this kind of cancer and she didn't have to have the treatment that made her go bald. Why not?"

Try to Understand Where Your Child Is Coming From

Leslie Gebhart recalls that her niece's first question to her mother after the initial news was delivered was: "Will anything bad happen to you?" At age 8, the question was really, "Am I going to be OK?"

While even young children are concerned about their mother having cancer, their life still revolves around themselves. In other words, it may be your cancer, but if you have young children, it's still all about them.

And that's normal, says Ellen Zahlis, M.N., a researcher at the University of Washington, Seattle, who studies the impact of cancer on families. Young children, and even some older ones, are likely to ask, "Can I still go to my games?" "Will I still get to have my birthday?"

It's OK, she adds, to say you don't know, especially if you don't know the toll treatment will take on you. It's OK to tell your kids their events will go on whenever possible and you'll do your best.

What Do Kids Worry About?

When Zahlis interviewed 16 children whose mothers had breast cancer, she found some key worries:

611

- Worrying about death

- Worrying something bad would happen, such as the cancer spreading or an allergic reaction to one of the treatment drugs

- Worrying about the family and how they would cope

- Worrying when the mom did not look good

- Worrying mom would never be her old self

- Worrying that financial cutbacks would be necessary

- Worrying about talking to others about the cancer

- Worrying that the child herself or himself would get cancer

As you discuss the treatment and progress with your kids, bear in mind that some of their questions may reflect these common worries.

Give Your Child Some Control Over the Situation

Leslie Gebhart recalls her niece's reaction when her sister said she would go bald. "She burst into tears."

Leslie Ann decided she didn't want to see her mother bald, so Carolyn Ingram agreed to honor that wish, asking her little daughter to knock on the bedroom door before their morning cuddle session, giving her enough time to grab a scarf or a wig.

Weeks later, after Leslie Ann was used to seeing her mother in a wig or a hat, she changed her mind. "The openness with which my sister talked to her helped her change her mind," Leslie Gebhart says.

When Leslie Ann saw her mom bald for the first time, she told her, lovingly, "Mom, you look like a little baby." And months later, as Carolyn's hair began to grow back, Leslie Ann told her she'd miss the bald head.

Allow your child to decide how he or she wants to handle feelings—Talk to another adult? Talk to you when they want to? Journal their feelings and keep it private? The feeling of control, however slight, will help them cope.

Avoid Role Reversal

Don't look to your child to nurture you, says Brandt. There's bound to be some degree of natural role reversal, but it shouldn't be a complete role reversal. "Let them do nice things for you, like get you

presents or bring you water when you are resting," she says. "A teen might stop by the video store and pick up a DVD that is your favorite, bring it home and watch it with you."

But remember, you're still the mom and you're still mothering, though understandably with less energy than before. Get your emotional needs and care giving mostly from other adults, not your kids.

Put It in Perspective

Unless the outlook is terribly uncertain, reassure your children that life will get back to normal. You might say, for instance, "Mom's treatment will be done by the time two more soccer games are over." Or you might plan something when treatment is finished—a trip to the beach or mountains, a day at the amusement park.

"Cancer is not something any of us would choose," Gebhart says. "As odd as it is to say this, this really is an opportunity to grow closer together."

Special Advice for Single Mothers

When a divorced, widowed, separated or single mom gets cancer, she's lacking the in-house support of another adult that married women can usually rely on.

"The challenges are greater for the single mom," says Ellen Zahlis, a researcher at the University of Washington, Seattle, who studies the impact of cancer on the family.

"She's just one person and she is ill. So presumably there is no well adult in the family who is also a caretaker. A lot of stuff falls on her when she is already depleted physically and emotionally."

Lack of energy to deal with day-to-day problems is a challenge for any mother dealing with cancer. For single moms, it might be doubly true.

Here, tips on how to tell your kids the news, how to cope, and how to keep the communication open.

First, Find Someone Outside to Lean On

"In the long run, it's better for both [mom and kids] if she finds someone else who can be the epicenter of her emotions, her feelings," Zahlis says. "Think about the people in your life who are good listeners, not the people who need to fix it for you, or who are the advice givers. There are many people with no [professional] training who are wonderful, gifted listeners."

Before hosting your family meeting to discuss the diagnosis, consider running your "script" by someone you trust, perhaps a friend who has children of the same age as yours. He or she might point out how to be more effective, alter the discussion to make it more age appropriate, or suggest you give the information in smaller bytes.

Let Go of the Super-Mom Image

"Single moms are more reticent to ask for help," says Zahlis, reiterating the feedback she got in one study. "They are more fiercely independent," she says. And if they do ask for outside help, many single moms worry about how they will return the favor.

One way Zahlis has persuaded single moms to drop the I-can-do-it-all-myself mantra is to frame it as this: "I need to ask someone else to listen or help me in this way, because it will provide the best outcome for my child."

Chapter 53

Sexuality and Reproductive Issues among Women with Cancer

Chapter Contents

Section 53.1

Renewing Intimacy and Sexuality after Gynecologic Cancer

Over 80,000 women a year are diagnosed with a gynecologic cancer each year.

The challenge for the woman with cancer and her healthcare team is to balance the desire for the best possible treatment while maintaining quality of life. When describing "quality of life" most adult women include desires for intimacy and satisfying sexual relationships as part the vibrant full life that they hope to preserve or regain. Cancer affects an individual's total being, including physical, emotional, spiritual, and sexual wellness. Many types of cancer treatment can affect a woman's response to intimacy and sexuality. Sexual functioning can be affected by illness, pain, anxiety, anger, stressful relationships, medications, and cultural norms. Sexuality not only refers to sexual intercourse, but other means of sexual expression, such as touching and kissing. Intimacy refers to the physical or emotional closeness shared with another individual. Self-esteem and body image are important factors that define how a woman feels about herself. Sexuality is important to one's identity. Cancer treatment may interfere with desire and functioning, but it cannot take away an individual's sexual self. This section will offer some general information that can be discussed further with your healthcare provider. Effective communication is important for the woman, her partner, and her healthcare team.

How will surgery affect my sexual functioning?

There are different treatments depending on the type of cancer diagnosis. The three most common gynecologic cancers are endometrial (also called uterine), ovarian, and cervical cancers. Most sexual disruption from these types of cancers are related to surgical interventions, such as hysterectomy (removal of uterus), bilateral salpingectomy-oophorectomy (removal of both fallopian tubes and ovaries, or BSO), and

vaginal resection. Abdominal scars and surgical incisions can interfere with how a woman views her body, making her uncomfortable in an intimate situation. The vaginal canal may be shorter after a hysterectomy causing discomfort with sexual intercourse. However, the elasticity of the vagina gives it the ability to stretch during intercourse.

The removal of both ovaries in a premenopausal woman will cause menopause or the lack of ovarian function. If estrogen is not replaced, vaginal dryness and vaginal atrophy (shrinkage) may occur causing discomfort with intercourse and pelvic examinations. The use of water-soluble vaginal lubricants and moisturizers often improves comfort. Regular vaginal intercourse will help to preserve normal vaginal length.

Special Surgical Considerations

A colostomy (a surgical diversion from the intestine that creates a pouch outside the skin) is indicated in rare situations for advanced cancer. This will not interfere with the woman's sexual functioning but may affect body image. Feeling comfortable with your body, is part of feeling sexual. Some women use sexy clothing to cover areas that makes them feel unattractive. For more specific information on sex with ostomies, talk to an enterostomal nurse who has advanced training on ostomy care and sexuality issues.

In addition to colostomies, certain other surgical procedures can cause special challenges for a woman seeking to regain sexual function. Surgical diversion of the urine flow, vulvectomy, surgical removal of the clitoris, and vaginal reconstruction are included in this group. Women recovering from these procedures will want to ask their surgeon frank questions about sexual recovery. Whenever possible, include your partner in these discussions.

How soon after a hysterectomy can I have sex?

Most patients can resume sexual intercourse in approximately four to six weeks after an abdominal or vaginal hysterectomy. It is important for the surgical incision at the top of the vagina (often called the vaginal cuff) to have adequate healing and cessation of vaginal spotting and discharge.

Will there be pain the first time I have sex after a hysterectomy?

The fear of pain after surgery is a common concern for a woman and her partner. After surgery there may still be pain and discomfort,

in addition to fatigue that can interfere with sexual pleasure. Finding a comfortable position to reduce discomfort is important. Some recommendations are positioning the woman on top or in a side-lying position to control depth of penetration, and decrease abdominal discomfort at the incision site. Placing pillows under the knees or behind the small of the back may increase comfort. Dilators are recommended for women with narrowing of the vagina, if intercourse is not an option. For women not interested in sexual intercourse, other forms of pleasure include self or manual stimulation, and oral sex.

The use of water based lubricants, which can be purchased without a prescription, and/or vaginal estrogens (prescribed by your physician) may reduce discomfort from vaginal dryness. If a woman is having post-operative pain from surgery or cancer related-pain, pain medication prior to sex may ease discomfort.

Will sex feel any differently to my partner after surgery?

Your partner will not be able to determine that you had a hysterectomy. The vagina is quite elastic and comfort can be achieved even if the vagina is shortened from surgery. Lubrication to the vagina will make penetration more gentle and pleasurable.

Will the ability to have an orgasm be affected by the surgery?

The nerves responsible for having an orgasm will not be affected by having a hysterectomy. Some of the physical changes associated with arousal, such as fullness in the labia and vaginal lubrication may not be as prominent or easily triggered if hormone levels are low or after radiation treatment. Talk to your partner; provide assurance that these changes are caused by your surgery and that they do not mean that you have lost interest in sex or that you do not find your partner desirable. Together you can find ways to adjust to these changes. Women who were able to achieve an orgasm prior to removal of their uterus, cervix, and ovaries should expect to achieve orgasm after most cancer treatments.

How will radiation affect my sexual functioning?

The effects of radiation are specific to each individual and depend on the dose and the area treated. Radiation to the pelvis or abdomen may cause side effects such as fatigue, nausea, diarrhea, bladder inflammation, and vaginal swelling that may interfere with sexual desire. Delayed side effects may include diarrhea, vaginal discharge, swelling

of the legs, and vaginal narrowing. Frequent intercourse is an excellent way to minimize the vaginal narrowing and maintain the elasticity of the tissues lining the vagina.

Other than intercourse, vaginal dilators can be used to maintain normal vaginal size. Water soluble vaginal lubricants may be needed for vaginal dryness.

Is it safe to have sex while I am still receiving radiation treatments?

Radiation is not contagious, nor will you or your partner become radioactive if you have sex during this time. During pelvic radiation, the vagina may be temporarily tender to touch, or swollen, due to sunburn-like effect. The use of lubricants may increase comfort. Many women find that they need to take a temporary break from vaginal intercourse during and shortly following radiation treatment. After a short time of healing (commonly two to four weeks) be reassured that sexual relations will be comfortable again.

How will chemotherapy affect my sexual functioning?

Chemotherapy does not directly cause sexual dysfunction, however side effects from treatment such as fatigue, nausea, mouth sores, and diarrhea, may interfere with mood and desire. Not all chemotherapy causes the same side effects and the treatment prescribed will depend on the specific cancer diagnosis and stage. Chemotherapy may cause low white blood counts seven to ten days after treatment, resulting in an increased risk for infection. Women may be more vulnerable to infections (i.e., respiratory, gastrointestinal, and vaginal) during the seven to ten day period after receiving chemotherapy. Your healthcare provider may recommend individual strategies to reduce your risk. Intimacy with a partner who has a sore throat or a cold sore should be limited during this time due to possible spread of infection. Fatigue, due to low red blood counts, is a common side effect of chemotherapy and may affect libido. Medications are available to help reduce or relieve many of the side effects of chemotherapy. Be sure that your doctor knows about the side effects that are troublesome for you. Loss of hair and skin rash can affect self-esteem and body image. Some women may feel more comfortable wearing a head covering or wig for hair loss, or a nightgown to cover wounds or scars. Being comfortable with one's self is the first step to a healthy sexual self.

The following are recommendations for improving libido and intimacy during chemotherapy:

619

1. Plan for it, by scheduling a "date night."

2. Set the mood for intimacy (i.e., candles, bubble bath, soft music, romantic movies).

3. To reduce fatigue, plan a nap prior to the occasion.

4. If symptoms such as nausea or pain occur from treatment, take medication an hour before having sex.

5. Discuss with your physician the use of testosterone and/or estrogen based products (i.e., creams) as an option to enhance your libido.

6. Touching, kissing, cuddling, or using massage and/or oils may be more desired and fulfilling than intercourse.

7. Ask your doctor about medications to reduce anemia and white blood cell depletion or to combat depression, anxiety, or severe fatigue.

8. Experiment with your partner finding means of sexual pleasuring that may or may not result in orgasm or sexual intercourse. The goal is to keep the sexual part of your relationship alive during a time when you might not be able to participate in sexual intercourse.

9. Play communication games with your partner. For example, take turns asking each other what types of touch is most pleasing. Practice touching parts of the body such as neck, ear, fingers, or inside of thigh, to discover what each other enjoys.

Communication

Women who are concerned about potential or actual sexual dysfunction should discuss these issues with the healthcare team, which may include their physician, oncology nurse, or social worker. A discussion with both the woman and her partner is encouraged to help reduce fears by the partner. Often partners are afraid that sex will be painful or even afraid that they may "catch" cancer. Single women who are dating or not yet involved in a relationship have concerns about when to disclose their cancer diagnosis to a potential partner. Support groups through the hospital or in the community can help women network with other patients who are dealing with similar issues. Effective communication is important for the woman, her healthcare team, and her partner, to understand that sexuality is part of her total return to wellness.

Special Experts Are Available

Cancer experts have variable levels of comfort and expertise in dealing with issues of sexual function. If you and your partner are not recovering intimacy, don't give up and don't assume that you are asking for too much. Don't assume that your problem is unheard of or hopeless. Ask for a referral to an expert in sexual counseling. Your recovery to full living is worth the extra effort.

Section 53.2

Cancer and Fertility Preservation

Excerpted from "What to Know: ASCO's Guideline on Fertility Preservation." Reprinted with permission. © 2010 American Society of Clinical Oncology. All rights reserved.

Cancer Treatment and Fertility

Some types of cancer treatment can affect a person's fertility, the ability to conceive a child or maintain a pregnancy. Infertility may be temporary or permanent. Whether treatment causes infertility depends on the following:

- The type and dose of the drug and how it's given (by mouth, injection, or intravenously [through a vein])

- The dose of radiation given and the area being irradiated

- The type of cancer

- The patient's age and gender

- Whether a patient had fertility problems before cancer treatment

Fertility in a woman may be decreased even if regular menstrual periods continue during treatment or return after treatment. In addition, cancer treatment can cause premature menopause, which shortens the length of time a woman is fertile. Learn more about pregnancy and cancer at www.cancer.net/features.

If you are concerned that your cancer treatment will affect your fertility, talk with your doctor. Not all cancer treatments harm fertility, but if the treatment you are receiving does include a risk of infertility, fertility preservation treatments are available. Your chances for maintaining your fertility are greatest if you discuss and think about your options as early as possible.

Options for Preserving Fertility before Cancer Treatment

This guide focuses on fertility preservation options that are available before cancer treatment. A patient's type of cancer and other personal preferences and circumstances may affect the available options. Many of these methods are investigational, which means that they are still being tested and may not be available to all patients.

For Women

- Embryo cryopreservation: The harvesting of eggs followed by in vitro fertilization and freezing of embryos for later use

- Radical trachelectomy: Surgery to remove the cervix that leaves the uterus intact

- Oophoropexy or ovarian transposition: Surgically moving the ovaries out of the field of radiation

- Other organ-preserving surgery and radiation therapy

- Oocyte (egg) cryopreservation: The collection and freezing of unfertilized eggs (investigational)

- Ovarian tissue cryopreservation: The freezing of ovarian tissue for reimplantation after cancer treatment (investigational)

- Ovarian suppression: The use of hormone therapy to protect ovarian tissue during chemotherapy or radiation therapy (investigational)

What This Means for Patients

Making decisions about potential options for preserving fertility at the time of a cancer diagnosis can be difficult. It is important to keep the following in mind:

- When discussing cancer treatment with your doctor, it is important to determine if you are at risk for treatment-related fertility

problems and whether you are concerned about preserving your fertility. Not all cancer treatments cause infertility.

- This discussion should take place as early as possible, as many of the available fertility preservation options require time to perform before cancer therapy begins. For example, some treatments for women depend on the phase of a woman's menstrual cycle and can only be started at monthly intervals.

- Although data so far are limited, most fertility preservation methods do not appear to increase the risk of recurrence (return of the cancer), even in cancers that are sensitive to hormones.

- Having a history of cancer, cancer treatment, or fertility preservation treatment does not appear to increase the risk of cancer or birth defects for future children. However, patients with a hereditary genetic syndrome and women whose children were exposed to chemotherapy while in the uterus (womb) may be at higher risk for developing cancer or birth defects. Talk with your doctor for more information.

- Talk with your doctor about referrals for counseling or other means of support if treatment-related infertility is a source of anxiety.

Section 53.3

Pregnancy and Cancer

Cancer during pregnancy is rare and little research is available to guide women and doctors. It is known that a pregnant woman with cancer is capable of giving birth to a healthy baby and that some cancer treatments are safe during pregnancy.

Cancer occurs in approximately one out of every 1,000 pregnancies. However, pregnancy itself does not cause cancer, and pregnant women are not more likely to get cancer than other women. The cancers that tend to occur during pregnancy are those that are more common in younger people, such as cervical cancer and breast cancer, Hodgkin lymphoma, malignant melanoma, and thyroid cancer. Because age is the most significant risk factor for cancer, doctors expect the rate of cancer during pregnancy to increase as more women are waiting until they are older to have children.

Diagnosis

Being pregnant can delay a cancer diagnosis. Symptoms such as abdominal bloating, frequent headaches, or rectal bleeding might suggest ovarian, brain, or colon cancer. These symptoms are also common during pregnancy and are not considered suspicious. If these symptoms are related to cancer, diagnosis of the cancer is likely to be delayed.

Breast cancer is the most common cancer in pregnant women, affecting approximately one in 3,000 pregnancies. Pregnancy-related breast enlargement makes it difficult to detect small breast tumors, and mammograms are not regularly done during pregnancy.

If cancer is suspected during pregnancy, women and their doctors may be concerned about diagnostic tests such as x-rays. However, research has shown that the level of radiation in diagnostic x-rays is too low to harm the fetus (unborn baby). When possible, a lead shield covering the abdomen offers extra protection. Other diagnostic tests,

such as magnetic resonance imaging test (MRI), ultrasound, and biopsy, are also considered safe during pregnancy because they don't use radiation.

Sometimes, pregnancy can uncover cancer that had previously gone undetected. For example, a Pap test performed as part of standard, early prenatal care can detect cervical cancer. Similarly, an ultrasound performed during pregnancy can often find ovarian cancer that might otherwise go undiagnosed.

Treatment

Treatment for cancer during pregnancy means balancing the best treatment for the mother with the possible risk to the fetus. The type of treatment given depends on many factors, including how far along the pregnancy is; the type, location, size, and stage of the cancer; and the wishes of the expectant mother and family. Because some cancer treatments can harm the fetus, especially during the first trimester (the first three months of pregnancy), treatment may be delayed until the second or third trimesters. When cancer is diagnosed later in pregnancy, doctors may wait to start treatment until after the baby is born, or they may consider inducing labor early. In some cases, such as early stage (stage 0 or IA) cervical cancer, doctors may wait to treat the cancer until after delivery.

Cancer treatments used during pregnancy may include surgery, chemotherapy, and possibly, radiation therapy, but only after careful consideration and treatment planning to optimize the safety of the mother and the unborn baby.

Surgery poses little risk to the fetus and is considered the safest cancer treatment option during pregnancy. In some instances, more extensive surgery can be done to avoid having to use chemotherapy or radiation therapy.

Chemotherapy is the use of drugs to kill cancer cells. Chemotherapy is capable of harming the fetus, particularly if given during the first trimester of pregnancy when the fetus' organs are still developing. Chemotherapy during the first trimester can cause birth defects or even the loss of the unborn baby. During the second and third trimesters, some types of chemotherapy can be taken without necessarily harming the fetus. The placenta (the organ that develops during pregnancy) acts as a barrier between the mother and the fetus, and the drugs cannot pass through the barrier (or they pass through only minimally). If the planned chemotherapy includes a drug that is not safe during any stage of pregnancy, another drug can usually be substituted.

Although chemotherapy later in pregnancy may not directly harm the fetus, chemotherapy can cause health problems for the mother that can indirectly harm the fetus, such as malnutrition and anemia (low red blood cell count). Chemotherapy given during the second and third trimesters can cause early labor and low birth weight, both of which may lead to further health concerns for the mother, such as weight gain and problems with breast-feeding and fighting infections.

Radiation therapy involves high energy x-rays to destroy cancer cells and shrink cancerous tumors. Because radiation therapy can harm the fetus, particularly during the first trimester, this treatment is generally not recommended. The use of radiation therapy in the second or third trimesters depends on the dose of radiation and the area of the body being treated.

The Effects of Cancer on the Pregnancy

The prognosis (chance of recovery) for a pregnant woman with cancer is often the same as for another woman of the same age with the same type and stage of cancer. However, if a woman's diagnosis is delayed during pregnancy, she will tend to have a worse, overall prognosis than a non-pregnant woman diagnosed with cancer. In addition, pregnancy can affect the behavior of some cancers. For example, there is some evidence to suggest that the hormonal changes of pregnancy may stimulate the growth of malignant melanoma.

Cancer rarely affects the fetus directly. Although some cancers can spread to the placenta, most cancers cannot spread to the fetus itself.

Breastfeeding

Although cancer cells cannot pass to the infant through breast milk, women who are being treated for cancer are generally advised not to breastfeed. Chemotherapy can be especially dangerous as it can build up in breast milk and harm the infant. Similarly, radioactive components that are taken internally, such as radioactive iodine used in treating thyroid cancer, also cross into breast milk and can harm the infant.

Pregnancy after Cancer

As more young people are surviving cancer, more women are considering whether they should have a baby after having cancer. In general,

pregnancy after cancer is considered safe for both the mother and the baby, and pregnancy does not appear to increase the chances of cancer recurring (coming back). However, since some cancers do recur, women are usually advised to wait a number of years after completing cancer treatment until the risk of recurrence has decreased. The amount of time you will be advised to wait before becoming pregnant depends on the type and stage of cancer and course of treatment.

Sometimes, cancer treatments can damage specific areas of the body such as the heart or lungs. Before becoming pregnant, your doctor may need to evaluate these organs to be sure that the pregnancy will be safe.

Unfortunately, some cancer treatments can also cause infertility, making it difficult or impossible for some women to have children.

Chapter 54

Taking Charge of Your Follow-Up Care

Every cancer patient looks forward to the day when the doctor says that treatment is finally complete. At that point, the end of cancer treatment signals the beginning of a new journey: survivorship.

Although you and your doctor may talk about the risk of a cancer recurrence down the road, it is also important to talk about "late effects" of treatment—side effects that may not become apparent until years later—and your overall plan for follow-up visits and cancer prevention.

Write It Down

Health care professionals now recognize that they need to better prepare patients for this next phase of life. Yet patients may need to take the reins in this area until formal survivorship plans are developed. This means they will need to schedule appointments for follow-up testing, communicate appropriate information to each of their doctors, and engage in healthy lifestyle practices.

Pediatric oncologists are leading the way in survivorship initiatives, thanks to the long-term survival of children with cancer. While the experts work out the details, make sure you document the following to start building your own survivorship plan:

Adapted with permission from the NCCN Living with Cancer Articles posted on www.nccn.com. © 2009 National Comprehensive Cancer Network. Available at: http://www.nccn.com. Accessed August 1, 2009. To view the most recent and complete version of these articles, go online to www.nccn.com.

- What type of cancer you had
- The names of the treatments you received
- The names of the drugs you took and/or were administered
- What follow-up tests and appointments are required and at what intervals

"If you don't know the answers, call your physicians and get them," urges Lidia Schapira, MD, medical oncologist at the Gillette Center for Breast Cancer at Massachusetts General Hospital Cancer Center in Boston and assistant professor of medicine at Harvard Medical School. The more details you can get, the better, she says.

Create Your Own Medical Record

Electronic medical records are still not widely used or required by the federal government, but you can improvise by creating your own. In addition to documenting the basics, you may want to create more detail. This includes the following:

- Your cancer diagnosis; treatment dates; drug names and doses, including chemotherapy; surgeries performed; and, if you received radiation, the specific areas of the body that were radiated, including organs in the path of exposure
- What doctor to see—and when—for future tests and check ups
- Contact Information for all physicians involved in your treatment—oncologists, surgeons, radiation therapists, and other specialists, as well as your primary care physician
- Facilities where x-rays, MRIs, CAT scans, and other studies were performed and where these records are stored
- Results of key lab tests and/or diagnostic studies

You may also choose to include this additional data:

- Other relevant data about your medical history
- Your blood type
- Current medications

To protect your privacy, do not record your Social Security number on any of the documents.

Collect this information on an ongoing basis. Near the end of your treatment, ask the doctor or nurse practitioner who is handling your care if he or she would review your "medical record" and notes for accuracy.

Here are some additional steps you may want to take:

- Print out copies of the documents or photocopy your handwritten documents.

- Download the electronic data to a flash drive or CD and have the handwritten documents scanned and save them to the same media.

- Store the flash drive or CD in a safe location.

- Give copies to trusted family members or friends in case you are hospitalized.

- Take the flash drive, CD, or printouts with you to all doctors' appointments.

- Take documentation with you when you travel—particularly overseas.

Just as patients with allergies or certain diseases wear bracelets to alert medical personnel, your record provides valuable details to better manage your medical care, prevent complications, or save your life.

For example, patients who once received the chemotherapy drug bleomycin may have developed diminished lung capacity, which would need to be communicated to an anesthesiologist before any future surgery. And because the drug doxorubicin can affect cardiac function, former cancer patients need to relay this information to both their primary care doctor and specialists.

Make a Plan

Because cancer treatment usually involves multiple medical professionals, people may be confused about whom to see for follow-up care. Do they return to their primary care physician or schedule visits with specialists or their oncologist?

Start by asking your oncologist if you should schedule follow-up appointments with him or her and, if so, for how many months or years. Ask if and when your care should be turned over to your primary care physician or nurse practitioner.

If your care is assigned to your primary care professional, provide him or her with the medical record you created, as described above.

Professional associations including the Institute of Medicine and the American Society of Clinical Oncology, as well as the Lance Armstrong Foundation, are working to create formal guidance to physicians on creating survivorship plans.

The National Comprehensive Cancer Network (NCCN) Clinical Practice Guidelines in Oncology™ (available through the NCCN website at www.nccn.org) have provided information to doctors about surveillance following completion of therapy, but NCCN is now expanding many of the NCCN Guidelines to include continuing and late effects of various treatments.

Until formal survivorship plans are widely adopted, people who arm themselves with information and documentation about their care will be in a good position to make a smooth transition from cancer patient to survivor.

Part Eight

Additional Help
and Information

Chapter 55

Glossary of Cancer Terms

adjuvant therapy: Additional cancer treatment given after the primary treatment to lower the risk that the cancer will come back. Adjuvant therapy may include chemotherapy, radiation therapy, hormone therapy, targeted therapy, or biological therapy.

alopecia: The lack or loss of hair from areas of the body where hair is usually found. Alopecia can be a side effect of some cancer treatments.

angiogenesis inhibitor: A substance that may prevent the formation of blood vessels. In anticancer therapy, an angiogenesis inhibitor may prevent the growth of new blood vessels that tumors need to grow.

antiestrogen: A substance that keeps cells from making or using estrogen (a hormone that plays a role in female sex characteristics, the menstrual cycle, and pregnancy). Antiestrogens may stop some cancer cells from growing and are used to prevent and treat breast cancer. They are also being studied in the treatment of other types of cancer. An antiestrogen is a type of hormone antagonist. Also called estrogen blocker.

atypical hyperplasia: A benign (not cancer) condition in which cells look abnormal under a microscope and are increased in number.

axilla: The underarm or armpit.

Excerpted from "Dictionary of Cancer Terms," National Cancer Institute (www.cancer.gov/dictionary), 2010.

axillary lymph node dissection: Surgery to remove lymph nodes found in the armpit region. Also called axillary dissection.

basal cell carcinoma: Cancer that begins in the lower part of the epidermis (the outer layer of the skin). It may appear as a small white or flesh-colored bump that grows slowly and may bleed. Basal cell carcinomas are usually found on areas of the body exposed to the sun. Basal cell carcinomas rarely metastasize (spread) to other parts of the body. They are the most common form of skin cancer. Also called basal cell cancer.

benign: Not cancerous. Benign tumors may grow larger but do not spread to other parts of the body. Also called nonmalignant.

bilateral cancer: Cancer that occurs in both paired organs, such as both breasts or both ovaries.

bilateral salpingo-oophorectomy: Surgery to remove both ovaries and both fallopian tubes.

biological therapy: Treatment to boost or restore the ability of the immune system to fight cancer, infections, and other diseases. Also used to lessen certain side effects that may be caused by some cancer treatments. Agents used in biological therapy include monoclonal antibodies, growth factors, and vaccines. These agents may also have a direct antitumor effect. Also called biological response modifier therapy, biotherapy, BRM therapy, and immunotherapy.

biopsy: The removal of cells or tissues for examination by a pathologist. The pathologist may study the tissue under a microscope or perform other tests on the cells or tissue. There are many different types of biopsy procedures. The most common types include: (1) incisional biopsy, in which only a sample of tissue is removed; (2) excisional biopsy, in which an entire lump or suspicious area is removed; and (3) needle biopsy, in which a sample of tissue or fluid is removed with a needle. When a wide needle is used, the procedure is called a core biopsy. When a thin needle is used, the procedure is called a fine-needle aspiration biopsy.

bone marrow: The soft, sponge-like tissue in the center of most bones. It produces white blood cells, red blood cells, and platelets.

BRCA-1: A gene on chromosome 17 that normally helps to suppress cell growth. A person who inherits certain mutations (changes) in a BRCA1 gene has a higher risk of getting breast, ovarian, prostate, and other types of cancer.

BRCA-2: A gene on chromosome 13 that normally helps to suppress cell growth. A person who inherits certain mutations (changes) in a BRCA2 gene has a higher risk of getting breast, ovarian, prostate, and other types of cancer.

breast-conserving surgery: An operation to remove the breast cancer but not the breast itself. Types of breast-conserving surgery include lumpectomy (removal of the lump), quadrantectomy (removal of one quarter, or quadrant, of the breast), and segmental mastectomy (removal of the cancer as well as some of the breast tissue around the tumor and the lining over the chest muscles below the tumor). Also called breast-sparing surgery.

CA-125: A substance that may be found in high amounts in the blood of patients with certain types of cancer, including ovarian cancer. CA-125 levels may also help monitor how well cancer treatments are working or if cancer has come back. Also called cancer antigen 125.

cancer of unknown primary origin: A case in which cancer cells are found in the body, but the place where the cells first started growing (the origin or primary site) cannot be determined. Also called carcinoma of unknown primary and CUP.

carcinoma: Cancer that begins in the skin or in tissues that line or cover internal organs.

carcinoma in situ: A group of abnormal cells that remain in the place where they first formed. They have not spread. These abnormal cells may become cancer and spread into nearby normal tissue. Also called stage 0 disease.

cervical intraepithelial neoplasia (CIN): Growth of abnormal cells on the surface of the cervix. Numbers from 1 to 3 may be used to describe how abnormal the cells are and how much of the cervical tissue is involved. Also called CIN.

cervix: The lower, narrow end of the uterus that forms a canal between the uterus and vagina.

chemotherapy: Treatment with drugs that kill cancer cells.

clinical breast exam: A physical exam of the breast performed by a health care provider to check for lumps or other changes. Also called CBE.

clinical trial: A type of research study that tests how well new medical approaches work in people. These studies test new methods of

screening, prevention, diagnosis, or treatment of a disease. Also called clinical study.

colon: The longest part of the large intestine, which is a tube-like organ connected to the small intestine at one end and the anus at the other. The colon removes water and some nutrients and electrolytes from partially digested food. The remaining material, solid waste called stool, moves through the colon to the rectum and leaves the body through the anus.

colonoscopy: Examination of the inside of the colon using a colonoscope, inserted into the rectum. A colonoscope is a thin, tube-like instrument with a light and a lens for viewing. It may also have a tool to remove tissue to be checked under a microscope for signs of disease.

colostomy: An opening into the colon from the outside of the body. A colostomy provides a new path for waste material to leave the body after part of the colon has been removed.

colposcopy: Examination of the vagina and cervix using a lighted magnifying instrument called a colposcope.

complementary and alternative medicine (CAM): Forms of treatment that are used in addition to (complementary) or instead of (alternative) standard treatments. These practices generally are not considered standard medical approaches. Standard treatments go through a long and careful research process to prove they are safe and effective, but less is known about most types of CAM. CAM may include dietary supplements, megadose vitamins, herbal preparations, special teas, acupuncture, massage therapy, magnet therapy, spiritual healing, and meditation. Also called CAM.

computed tomography (CT scan): A series of detailed pictures of areas inside the body taken from different angles. The pictures are created by a computer linked to an x-ray machine. Also called CAT scan, computerized axial tomography scan, computerized tomography, and CT scan.

conization: Surgery to remove a cone-shaped piece of tissue from the cervix and cervical canal. Conization may be used to diagnose or treat a cervical condition. Also called cone biopsy.

cryosurgery: A procedure in which tissue is frozen to destroy abnormal cells. Liquid nitrogen or liquid carbon dioxide is used to freeze the tissue. Also called cryoablation and cryosurgical ablation.

cyst: A sac or capsule in the body. It may be filled with fluid or other material.

diethylstilbestrol (DES): A synthetic form of the hormone estrogen that was prescribed to pregnant women between about 1940 and 1971 because it was thought to prevent miscarriages. Diethylstilbestrol may increase the risk of uterine, ovarian, or breast cancer in women who took it. It also has been linked to an increased risk of clear cell carcinoma of the vagina or cervix in daughters exposed to diethylstilbestrol before birth. Also called DES.

dilation and curettage (D&C): A procedure to remove tissue from the cervical canal or the inner lining of the uterus. The cervix is dilated (made larger) and a curette (spoon-shaped instrument) is inserted into the uterus to remove tissue. Also called D&C and dilatation and curettage.

dilator: A device used to stretch or enlarge an opening.

dose-dense chemotherapy: A chemotherapy treatment plan in which drugs are given with less time between treatments than in a standard chemotherapy treatment plan.

ductal carcinoma in situ (DCIS): A noninvasive condition in which abnormal cells are found in the lining of a breast duct. The abnormal cells have not spread outside the duct to other tissues in the breast. In some cases, ductal carcinoma in situ may become invasive cancer and spread to other tissues, although it is not known at this time how to predict which lesions will become invasive. Also called DCIS and intraductal carcinoma.

dysplasia: Cells that look abnormal under a microscope but are not cancer.

dysplastic nevus: A type of nevus (mole) that looks different from a common mole. A dysplastic nevus is often larger with borders that are not easy to see. Its color is usually uneven and can range from pink to dark brown. Parts of the mole may be raised above the skin surface. A dysplastic nevus may develop into malignant melanoma (a type of skin cancer).

early-stage breast cancer: Breast cancer that has not spread beyond the breast or the axillary lymph nodes. This includes ductal carcinoma in situ and stage I, stage IIA, stage IIB, and stage IIIA breast cancers.

endometriosis: A benign condition in which tissue that looks like endometrial tissue grows in abnormal places in the abdomen.

endometrium: The layer of tissue that lines the uterus.

epithelial carcinoma: Cancer that begins in the cells that line an organ.

estrogen: A type of hormone made by the body that helps develop and maintain female sex characteristics and the growth of long bones. Estrogens can also be made in the laboratory. They may be used as a type of birth control and to treat symptoms of menopause, menstrual disorders, osteoporosis, and other conditions.

excisional biopsy: A surgical procedure in which an entire lump or suspicious area is removed for diagnosis. The tissue is then examined under a microscope.

fallopian tube: A slender tube through which eggs pass from an ovary to the uterus. In the female reproductive tract, there is one ovary and one fallopian tube on each side of the uterus.

fibrocystic breast changes: A common condition marked by benign (not cancer) changes in breast tissue. These changes may include irregular lumps or cysts, breast discomfort, sensitive nipples, and itching. These symptoms may change throughout the menstrual cycle and usually stop after menopause. Also called benign breast disease, fibrocystic breast disease, and mammary dysplasia.

fibroid: A benign smooth-muscle tumor, usually in the uterus or gastrointestinal tract. Also called leiomyoma.

fine-needle aspiration: The removal of tissue or fluid with a thin needle for examination under a microscope. Also called FNA biopsy.

gestational trophoblastic tumor: Any of a group of tumors that develops from trophoblastic cells (cells that help an embryo attach to the uterus and help form the placenta) after fertilization of an egg by a sperm. The two main types of gestational trophoblastic tumors are hydatidiform mole and choriocarcinoma. Also called gestational trophoblastic disease.

grade: A description of a tumor based on how abnormal the cancer cells look under a microscope and how quickly the tumor is likely to grow and spread. Grading systems are different for each type of cancer.

graft: Healthy skin, bone, or other tissue taken from one part of the body and used to replace diseased or injured tissue removed from another part of the body.

gynecologic cancer: Cancer of the female reproductive tract, including the cervix, endometrium, fallopian tubes, ovaries, uterus, and vagina.

gynecologic oncologist: A doctor who specializes in treating cancers of the female reproductive organs.

Herceptin: A monoclonal antibody that binds to HER2 (human epidermal growth factor receptor 2), and can kill HER2-positive cancer cells. Monoclonal antibodies are made in the laboratory and can locate and bind to substances in the body, including cancer cells. Herceptin is used to treat breast cancer that is HER2-positive and has spread after treatment with other drugs. It is also used with other anticancer drugs to treat HER2-positive breast cancer after surgery. Herceptin is also being studied in the treatment of other types of cancer. Also called trastuzumab.

hormone: One of many chemicals made by glands in the body. Hormones circulate in the bloodstream and control the actions of certain cells or organs. Some hormones can also be made in the laboratory.

hormone receptor test: A test to measure the amount of certain proteins, called hormone receptors, in cancer tissue. Hormones can attach to these proteins. A high level of hormone receptors may mean that hormones help the cancer grow.

hormone replacement therapy (HRT): Hormones (estrogen, progesterone, or both) given to women after menopause to replace the hormones no longer produced by the ovaries. Also called HRT and menopausal hormone therapy.

human papillomavirus (HPV): A type of virus that can cause abnormal tissue growth (for example, warts) and other changes to cells. Infection for a long time with certain types of human papillomavirus can cause cervical cancer. Human papillomavirus can also play a role in some other types of cancer, such as anal, vaginal, vulvar, penile, and oropharyngeal cancers. Also called HPV.

hysterectomy: Surgery to remove the uterus and, sometimes, the cervix. When the uterus and the cervix are removed, it is called a total hysterectomy. When only the uterus is removed, it is called a partial hysterectomy.

immunotherapy: Treatment to boost or restore the ability of the immune system to fight cancer, infections, and other diseases. Also used to lessen certain side effects that may be caused by some cancer treatments. Agents used in immunotherapy include monoclonal antibodies, growth factors, and vaccines. These agents may also have a direct antitumor effect. Also called biological response modifier therapy, biological therapy, biotherapy, and BRM therapy.

in vitro: In the laboratory (outside the body). The opposite of in vivo (in the body).

in vivo: In the body. The opposite of in vitro (outside the body or in the laboratory).

infiltrating ductal carcinoma: The most common type of invasive breast cancer. It starts in the cells that line the milk ducts in the breast, grows outside the ducts, and often spreads to the lymph nodes.

intraductal carcinoma: A noninvasive condition in which abnormal cells are found in the lining of a breast duct. The abnormal cells have not spread outside the duct to other tissues in the breast. In some cases, intraductal carcinoma may become invasive cancer and spread to other tissues, although it is not known at this time how to predict which lesions will become invasive. Also called DCIS and ductal carcinoma in situ.

intraepithelial: Within the layer of cells that form the surface or lining of an organ.

invasive cancer: Cancer that has spread beyond the layer of tissue in which it developed and is growing into surrounding, healthy tissues. Also called infiltrating cancer.

invasive hydatidiform mole: A type of cancer that grows into the muscular wall of the uterus. It is formed after conception (fertilization of an egg by a sperm). It may spread to other parts of the body, such as the vagina, vulva, and lung. Also called chorioadenoma destruens.

laser therapy: Treatment that uses intense, narrow beams of light to cut and destroy tissue, such as cancer tissue. Laser therapy may also be used to reduce lymphedema (swelling caused by a buildup of lymph fluid in tissue) after breast cancer surgery.

lobular carcinoma in situ (LCIS): A condition in which abnormal cells are found in the lobules of the breast. Lobular carcinoma in situ seldom becomes invasive cancer; however, having it in one breast increases the risk of developing breast cancer in either breast. Also called LCIS.

local cancer: An invasive malignant cancer confined entirely to the organ where the cancer began.

locally advanced cancer: Cancer that has spread from where it started to nearby tissue or lymph nodes.

loop electrosurgical excision procedure (LEEP): A technique that uses electric current passed through a thin wire loop to remove abnormal tissue. Also called LEEP and loop excision.

low grade: A term used to describe cells that look nearly normal under a microscope. These cells are less likely to grow and spread more quickly than cells in high-grade cancer or in growths that may become cancer.

lumpectomy: Surgery to remove abnormal tissue or cancer from the breast and a small amount of normal tissue around it. It is a type of breast-sparing surgery.

lymph node: A rounded mass of lymphatic tissue that is surrounded by a capsule of connective tissue. Lymph nodes filter lymph (lymphatic fluid), and they store lymphocytes (white blood cells). They are located along lymphatic vessels. Also called lymph gland.

lymphatic system: The tissues and organs that produce, store, and carry white blood cells that fight infections and other diseases. This system includes the bone marrow, spleen, thymus, lymph nodes, and lymphatic vessels (a network of thin tubes that carry lymph and white blood cells). Lymphatic vessels branch, like blood vessels, into all the tissues of the body.

lymphedema: A condition in which extra lymph fluid builds up in tissues and causes swelling. It may occur in an arm or leg if lymph vessels are blocked, damaged, or removed by surgery.

magnetic resonance imaging (MRI): A procedure in which radio waves and a powerful magnet linked to a computer are used to create detailed pictures of areas inside the body. These pictures can show the difference between normal and diseased tissue. Magnetic resonance imaging makes better images of organs and soft tissue than other scanning techniques, such as computed tomography (CT) or x-ray. Magnetic resonance imaging is especially useful for imaging the brain, the spine, the soft tissue of joints, and the inside of bones. Also called MRI, NMRI, and nuclear magnetic resonance imaging.

malignant: Cancerous. Malignant tumors can invade and destroy nearby tissue and spread to other parts of the body.

mammography: The use of film or a computer to create a picture of the breast.

mastectomy: Surgery to remove the breast (or as much of the breast tissue as possible).

menopause: The time of life when a woman's ovaries stop producing hormones and menstrual periods stop. Natural menopause usually occurs around age 50. A woman is said to be in menopause when she

hasn't had a period for 12 months in a row. Symptoms of menopause include hot flashes, mood swings, night sweats, vaginal dryness, trouble concentrating, and infertility.

metastasis: The spread of cancer from one part of the body to another. A tumor formed by cells that have spread is called a metastatic tumor or a metastasis. The metastatic tumor contains cells that are like those in the original (primary) tumor. The plural form of metastasis is metastases (meh-TAS-tuh-SEEZ).

microcalcification: A tiny deposit of calcium in the breast that cannot be felt but can be detected on a mammogram. A cluster of these very small specks of calcium may indicate that cancer is present.

mutation: Any change in the DNA of a cell. Mutations may be caused by mistakes during cell division, or they may be caused by exposure to DNA-damaging agents in the environment. Mutations can be harmful, beneficial, or have no effect. If they occur in cells that make eggs or sperm, they can be inherited; if mutations occur in other types of cells, they are not inherited. Certain mutations may lead to cancer or other diseases.

neoadjuvant therapy: Treatment given as a first step to shrink a tumor before the main treatment, which is usually surgery, is given. Examples of neoadjuvant therapy include chemotherapy, radiation therapy, and hormone therapy. It is a type of induction therapy.

occult primary tumor: Cancer in which the site of the primary (original) tumor cannot be found. Most metastases from occult primary tumors are found in the head and neck.

oncologist: A doctor who specializes in treating cancer. Some oncologists specialize in a particular type of cancer treatment. For example, a radiation oncologist specializes in treating cancer with radiation.

oophorectomy: Surgery to remove one or both ovaries.

ostomy: An operation to create an opening (a stoma) from an area inside the body to the outside. Colostomy and urostomy are types of ostomies.

ovarian ablation: Surgery, radiation therapy, or a drug treatment to stop the functioning of the ovaries. Also called ovarian suppression.

ovary: One of a pair of female reproductive glands in which the ova, or eggs, are formed. The ovaries are located in the pelvis, one on each side of the uterus.

palliative care: Care given to improve the quality of life of patients who have a serious or life-threatening disease. The goal of palliative care is to prevent or treat as early as possible the symptoms of a disease, side effects caused by treatment of a disease, and psychological, social, and spiritual problems related to a disease or its treatment. Also called comfort care, supportive care, and symptom management.

palpation: Examination by pressing on the surface of the body to feel the organs or tissues underneath.

Pap test: A procedure in which cells are scraped from the cervix for examination under a microscope. It is used to detect cancer and changes that may lead to cancer. A Pap test can also show conditions, such as infection or inflammation, that are not cancer. Also called Pap smear and Papanicolaou test.

pathologist: A doctor who identifies diseases by studying cells and tissues under a microscope.

polyp: A growth that protrudes from a mucous membrane.

positron emission tomography scan (PET scan): A procedure in which a small amount of radioactive glucose (sugar) is injected into a vein, and a scanner is used to make detailed, computerized pictures of areas inside the body where the glucose is used. Because cancer cells often use more glucose than normal cells, the pictures can be used to find cancer cells in the body. Also called PET scan.

precancerous: A term used to describe a condition that may (or is likely to) become cancer. Also called premalignant.

progesterone: A type of hormone made by the body that plays a role in the menstrual cycle and pregnancy. Progesterone can also be made in the laboratory. It may be used as a type of birth control and to treat menstrual disorders, infertility, symptoms of menopause, and other conditions.

progestin: Any natural or laboratory-made substance that has some or all of the biologic effects of progesterone, a female hormone.

prophylactic mastectomy: Surgery to reduce the risk of developing breast cancer by removing one or both breasts before disease develops. Also called preventive mastectomy.

prophylactic oophorectomy: Surgery intended to reduce the risk of ovarian cancer by removing the ovaries before disease develops.

radiation therapy: The use of high-energy radiation from x-rays, gamma rays, neutrons, protons, and other sources to kill cancer cells and shrink tumors. Radiation may come from a machine outside the body (external-beam radiation therapy), or it may come from radioactive material placed in the body near cancer cells (internal radiation therapy). Systemic radiation therapy uses a radioactive substance, such as a radiolabeled monoclonal antibody, that travels in the blood to tissues throughout the body. Also called irradiation and radiotherapy.

radical mastectomy: Surgery for breast cancer in which the breast, chest muscles, and all of the lymph nodes under the arm are removed. For many years, this was the breast cancer operation used most often, but it is used rarely now. Doctors consider radical mastectomy only when the tumor has spread to the chest muscles. Also called Halsted radical mastectomy.

raloxifene: The active ingredient in a drug used to reduce the risk of invasive breast cancer in postmenopausal women who are at high risk of the disease or who have osteoporosis. It is also used to prevent and treat osteoporosis in postmenopausal women. It is also being studied in the prevention of breast cancer in certain premenopausal women and in the prevention and treatment of other conditions. Raloxifene blocks the effects of the hormone estrogen in the breast and increases the amount of calcium in bone. It is a type of selective estrogen receptor modulator (SERM).

recurrent cancer: Cancer that has recurred (come back), usually after a period of time during which the cancer could not be detected. The cancer may come back to the same place as the original (primary) tumor or to another place in the body. Also called recurrence.

salpingo-oophorectomy: Surgical removal of the fallopian tubes and ovaries.

sarcoma: A cancer of the bone, cartilage, fat, muscle, blood vessels, or other connective or supportive tissue.

selective estrogen receptor modulator: A drug that acts like estrogen on some tissues but blocks the effect of estrogen on other tissues. Tamoxifen and raloxifene are selective estrogen receptor modulators. Also called SERM.

sigmoidoscopy: Examination of the lower colon using a sigmoidoscope, inserted into the rectum. A sigmoidoscope is a thin, tube-like instrument with a light and a lens for viewing. It may also have a tool

to remove tissue to be checked under a microscope for signs of disease. Also called proctosigmoidoscopy.

speculum: An instrument used to widen an opening of the body to make it easier to look inside.

squamous cell: Flat cell that looks like a fish scale under a microscope. These cells cover inside and outside surfaces of the body. They are found in the tissues that form the surface of the skin, the lining of the hollow organs of the body (such as the bladder, kidney, and uterus), and the passages of the respiratory and digestive tracts.

squamous intraepithelial lesion (SIL): A general term for the abnormal growth of squamous cells on the surface of the cervix. The changes in the cells are described as low grade or high grade, depending on how much of the cervix is affected and how abnormal the cells appear. Also called SIL.

stage: The extent of a cancer in the body. Staging is usually based on the size of the tumor, whether lymph nodes contain cancer, and whether the cancer has spread from the original site to other parts of the body.

stem cell transplant: A method of replacing immature blood-forming cells in the bone marrow that have been destroyed by drugs, radiation, or disease. Stem cells are injected into the patient and make healthy blood cells. A stem cell transplant may be autologous (using a patient's own stem cells that were saved before treatment), allogeneic (using stem cells donated by someone who is not an identical twin), or syngeneic (using stem cells donated by an identical twin).

tamoxifen: A drug used to treat certain types of breast cancer in women and men. It is also used to prevent breast cancer in women who have had ductal carcinoma in situ (abnormal cells in the ducts of the breast) and in women who are at a high risk of developing breast cancer. Tamoxifen is also being studied in the treatment of other types of cancer. It blocks the effects of the hormone estrogen in the breast. Tamoxifen is a type of antiestrogen. Also called tamoxifen citrate.

taxane: A type of drug that blocks cell growth by stopping mitosis (cell division). Taxanes interfere with microtubules (cellular structures that help move chromosomes during mitosis). They are used to treat cancer. A taxane is a type of mitotic inhibitor and antimicrotubule agent.

tumor: An abnormal mass of tissue that results when cells divide more than they should or do not die when they should. Tumors may be benign (not cancer), or malignant (cancer). Also called neoplasm.

ultrasound: A procedure in which high-energy sound waves are bounced off internal tissues or organs and make echoes. The echo patterns are shown on the screen of an ultrasound machine, forming a picture of body tissues called a sonogram. Also called ultrasonography.

uterus: The small, hollow, pear-shaped organ in a woman's pelvis. This is the organ in which a fetus develops. Also called womb.

vagina: The muscular canal extending from the uterus to the exterior of the body. Also called birth canal.

vulva: The external female genital organs, including the clitoris, vaginal lips, and the opening to the vagina.

Chapter 56

Resources for More Information about Cancer in Women

General Cancer Information

Agency for Healthcare Research and Quality
540 Gaither Road
Rockville, MD 20850
Clearinghouse Toll-Free:
800-358-9295
Clearinghouse TTY:
888-586-6340
Phone: 301-427-1364
Website: http://www.ahrq.gov
E-mail: info@ahrq.gov

American Association for Cancer Research
615 Chestnut Street, 17th Floor
Philadelphia, PA 19106-4404
Toll-Free: 866-423-3965
Phone: 215-440-9300
Fax: 215-440-9313
Website: http://www.aacr.org
E-mail: aacr@aacr.org

American Cancer Society
1599 Clifton Road NE
Atlanta, GA 30329
Toll-Free: 800-ACS-2345
(227-2345)
TTY: 866-228-4327
Website: http://www.cancer.org

American College of Surgeons
Website: http://www.facs.org

Information in this chapter was compiled from many sources deemed reliable. Inclusion does not constitute endorsement and there is no implication associated with omission. All contact information was updated and verified in May 2010.

649

American Institute for Cancer Research
1759 R Street NW
Washington, DC 20009
Toll-Free: 800-843-8114
Phone: 202-328-7744
Fax: 202-328-7226
Website: http://www.aicr.org
E-mail: aicrweb@aicr.org

American Society of Clinical Oncology
2318 Mill Road, Suite 800
Alexandria, VA 22314
Toll-Free: 888-282-2552
Phone: 571-483-1300
Fax: 703-299-1044
Website: http://www.asco.org

Association of Community Cancer Centers
11600 Nebel Street, Suite 201
Rockville, MD 20852-2557
Phone: 301-984-9496
Fax: 301-770-1949
Website: http://www.accc-cancer
.org

Bloch (R.A.) Cancer Foundation, Inc.
One H&R Block Way
Kansas City, MO 64105
Toll-Free: 800-433-0464
Phone: 816-WE BUILD
(932-8453)
Fax: 816-931-7486
Website: http://www.blochcancer
.org

Canadian Cancer Society
565 W. 10th Ave.
Vancouver, BC V5Z 4J4
Tel: 604-872-4400
Website: www.bc.cancer.ca
E-mail: inquiries@bc.cancer.ca

Cancer and Careers.org
Phone: 212-685-5955
Website: http://www
.cancerandcareers.org

Cancer Hope Network
2 North Road, Suite A
Chester, NJ 07930
Toll-Free: 877-HOPENET
(877-467-3638)
Phone: 908-879-4039 (Local)
Fax: 908-879-6518
Website: http://www
.cancerhopenetwork.org
E-mail: info@cancerhopenetwork
.org

Cancer Project
5100 Wisconsin Avenue
Suite 400
Washington, DC 20016
Phone: 202-244-5038
Website: http://www
.CancerProject.org
E-mail: info@CancerProject.org

Cancer Research UK
Website: http://www.cancerhelp
.org.uk

CancerCare
275 Seventh Avenue
New York, NY 10001
Toll-Free: 800-813-HOPE
(813-4673)
Phone: 212-712-8400
Website: http://www.cancercare
.org
E-mail: info@cancercare.org

Centers for Disease Control and Prevention
1600 Clifton Road
Atlanta, GA 30333
Toll-Free: 800-CDC-INFO
(800-232-4636)
Phone: 404-639-3311
Website: http://www.cdc.gov
E-mail: cdcinfo@cdc.gov

Cleveland Clinic
9500 Euclid Avenue, NA31
Cleveland, OH 44195
Toll-Free: 800-223-2273
Phone: 216-444-2200
TTY: 216-444-0261
Website: http://www
.clevelandclinic.org
E-mail: healthl@ccf.org

Dana-Farber Cancer Institute
44 Binney Street
Boston, MA 02115
Phone: 866-408-DFCI (408-3324)
TDD: 617-632-5330
Website: http://www.dfci.harvard
.edu
E-mail: Dana-FarberContactUs
@dfci.harvard.edu

Facing Our Risk of Cancer Empowered (FORCE)
16057 Tampa Palms Blvd. W
PMB #373
Tampa, FL 33647
Toll-Free: 866-824-RISK (7475)
Phone: 954-255-8732
Website: www.facingourrisk.org
E-mail: info@facingourrisk.org

Intercultural Cancer Council
Bayor College of Medicine
Suite 1025
1720 Dryden, PMB 25
Houston, TX 77030
Phone: 713-798-4617
Website: http://iccnetwork.org
E-mail: info@iccnetwork.org

International Union Against Cancer
Website: http://www.uicc.org

Lesbian Community Cancer Project
4025 N. Sheridan Road
Chicago, IL 60613
Phone: 773-388-1600
Fax: 773-388-8887
Website: http://www.lccp.org
E-mail: info@lccp.com

Macmillan Cancer Support
Phone: (+44)0808-88-00-00
Website: www.macmillan.org
E-mail: webmanager@macmillan
.org.uk

Mayo Foundation for Medical Education and Research
200 First Street SW
Rochester, MN 55905
Website: http://www
.mayoclinic.com
E-mail: comments@mayoclinic
.com

Memorial Sloan-Kettering Cancer Center
1275 York Avenue
New York, NY 10021
Toll-Free: 800-525-2225 (referral service)
Phone: 212-639-2000
Website: www.mskcc.org

Moores Cancer Center
University of California
San Diego
Website: http://health.ucsd.edu
/cancer

National Association for Proton Therapy
1301 Highland Drive
Silver Spring, MD 20910
Phone: 301-587-6100
Website: http://www
.proton-therapy.org

National Cancer Institute
Public Inquiries Office
Suite 3036A
6116 Executive Boulevard
MSC8322
Bethesda, MD 20892-8322
Toll-Free: 800-4-CANCER
(800-422-6237)
TTY: 800-332-8615
Website: http://www.cancer.gov

National Center for Complementary and Alternative Medicine
NCCAM Clearinghouse
P.O. Box 7923
Gaithersburg, MD 20898-7923
Toll-Free: 888-644-6226
TTY: 866-464-3615
Fax: 866-464-3616
Website: http://nccam.nih.gov
E-mail: info@nccam.nih.gov

National Coalition for Cancer Survivorship
1010 Wayne Avenue, Suite 770
Silver Spring, MD 20910
Toll-Free: 888-650-9127
Phone: 301-650-9127
Fax: 301-565-9670
Website: http://www
.canceradvocacy.org
E-mail: info@canceradvocacy.org

National Comprehensive Cancer Network
275 Commerce Drive, Suite 300
Fort Washington, PA 19034
Phone: 215-690-0300
Fax: 215-690-0280
Website: http://www.nccn.org

National Foundation for Cancer Research
4600 East West Highway
Suite 525
Bethesda, MD 20814
Toll-Free: 800-321-CURE
(321-2873)
Phone: 301-654-1250
Fax: 301-654-5824
Website: http://www.nfcr.org

National Heart, Lung, and Blood Institute
NHLBI Health Information Center
P.O. Box 30105
Bethesda, MD 20824-0105
Phone: 301-592-8573
TTY: 240-629-3255
Fax: 240-629-3246
Website: http://www.nhlbi.nih
.gov
E-mail: nhlbiinfo@nhlbi.nih.gov

National Hospice and Palliative Care Organization
1731 King St., Suite 100
Alexandria, VA 22314
Toll-Free: 800-658-8898
Phone: 703-837-1500
Fax: 703-837-1233
Website: http://www.nhpco.org
E-mail: nhpco_info@nhpco.org

National Institute on Aging
Building 31C, Room 5C27
31 Center Drive, MSC 2292
Bethesda, MD 20892
Publications Toll-Free:
800-222-2225
Phone: 301-496-1752
TTY: 800-222-4225
Fax: 301-496-1072
Website: http://www.nia.nih.gov
Publications Website: http://
www.niapublications.org
E-mail: niainfo@nia.nih.gov

National Marrow Donor Program
3001 Broadway Street Northeast
Suite 500
Minneapolis, MN 55413-1753
Be the Match Registry:
800-MARROW2 (627-7692)
Website: http://www
.marrow-donor.org

National Women's Health Information Center
8270 Willow Oaks Corporate Dr.
Fairfax, VA 22031
Toll-Free: 800-994-WOMAN
(994-9662)
TTY: 888-220-5446
Website: http://www.4woman.gov

Native American Cancer Research
Phone: 303-838-9359
Website: http://natamcancer.org

Novartis Oncology
Novartis Pharmaceuticals
Corporation
One Health Plaza
East Hanover, NJ 07936-1080
Toll-Free: 888-669-6682
Website: http://www.
us.novartisoncology.com

OncoLink
Abramson Cancer Center of the
University of Pennsylvania
3400 Spruce Street, 2 Donner
Philadelphia, PA 19104-4283
Fax: 215-349-5445
Website: http://www.oncolink
.com

Pregnant With Cancer Network
P.O. Box 1243
Buffalo, NY 14220
Website: http://www
.pregnantwithcancer.org

Prevent Cancer Foundation
1600 Duke Street, Suite 500
Alexandria, VA 22314
Toll-Free: 800-227-2732
Phone: 703-836-4412
Fax: 703-836-4413
Website: http://www
.preventcancer.org

Society of Laparoendoscopic Surgeons
Website: http://www.sls.org

Society of Surgical Oncology
85 West Algonquin Road
Suite 550
Arlington Heights, IL 60005
Phone: 847-427-1400
Fax: 847-427-9656
Website: http://www.surgonc.org
E-mail: webmaster@surgonc.org

University of Texas
M.D. Anderson Cancer Center
1515 Holcombe Blvd.
Houston, TX 77030
Toll-Free: 800-392-1611
Phone: 713-792-6161
Website: http://www.mdanderson
.org

U.S. Food and Drug Administration
10903 New Hampshire Ave.
Silver Spring, MD 20993
Toll-Free: 888-463-6332
Website: http://www.fda.gov

Women's Cancer Resource Center
5741 Telegraph Avenue
Oakland, CA 94609
Toll-Free: 888-421-7900
Phone: 510-601-4040
Fax: 510-601-4045
Website: http://www.wcrc.org

Breast Cancer Resources

African American Breast Cancer Alliance
P.O. Box 8981
Minneapolis, MN 55408
Phone: 612-825-3675
Fax: 612-827-2977
Website: http://aabcainc.org

American Breast Cancer Foundation
1220 B East Joppa Road
Suite 332
Baltimore, MD 21286
Toll-Free: 877-KEY-2-LIFE
(539-2543)
Phone: 410-825-9388
Fax: 410-825-4395
Website: http://www.abcf.org
E-mail: contact@abcf.org

American Society of Breast Disease
P.O. Box 140186
Dallas, TX 75214
Phone: 214-368-6836
Fax: 214-368-5719
Website: http://www.asbd.org
E-mail: info@asbd.org

Avon Foundation Breast Cancer Crusade
1345 Avenue of the Americas
New York, NY 10105
Phone: 866-505-AVON (505-2866)
Website: http://www.avoncompany
.com/women/avoncrusade
E-mail: info@avonfoundation.org

Breast Cancer Action
55 New Montgomery, Suite 323
San Francisco, CA 94105
Toll-Free: 877-2STOPBC
(278-6722)
Phone: 415-243-9301
Fax: 415-243-3996
Website: http://www.bcaction.org
E-mail: info@bcaction.org

Breast Cancer Fund
1388 Sutter Street, Suite 400
San Francisco, CA 94109-5400
Toll-Free: 866-760-8223
Phone: 415-346-8223
Fax: 415-346-2975
Website: http://www
.breastcancerfund.org
E-mail: info@breastcancerfund
.org

Breast Cancer Network of Strength
135 S. LaSalle St., Suite 2000
Chicago, IL 60603
Toll-Free: 800-221-2141 (24 hour
hotline and resources)
Phone: 312-986-8338
Website: http://www
.networkofstrength.org

Breast Cancer Research Foundation
60 East 56th Street, 8th Floor
New York, NY 10022
Toll-Free: 866-FIND-A-CURE
(346-3228)
Phone: 646-497-2600
Fax: 646-497-0890
Website: http://www.bcrfcure.org
E-mail: bcrf@bcrfcure.org

Healthy Women
157 Broad Street, Suite 106
Red Bank, NJ 07701
Phone: 1-877-986-9472
Fax: 732-530-3347
Website: http://www
.healthywomen.org
E-mail: mail@winabc.org

Imaginis: The Breast Cancer Resource
P.O. Box 27018
Greenville, SC 29616
Website: http://www.imaginis.com
E-mail: learnmore@imaginis.com

Johns Hopkins Breast Cancer Center
601 North Caroline Street
Room 4161
Baltimore, MD 21287
Phone: 4410-955-5000
Fax: 410-614-1947
Website: http://www
.hopkinsbreastcenter.org

Komen (Susan G.) Breast Cancer Foundation
5005 LBJ Freeway, Suite 250
Dallas, TX 75244
Toll-Free: 800-I'M AWARE
(462-9273)
Phone: 972-855-1600
Fax: 972-855-1605
Website: http://www.komen.org

Living Beyond Breast Cancer
354 West Lancaster Avenue
Suite 224
Haverford, PA 19041
Phone: 610-645-4567;
484-708-1550
Survivors' Helpline:
888-753-LBBC (5222)
Fax: 610-645-4573
Website: http://www.lbbc.org
E-mail: mail@lbbc.org

Mayors' Campaign Against Breast Cancer
U.S. Conference of Mayors
1620 Eye Street, NW, 3rd Floor
Washington, DC 20006
Phone: 202-293-7330
Fax: 202-293-2352
Website: http://www.usmayors
.org/cancer
E-mail: info@usmayors.org

National Breast and Cervical Cancer Early Detection Program
Website: http://www.cdc
.gov/cancer/nbccedp/index.htm

National Breast and Ovarian Cancer Centre
Phone (Australia): 02-9357-9400
Fax (Australia): 02-9357-9477
International Phone:
(+61) 2-9357-9400
International Fax:
(+61) 2-9357-9477
Website: http://www.nbocc.org.au
E-mail: directorate@nbocc.org.au

National Breast Cancer Awareness Month
P.O. Box 15437
Wilmington, DE 19850-5437
Phone: 877-88-NBCAM
(886-2226)
Website: http://www.nbcam.org

National Breast Cancer Coalition
1101 17th Street, NW
Suite 1300
Washington, DC 20036
Toll-Free: 800-622-2838
Phone: 202-296-7477
Website: http://www
.stopbreastcancer.org
E-mail: info@stopbreastcancer.org

National Breast Cancer Foundation
2600 Network Blvd., Suite 300
Frisco, TX 75034
Website: http://www
.nationalbreastcancer.org

Program on Breast Cancer and Environmental Risk Factors

Cornell University, College of
Veterinary Medicine
Vet Box 31
Ithaca, NY 14853-6401
Fax: 607-254-4730
Website: http://envirocancer
.cornell.edu
E-mail: breastcancer@cornell
.edu

SHARE: Self-Help for Women with Breast or Ovarian Cancer

1501 Broadway, Suite 704A
New York, NY 10036
Toll-Free: 866-891-2392
Phone: 212-719-0364
Fax: 212-869-3431
Website: http://www
.sharecancersupport.org
E-mail:
info@sharecancersupport.org

Gynecologic Cancer Resources

Alliance for Cervical Cancer Prevention

Website: http://www
.alliance-cxca.org
E-mail: accp@path.org

American College of Obstetricians and Gynecologists

P.O. Box 96920
Washington, DC 20090-6920
Phone: 202-638-5577
Website: http://www.acog.org

American Society for Colposcopy and Cervical Pathology

150 West Washington Street
Suite 1
Hagerstown, MD 21740
Toll-Free: 800-787-7227
Phone: 301-733-3640
Fax: 301-733-5775
Website: http://www.asccp.org

Gynecologic Cancer Foundation

Phone: 312-578-1439
Website: http://www.thegcf.org

Gynecologic Cancer Foundation/Women's Cancer Network

230 W. Monroe, Suite 2528
Chicago, IL 60606
Phone: 312-578-1439
Website: http://www.wcn.org
E-mail: info@thegcf.org

International Gynecologic Cancer Society

P.O. Box 6387
Louisville, KY 40206
Phone: 502-981-4575
Fax: 502-891-4576
Website: http://www.igcs.org
E-mail: adminoffice@igcs.org

National Cervical Cancer Coalition
6520 Platt Ave. #693
West Hills, CA 91307
Toll-Free: 800-685-5531
Phone: 818-909-3849
Fax: 818-780-8199
Website: http://www.nccc-online
.org
E-mail: info@nccc-online.org

National HPV and Cervical Cancer Prevention Resource Center
P.O. Box 13827
Research Triangle Park, NC 27713
Website: http://www.ashastd
.org/hpvccrc

National Ovarian Cancer Association
101-145 Front Street East
Toronto, Ontario M5A 1E3
Canada
Toll-Free: 877-413-7970 (Canada only)
Phone: 416-962-2700
Fax: 416-962-2701
Website: http://www
.ovariancanada.org
E-mail: noca@ovariancanada.org

National Ovarian Cancer Coalition
2501 Oak Lawn Avenue, Suite 435
Dallas, TX 75219
Toll-Free: 888-OVARIAN (682-7426) (Helpline)
Phone: 561-393-0005 (Helpline)
Fax: 561-393-7275
Website: http://www.ovarian.org
E-mail: NOCC@ovarian.org

Ovarian Cancer National Alliance
910 17th Street, NW, Suite 1190
Washington, DC 20006
Phone: 202-331-1332
Fax: 202-331-2292
Website: http://www
.ovariancancer.org
E-mail: ocna@ovariancancer.org

Ovarian Cancer Research Fund, Inc.
14 Pennsylvania Plaza
Suite 1400
New York, NY 10122
Toll-Free: 800-873-9569
Phone: 212-268-1002
Fax: 212-947-5652
Website: http://www.ocrf.org
E-mail: info@ocrf.org

Resources for Other Types of Cancer

American Gastroenterological Association
4930 Del Ray Avenue
Bethesda, MD 20814
Phone: 301-654-2055
Fax: 301-654-5920
Website: http://www.gastro.org
E-mail: member@gstro.org

American Liver Foundation
75 Maiden Lane, Suite 603
New York, NY 10038
Toll-Free: 800-GO-Liver
(465-4837)
Phone: 212-668-1000
Fax: 212-483-8179
Website: http://www
.liverfoundation.org

American Lung Association
1301 Pennsylvania Avenue, NW
Washington, DC 20004
Toll-Free: 800-LUNGUSA
(586-4872)
Website: http://www.lungusa.org

American Melanoma Foundation
4150 Regents Park Row, Suite 300
La Jolla, CA 92037
Phone: 858-882-7712
Fax: 619-448-2902
Website: http://www
.melanomafoundation.org
E-mail: sunsmartz
@melanomafoundation.org

American Society for Gastrointestinal Endoscopy
1520 Kensington Road
Suite 202
Oak Brook, IL 60523
Phone: 630-573-0600
Fax: 630-573-0691
Website: http://www.asge.org
E-mail: info@asge.org

American Society of Colon and Rectal Surgeons
85 W. Algonquin Road
Suite 550
Arlington Heights, IL 60005
Phone: 847-290-9184
Fax: 847-290-9203
Website: http://www.fascrs.org
E-mail: ascrs@fascrs.org

C3: Colorectal Cancer Coalition
1414 Prince Street, Suite 204
Alexandria, VA 22314
Phone: 202-244-2906
Website: http://www.c-three.org
E-mail: info@c-three.org

Colon Cancer Alliance
1200 G Street, NW, Suite 800
Washington, DC 20005
Toll-Free: 877-422-2030
Website: http://www.ccalliance
.org
E-mail: info@ccalliance.org

Kidney Cancer Association
1234 Sherman Avenue
Suite 203
Evanston, IL 60202-1375
Phone: 847-332-1051
Toll-Free: 800-850-9132
Website: http://www
.kidneycancer.org

Leukemia and Lymphoma Society
1311 Mamaroneck Avenue
White Plains, NY 10605-5221
Phone: 914-949-5213
Toll-Free: 800-955-4572
Website: http://www
.leukemia-lymphoma.org
E-mail: infocenter
@leukemia-lymphoma.org

Lung Cancer Alliance
888 16th Street, NW, Suite 150
Washington, DC 20006
Toll-Free: 800-298-2436
Website: http://www
.lungcanceralliance.org
E-mail: info@lungcanceralliance
.org

**Lung Cancer Online
Foundation**
Website: http://www
.lungcanceronline.org

**Lymphoma Foundation of
America**
1100 North Main Street
Ann Arbor, MI 48104
Phone: 734-222-1133 (Patient
Voicemail Hotline)
Toll-Free: 800-385-1060 (Patient
Voicemail Hotline)
Website: http://www
.lymphomahelp.org
E-mail: LFA@lymphomahelp.org

**Lymphoma Research
Foundation**
8800 Venice Boulevard
Suite 207
Los Angeles, CA 90034
Toll-Free: 800-500-9976
Phone: 310-204-7040
Website: http://www.lymphoma
.org
E-mail for general information:
LRF@lymphoma.org
E-mail for patient services:
helpline@lymphoma.org

**Melanoma Education
Foundation**
P.O. Box 2023
Peabody, MA 01960
Phone: 978-535-3080
Fax: 978-535-5602
Website: http://www.skincheck
.org
E-mail: mef@skincheck.org

**Multiple Myeloma Research
Foundation**
383 Main Avenue, 5th floor
Norwalk, CT 06851
Phone: 203-972-1250
Website: http://www
.multiplemyeloma.org
E-mail: info@themmrf.org

**National Brain Tumor
Foundation**
22 Battery Street, Suite 612
San Francisco, CA 94111-5520
Toll-Free: 800-934-CURE
(934-2873)
Website: http://www.braintumor
.org
E-mail: nbtf@braintumor.org

**National Lymphedema
Network**
116 New Montgomery Street
Suite 235
San Francisco, CA 94105
Toll-Free: 800-541-3259
Phone: 510-208-3200
Fax: 510-208-3110
Website: http://www.lymphnet
.org
E-mail: nln@lymphnet.org

Pancreatic Cancer Action Network
2141 Rosecrans Avenue
Suite 7000
El Segundo, CA 90245
Toll-Free: 877-272-6226
Phone: 310-725-0025
Fax: 310-725-0029
Website: http://www.pancan.org
E-mail: info@pancan.org

Skin Cancer Foundation
149 Maddison Avenue, Suite 901
New York, NY 10016
Toll-Free: 800-SKIN490
(754-6490)
Fax: 212-725-5751
Website: http://www.skincancer
.org
E-mail: info@skincancer.org

Thyroid Cancer Survivors' Association, Inc.
P.O. Box 1545
New York, NY 10159-1545
Toll-Free: 877-588-7904
Website: http://www.thyca.org
E-mail: thyca@thyca.org

Chapter 57

How to Find a Cancer Support Group

Support Groups

Cancer support groups are meetings for people with cancer and those touched by cancer. They can be in person, by phone, or on the Internet. These groups allow you and your loved ones to talk with others facing the same problems. Some support groups have a lecture as well as time to talk. Almost all groups have a leader who runs the meeting. The leader can be someone with cancer or a counselor or social worker.

You may think that a support group is not right for you. Maybe you think that a group won't help or that you don't want to talk with others about your feelings. Or perhaps you're afraid that the meetings will make you sad or depressed.

Support groups may not be for everyone. Some people choose to find support in other ways. But many people find them very helpful. People in the groups often benefit from these experiences:

- Talk about what it's like to have cancer

- Help each other feel better, more hopeful, and not so alone

- Learn about what's new in cancer treatment

- Share tips about ways to cope with cancer

Excerpted from "Taking Time: Support for People with Cancer," National Cancer Institute, 2009. The appended list of additional resources was compiled by the editor; all contact information was verified in June 2010.

Types of Support Groups

- Some groups focus on all kinds of cancer. Others talk about just one kind, such as a group for women with breast cancer or a group for men with prostate cancer.

- Groups can be open to everyone or just for people of a certain age, sex, culture, or religion. For instance, some groups are just for teens or young children.

- Some groups talk about all aspects of cancer. Others focus on only one or two topics such as treatment choices or self-esteem.

- Therapy groups focus on feelings such as sadness and grief. Mental health professionals often lead these types of groups.

- In some groups, people with cancer meet in one support group and their loved ones meet in another. This way, people can say what they really think and feel and not worry about hurting someone's feelings.

- In other groups, patients and families meet together. People often find that meeting in these groups is a good way for each to learn what the other is going through.

- Telephone support groups are where everyone dials in to a phone line and are linked together to talk. They can share and talk to others with similar experiences from all over the country. There is usually little or no charge.

- Online support groups are "meetings" that take place by computer. People meet through chat rooms, listservs, or moderated discussion groups and talk with each other over e-mail. People often like online support groups because they can take part in them any time of the day or night. They're also good for people who can't travel to meetings. The biggest problem with online groups is that you can't be sure if what you learn is correct. Always talk with your doctor about cancer information you learn from the internet.

If you have a choice of support groups, visit a few and see what they are like. See which ones make sense for you. Although many groups are free, some charge a small fee. Find out if your health insurance pays for support groups.

Where to Find a Support Group

Many hospitals, cancer centers, community groups, and schools offer cancer support groups. Here are some ways to find groups near you:

- Call your local hospital and ask about its cancer support programs.
- Ask your social worker to suggest groups.
- Do an online search for groups.
- Look in the health section of your local newspaper for a listing of cancer support groups.

The following resources can also help you get started on your search for support groups.

Support Helplines

American Cancer Society
Phone: 800-ACS-2345

CancerCare
Phone: 800-813-HOPE (4673);
212-302-2400 (outside North America)

Cancer Information and Counseling Line (CICL)
Phone: 800-525-3777

Cancer Research Foundations of America
Phone: 800-227-2732

Komen (Susan G.) Breast Cancer Foundation
Phone: 800-I'M-AWARE (462-9273)

Living Beyond Breast Cancer
Phone: 888-753-LBBC (5222)

National Cancer Institute's Cancer Information Service
Phone: 800-4-CANCER (422-6237)

SHARE: Self Help for Women with Breast or Ovarian Cancer
Phone: 866-891-2392

Online Support

Cancer Survivors Network
American Cancer Society
http://csn.cancer.org

LiveHelp
National Cancer Institute
www.cancer.gov/livehelp

OncoChat
www.oncochat.org

Support Organizations

Avon Breast Cancer Crusade
Avon Foundation
1345 Avenue of the Americas
New York, NY 10105
Phone: 866-505-AVON (2866)
Website: http://www
.avoncompany.com/women
/avoncrusade

Black Women's Health Imperative
1726 M Street NW. Suite 300
Washington, DC 20036
Phone: 202-548-4000
Website: http://www.
blackwomenshealth.org
E-mail:
Info@BlackWomensHealth.org

Breast Cancer Network of Strength™
135 S. LaSalle St. Suite 2000
Chicago, IL 60603
Toll-Free: 800-221-2141 (English);
800-986-9505 (Spanish)
Phone: 312-986-8338
Website: http://www
.networkofstrength.org

Cancer Support Community®
919 18th Street, NW, Suite 54
Washington, DC 20006
Toll-Free: 888-793-WELL
(888-793-9355)
Phone: 202-659-9709
Website: http://www
.thewellnesscommunity.org
E-mail: help
@thewellnesscommunity.org

Celebrating Life Foundation
12100 Ford Road, Suite 100
Dallas, TX 75234
Phone: 800-207-0992 ext 110
Website: http://www
.celebratinglife.org/Foundation
_Profile.htm
E-mail: info@celebratinglife.org

Look Good...Feel Better
c/o CTFA Foundation
American Cancer Society
Toll-Free: 800-395-LOOK (5665);
800-ACS-2345 (227-2345)
Phone: 202-331-1770
Website: http://www
.lookgoodfeelbetter.org

People Living with Cancer
American Society of Clinical
Oncology
2318 Mill Road
Alexandria, VA 22314
Toll-Free: 888-651-3038
Fax: 703-299-1044
Website: http://www.plwc.org

Reach to Recovery
American Cancer Society
Phone: 800-ACS-2345
(800-227-2345)
Website: http://www.cancer.org/
docroot/ESN/content/ESN_3_1x
_Reach_to_Recovery_5.asp

Sisters Network
2922 Rosedale St.
Houston, TX 77004
Phone: 713-781-0255
Website: http://www
.sistersnetworkinc.org

"TLC" Tender Loving Care®
American Cancer Society
P.O. Box 395
Louisiana, MO 63353
Phone: 800-850-9445 (Catalog
number)
Website: http://www.tlcdirect.org
E-mail:
customerservice@tlccatalog.org

Vital Options® International TeleSupport® Cancer Network
4419 Coldwater Canyon Avenue
Suite I
Studio City, CA 91604
Toll-Free: 800-GRP-ROOM
(800-477-7666)
Phone: 818-508-5657
Fax: 818-788-5260
Website: http://www.vitaloptions
.org
E-mail: info@vitaloptions.org

Young Survival Coalition
61 Broadway, Suite 2235
New York, NY 10006
Toll-Free 877-YSC-1011
(972-1011)
Phone: 646-257-3000
Fax: 646-257-3030
Website: www.youngsurvival.org
E-mail: info@youngsurvival.org

Index

Index

National HPV and Cervical Cancer
Prevention Resource Center, contact
information 658
National Institute on Aging,
contact information 653
National Lymphedema Network,
contact information 660
National Marrow Donor Program
(NMDP), contact information
442–43, 653
National Ovarian Cancer
Association, contact
information 658
National Ovarian Cancer
Coalition, contact information 658
National Women's Health Information
Center (NWHIC)
contact information 653
second opinions publication 349n
Native American Cancer Research,
contact information 653
naturopathic medicine,
described 462
nausea, overview 485–90
"Nausea and Vomiting (PDQ):
Patient Version" (NCI) 485n
Navelbine (vinorelbine) 550
NCI *see* National Cancer Institute
needle biopsy, described 636
neoadjuvant therapy, defined 644
neoplasm, described 647
nervous system, described 548
neuropathy, overview 547–55
neutropenia, overview 532–37
NHLBI *see* National Heart, Lung,
and Blood Institute
nipple aspiration, breast
cancer screening 127
NMDP *see* National Marrow
Donor Program
NMRI *see* nuclear magnetic
resonance imaging
noncancerous uterine
conditions, described 16–25
nonmalignant tumors, described 636
non-melanoma skin cancer
described 307
overview 313–17
nonopioids, described 511–12

non-small cell lung cancer
described 278
overview 283–88
"Non-Small Cell Lung Cancer
Treatment (PDQ): Patient
Version" (NCI) 283n
nonspecific immunomodulating
agents, described 451
nonsteroidal anti-inflammatory
drugs (NSAID)
described 511–12
fever 543–44
Novartis Oncology,
contact information 653
nuclear magnetic resonance
imaging (NMRI)
breast cancer 126
described 643
nutrition *see* diet and nutrition
NWHIC *see* National Women's
Health Information Center

O

obesity
breast cancer 88, 101, 119–20
endometrial cancer 170–71
occult primary tumor, defined 644
Office on Women's Health, cancer
publication 3n
olanzapine 489
omentectomy
ovarian germ cell tumors 204
ovarian low malignant potential
tumors 207
OncoChat, website address 664
OncoLink, contact information 653
oncologists, defined 644
oncology, described 337
Oncovin (vincristine) 550
ondansetron 489
1-800-QUIT-NOW, website address 44
oophorectomy
defined 644
ovarian cysts 22
overview 407–10
see also bilateral salpingo-oophorectomy; prophylactic oophorectomy;
salpingo-oophorectomy

Health Reference Series
Complete Catalog
List price $93 per volume. School and library price $84 per volume.

Adolescent Health Sourcebook, 3rd Edition

Basic Consumer Health Information about Adolescent Growth and Development, Puberty, Sexuality, Reproductive Health, and Physical, Emotional, Social, and Mental Health Concerns of Teens and Their Parents, Including Facts about Nutrition, Physical Activity, Weight Management, Acne, Allergies, Cancer, Diabetes, Growth Disorders, Juvenile Arthritis, Infections, Substance Abuse, and More

Along with Information about Adolescent Safety Concerns, Youth Violence, a Glossary of Related Terms, and a Directory of Resources

Edited by Amy L. Sutton. 600 pages. 2010. 978-0-7808-1140-9.

Adult Health Concerns Sourcebook

Basic Consumer Health Information about Medical and Mental Concerns of Adults, Including Facts about Choosing Healthcare Providers, Navigating Insurance Options, Maintaining Wellness, Preventing Cancer, Heart Disease, Stroke, Diabetes, and Osteoporosis, and Understanding Aging-Related Health Concerns, Including Menopause, Cognitive Changes, and Changes in the Coronary and Vascular Systems

Along with Tips on Caring for Aging Parents and Dealing with Health-Related Work and Travel Issues, a Glossary, and a Directory of Resources for Additional Help and Information

Edited by Sandra J. Judd. 648 pages. 2008. 978-0-7808-0999-4.

"Provides a thorough list of topics that are important to adult health and for caregivers."
—*CHOICE, Nov '08*

"Written in easy-to-understand language... the content is well-organized and is intended to aid adults in making health care-related decisions."
—*AORN Journal, Dec '08*

AIDS Sourcebook, 4th Edition

Basic Consumer Health Information about Human Immunodeficiency Virus (HIV) and Acquired Immunodeficiency Syndrome (AIDS), Featuring Updated Statistics and Facts about Risks, Prevention, Screening, Diagnosis, Treatments, Side Effects, and Complications, and Including a Section about the Impact of HIV/AIDS on the Health of Women, Children, and Adolescents

Along with Tips on Managing Life with AIDS, Reports on Current Research Initiatives and Clinical Trials, a Glossary of Related Terms, and Resource Directories for Further Help and Information

Edited by Ivy L. Alexander. 680 pages. 2008. 978-0-7808-0997-0.

SEE ALSO *Contagious Diseases Sourcebook, 2nd Edition*

Alcoholism Sourcebook, 3rd Edition

Basic Consumer Health Information about Alcohol Use, Abuse, and Dependence, Featuring Facts about the Physical, Mental, and Social Health Effects of Alcohol Addiction, Including Alcoholic Liver Disease, Pancreatic Disease, Cardiovascular Disease, Neurological Disorders, and the Effects of Drinking during Pregnancy

Along with Information about Alcohol Treatment, Medications, and Recovery Programs, in Addition to Tips for Reducing the Prevalence of Underage Drinking, Statistics about Alcohol Use, a Glossary of Related Terms, and Directories of Resources for More Help and Information

Edited by Joyce Brennfleck Shannon. 600 pages. 2010. 978-0-7808-1141-6.

SEE ALSO *Drug Abuse Sourcebook, 3rd Edition*

Allergies Sourcebook, 3rd Edition

Basic Consumer Health Information about Allergic Disorders, Such as Anaphylaxis, Hives,

Eczema, Rhinitis, Sinusitis, and Conjunctivitis, and Their Triggers, Including Pollen, Mold, Dust Mites, Animal Dander, Insects, Chemicals, Food, Food Additives, and Medications

Along with Advice about the Diagnosis and Treatment of Allergy Symptoms, a Glossary of Related Terms, a Directory of Resources for Help and Information, and Suggestions for Additional Reading

Edited by Amy L. Sutton. 588 pages. 2007. 978-0-7808-0950-5.

SEE ALSO Asthma Sourcebook, 2nd Edition

Alzheimer Disease Sourcebook, 4th Edition

Basic Consumer Health Information about Alzheimer Disease, Other Dementias, and Related Disorders, Including Multi-Infarct Dementia, Dementia with Lewy Bodies, Frontotemporal Dementia (Pick Disease), Wernicke-Korsakoff Syndrome (Alcohol-Related Dementia), AIDS Dementia Complex, Huntington Disease, Creutzfeldt-Jacob Disease, and Delirium

Along with Information about Coping with Memory Loss and Forgetfulness, Maintaining Skills, and Long-Term Planning for People with Dementia, and Suggestions Addressing Common Caregiver Concerns, Updated Information about Current Research Efforts, a Glossary of Related Terms, and Directories of Sources for Additional Help and Information

Edited by Karen Bellenir. 603 pages. 2008. 978-0-7808-1001-3.

"An invaluable resource for persons who have received a diagnosis, for caregivers, and for family members dealing with this insidious disease. It is recommended for public, community college, and ready-reference sections in academic libraries."
— *American Reference Books Annual, 2009*

SEE ALSO Brain Disorders Sourcebook, 3rd Edition

Arthritis Sourcebook, 3rd Edition

Basic Consumer Health Information about the Risk Factors, Symptoms, Diagnosis, and Treatment of Osteoarthritis, Rheumatoid Arthritis, Juvenile Arthritis, Gout, Infectious Arthritis, and Autoimmune Disorders Associated with Arthritis

Along with Facts about Medications, Surgeries, and Self-Care Techniques to Manage Pain and Disability, Tips on Living with Arthritis, a Glossary of Related Terms, and Resources for Additional Help and Information

Edited by Amy L. Sutton. 600 pages. 2010. 978-0-7808-1077-8.

Asthma Sourcebook, 2nd Edition

Basic Consumer Health Information about the Causes, Symptoms, Diagnosis, and Treatment of Asthma in Infants, Children, Teenagers, and Adults, Including Facts about Different Types of Asthma, Common Co-Occurring Conditions, Asthma Management Plans, Triggers, Medications, and Medication Delivery Devices

Along with Asthma Statistics, Research Updates, a Glossary, a Directory of Asthma-Related Resources, and More

Edited by Karen Bellenir. 581 pages. 2006. 978-0-7808-0866-9.

SEE ALSO Lung Disorders Sourcebook; Respiratory Disorders Sourcebook, 2nd Edition

Attention Deficit Disorder Sourcebook

Basic Consumer Health Information about Attention Deficit/Hyperactivity Disorder in Children and Adults, Including Facts about Causes, Symptoms, Diagnostic Criteria, and Treatment Options Such as Medications, Behavior Therapy, Coaching, and Homeopathy

Along with Reports on Current Research Initiatives, Legal Issues, and Government Regulations, and Featuring a Glossary of Related Terms, Internet Resources, and a List of Additional Reading Material

Edited by Dawn D. Matthews. 447 pages. 2002. 978-0-7808-0624-5.

"Recommended reference source."
— *Booklist, Jan '03*

SEE ALSO Learning Disabilities Sourcebook, 3rd Edition

Autism and Pervasive Developmental Disorders Sourcebook

Basic Consumer Health Information about Autism Spectrum and Pervasive Developmental Disorders, Such as Classical Autism, Asperger Syndrome, Rett Syndrome, and Childhood Disintegrative Disorder, Including Information about Related Genetic Disorders and Medical Problems and Facts about Causes, Screening Methods, Diagnostic Criteria, Treatments and Interventions, and Family and Education Issues

Along with a Glossary of Related Terms, Tips for Evaluating the Validity of Health Claims, and a Directory of Resources for Additional Help and Information

Edited by Sandra J. Judd. 603 pages. 2007. 978-0-7808-0953-6.

"This book provides a current overview of disorders on the autism spectrum and information about various therapies, educational resources, and help for families with practical issues such as workplace adjustments, living arrangements, and estate planning. It is a useful resource for public and consumer health libraries."
—*American Reference Books Annual, 2009*

SEE ALSO *Learning Disabilities Sourcebook, 3rd Edition*

Back and Neck Disorders Sourcebook, 2nd Edition

Basic Consumer Health Information about Spinal Pain, Spinal Cord Injuries, and Related Disorders, Such as Degenerative Disk Disease, Osteoarthritis, Scoliosis, Sciatica, Spina Bifida, and Spinal Stenosis, and Featuring Facts about Maintaining Spinal Health, Self-Care, Pain Management, Rehabilitative Care, Chiropractic Care, Spinal Surgeries, and Complementary Therapies

Along with Suggestions for Preventing Back and Neck Pain, a Glossary of Related Terms, and a Directory of Resources

Edited by Amy L. Sutton. 607 pages. 2004. 978-0-7808-0738-9.

"Recommended... An easy to use, comprehensive medical reference book."
—*E-Streams, Sep '05*

"For anyone who has back or neck problems, this book is ideal. Its easy-to-understand language and variety of topics makes this sourcebook a worthwhile read. The price... is reasonable for the amount of information contained in the book"
—*Occupational Therapy in Health Care, 2007*

Blood & Circulatory Disorders Sourcebook, 3rd Edition

Basic Consumer Health Information about Blood and Circulatory System Disorders, Such as Anemia, Leukemia, Lymphoma, Rh Disease, Hemophilia, Thrombophilia, Other Bleeding and Clotting Deficiencies, and Artery, Vascular, and Venous Diseases, Including Facts about Blood Types, Blood Donation, Bone Marrow and Stem Cell Transplants, Tests and Medications, and Tips for Maintaining Circulatory Health

Along with a Glossary of Related Terms and a List of Resources for Additional Help and Information

Edited by Sandra J. Judd. 600 pages. 2010. 978-0-7808-1081-5.

SEE ALSO *Leukemia Sourcebook*

Brain Disorders Sourcebook, 3rd Edition

Basic Consumer Health Information about Acquired and Traumatic Brain Injuries, Brain Tumors, Cerebral Palsy and Other Genetic and Congenital Brain Disorders, Infections of the Brain, Epilepsy, and Degenerative Neurological Disorders Such as Dementia, Huntington Disease, and Amyotrophic Lateral Sclerosis (ALS)

Along with Information on Brain Structure and Function, Treatment and Rehabilitation Options, a Glossary of Terms Related to Brain Disorders, and a Directory of Resources for More Information

Edited by Joyce Brennfleck Shannon. 600 pages. 2010. 978-0-7808-1083-9.

SEE ALSO *Alzheimer Disease Sourcebook, 4th Edition*

Breast Cancer Sourcebook, 3rd Edition

Basic Consumer Health Information about Breast Health and Breast Cancer, Including Facts about Environmental, Genetic, and Other Risk Factors, Prevention Efforts, Screening and Diagnostic Methods, Surgical Treatment Options and Other Care Choices, Complementary and Alternative Therapies, and Post-Treatment Concerns

Along with Statistical Data, News about Research Advances, a Glossary of Related Terms, and Directories of Resources for Additional Information and Support

Edited by Karen Bellenir. 606 pages. 2009. 978-0-7808-1030-3.

"A very useful reference for people wanting to learn more about breast cancer and how to negotiate their care or the care of a loved one. The third edition is necessary as information/treatment options continue to evolve."
—Doody's Review Service, 2009

SEE ALSO Cancer Sourcebook for Women, 3rd Edition, Women's Health Concerns Sourcebook, 3rd Edition

Breastfeeding Sourcebook

Basic Consumer Health Information about the Benefits of Breastmilk, Preparing to Breastfeed, Breastfeeding as a Baby Grows, Nutrition, and More, Including Information on Special Situations and Concerns Such as Mastitis, Illness, Medications, Allergies, Multiple Births, Prematurity, Special Needs, and Adoption

Along with a Glossary and Resources for Additional Help and Information

Edited by Jenni Lynn Colson. 367 pages. 2002. 978-0-7808-0332-9.

SEE ALSO Pregnancy and Birth Sourcebook, 3rd Edition

Burns Sourcebook

Basic Consumer Health Information about Various Types of Burns and Scalds, Including Flame, Heat, Cold, Electrical, Chemical, and Sun Burns

Along with Information on Short-Term and Long-Term Treatments, Tissue Reconstruction, Plastic Surgery, Prevention Suggestions, and First Aid

Edited by Allan R. Cook. 604 pages. 1999. 978-0-7808-0204-9.

"This is an exceptional addition to the series and is highly recommended for all consumer health collections, hospital libraries, and academic medical centers."
—E-Streams, Mar '00

"This key reference guide is an invaluable addition to all health care and public libraries in confronting this ongoing health issue."
—American Reference Books Annual, 2000

SEE ALSO Dermatological Disorders Sourcebook, 2nd Edition

Cancer Sourcebook, 5th Edition

Basic Consumer Health Information about Major Forms and Stages of Cancer, Featuring Facts about Head and Neck Cancers, Lung Cancers, Gastrointestinal Cancers, Genitourinary Cancers, Lymphomas, Blood Cell Cancers, Endocrine Cancers, Skin Cancers, Bone Cancers, Metastatic Cancers, and More

Along with Facts about Cancer Treatments, Cancer Risks and Prevention, a Glossary of Related Terms, Statistical Data, and a Directory of Resources for Additional Information

Edited by Karen Bellenir. 1105 pages. 2007. 978-0-7808-0947-5.

"The 5th, updated edition of Cancer Sourcebook should be in every public and health lending library collection... An unparalleled discussion essential for any health collections considering an all-in-one basic general reference."
—California Bookwatch, Aug '07

SEE ALSO Breast Cancer Sourcebook, 3rd Edition, Cancer Survivorship Sourcebook, Leukemia Sourcebook

Cancer Sourcebook for Women, 4th Edition

Basic Consumer Health Information about Gynecologic Cancers and Other Cancers of Special Concern to Women, Including Cancers of the Breast, Cervix, Colon, Lung, Ovaries, Thyroid, and Uterus

Along with Facts about Benign Conditions of the Female Reproductive System, Cancer Risk

Factors, Diagnostic and Treatment Procedures, Side Effects of Cancer and Cancer Treatments, Women's Issues in Cancer Survivorship, a Glossary of Related Terms, and a Directory of Resources for Additional Help and Information

Edited by Karen Bellenir. 600 pages. 2010. 978-0-7808-1139-3.

SEE ALSO Breast Cancer Sourcebook, 3rd Edition, Women's Health Concerns Sourcebook, 3rd Edition

Cancer Survivorship Sourcebook

Basic Consumer Health Information about the Physical, Educational, Emotional, Social, and Financial Needs of Cancer Patients from Diagnosis, through Cancer Treatment, and Beyond, Including Facts about Researching Specific Types of Cancer and Learning about Clinical Trials and Treatment Options, and Featuring Tips for Coping with the Side Effects of Cancer Treatments and Adjusting to Life after Cancer Treatment Concludes

Along with Suggestions for Caregivers, Friends, and Family Members of Cancer Patients, a Glossary of Cancer Care Terms, and Directories of Related Resources

Edited by Karen Bellenir. 633 pages. 2007. 978-0-7808-0985-7.

"Well organized and comprehensive in coverage, the book speaks to issues encountered both during and after cancer treatment. Recommended for consumer health and public libraries."
—Library Journal, Aug 1 '07

"Cancer Survivorship Sourcebook will be useful to anyone who has a friend or loved one with a cancer diagnosis."
—American Reference Books Annual, 2008

SEE ALSO Cancer Sourcebook, 5th Edition, Disease Management Sourcebook

Cardiovascular Disorders Sourcebook, 4th Edition

Basic Consumer Health Information about Heart and Blood Vessel Diseases and Disorders, Such as Angina, Heart Attack, Heart Failure, Cardiomyopathy, Arrhythmias, Valve Disease, Atherosclerosis, Aneurysms, and Congenital Heart Defects, Including Information about Cardiovascular Disease in Women, Men, Children, Adolescents, and Minorities

Along with Facts about Diagnosing, Managing, and Preventing Cardiovascular Disease, a Glossary of Related Medical Terms, and a Directory of Resources for Additional Information

Edited by Amy L. Sutton. 600 pages. 2010. 978-0-7808-1080-8.

Caregiving Sourcebook

Basic Consumer Health Information for Caregivers, Including a Profile of Caregivers, Caregiving Responsibilities and Concerns, Tips for Specific Conditions, Care Environments, and the Effects of Caregiving

Along with Facts about Legal Issues, Financial Information, and Future Planning, a Glossary, and a Listing of Additional Resources

Edited by Joyce Brennfleck Shannon. 583 pages. 2001. 978-0-7808-0331-2.

"Essential for most collections."
—Library Journal, Apr 1 '02

"An ideal addition to the reference collection of any public library. Health sciences information professionals may also want to acquire the Caregiving Sourcebook for their hospital or academic library for use as a ready reference tool by health care workers interested in aging and caregiving."
—E-Streams, Jan '02

Child Abuse Sourcebook, 2nd Edition

Basic Consumer Health Information about the Physical, Sexual, and Emotional Abuse of Children, Neglect, Münchhausen Syndrome by Proxy (MSBP), and Shaken Baby Syndrome, and Featuring Facts about Withholding Medical Care, Corporal Punishment, Child Maltreatment in Youth Sports, and Parental Substance Abuse

Along with Information about Child Protective Services, Foster Care, Adoption, Parenting Challenges, Abuse Prevention Programs, and Intervention, Treatment, and Recovery Guidelines, a Glossary of Related Terms, and Resources for Additional Help and Information

Edited by Joyce Brennfleck Shannon. 600 pages. 2009. 978-0-7808-1037-2.

SEE ALSO *Domestic Violence Sourcebook, 3rd Edition*

Childhood Diseases and Disorders Sourcebook, 2nd Edition

Basic Consumer Health Information about the Physical, Mental, and Developmental Health of Pre-Adolescent Children, Including Facts about Infectious Diseases, Asthma, Allergies, Diabetes, and Other Acute and Chronic Conditions Affecting the Gastrointestinal Tract, Ears, Nose, Throat, Liver, Kidneys, Heart, Blood, Brain, Muscles, Bones, and Skin

Along with Reports on Recommended Childhood Vaccinations, Wellness Guidelines, a Glossary of Related Medical Terms, and a List of Resources for Parents

Edited by Sandra J. Judd. 694 pages. 2009. 978-0-7808-1031-0.

"The strength of this source is the wide range of information given about childhood health issues... It is most appropriate for public libraries and academic libraries that field medical questions."
—*American Reference Books Annual, 2009*

SEE ALSO *Healthy Children Sourcebook*

Colds, Flu and Other Common Ailments Sourcebook

Basic Consumer Health Information about Common Ailments and Injuries, Including Colds, Coughs, the Flu, Sinus Problems, Headaches, Fever, Nausea and Vomiting, Menstrual Cramps, Diarrhea, Constipation, Hemorrhoids, Back Pain, Dandruff, Dry and Itchy Skin, Cuts, Scrapes, Sprains, Bruises, and More

Along with Information about Prevention, Self-Care, Choosing a Doctor, Over-the-Counter Medications, Folk Remedies, and Alternative Therapies, and Including a Glossary of Important Terms and a Directory of Resources for Further Help and Information

Edited by Chad T. Kimball. 622 pages. 2001. 978-0-7808-0435-7.

"A good starting point for research on common illnesses. It will be a useful addition to public and consumer health library collections."
—*American Reference Books Annual, 2002*

"Will prove valuable to any library seeking to maintain a current, comprehensive reference collection of health resources... Excellent reference."
—*The Bookwatch, Aug '01*

SEE ALSO *Contagious Diseases Sourcebook, 2nd Edition*

Communication Disorders Sourcebook

Basic Information about Deafness and Hearing Loss, Speech and Language Disorders, Voice Disorders, Balance and Vestibular Disorders, and Disorders of Smell, Taste, and Touch

Edited by Linda M. Ross. 533 pages. 1996. 978-0-7808-0077-9.

"This is skillfully edited and is a welcome resource for the layperson. It should be found in every public and medical library."
—*Booklist Health Sciences Supplement, Oct '97*

Complementary & Alternative Medicine Sourcebook, 4th Edition

Basic Consumer Health Information about Ayurveda, Acupuncture, Aromatherapy, Chiropractic Care, Diet-Based Therapies, Guided Imagery, Herbal and Vitamin Supplements, Homeopathy, Hypnosis, Massage, Meditation, Naturopathy, Pilates, Reflexology, Reiki, Shiatsu, Tai Chi, Traditional Chinese Medicine, Yoga, and Other Complementary and Alternative Medical Therapies

Along with Statistics, Tips for Selecting a Practitioner, Treatments for Specific Health Conditions, a Glossary of Related Terms, and a Directory of Resources for Additional Help and Information

Edited by Amy L. Sutton. 600 pages. 2010. 978-0-7808-1082-2.

Congenital Disorders Sourcebook, 2nd Edition

Basic Consumer Health Information about Nonhereditary Birth Defects and Disorders

Related to Prematurity, Gestational Injuries, Congenital Infections, and Birth Complications, Including Heart Defects, Hydrocephalus, Spina Bifida, Cleft Lip and Palate, Cerebral Palsy, and More

Along with Facts about the Prevention of Birth Defects, Fetal Surgery and Other Treatment Options, Research Initiatives, a Glossary of Related Terms, and Resources for Additional Information and Support

Edited by Sandra J. Judd. 619 pages. 2007. 978-0-7808-0945-1.

"Congenital Disorders Sourcebook provides an excellent, non-technical overview of many aspects of pregnancy with the focus on congenital disorders."
—*American Reference Books Annual, 2008*

"An excellent readable reference aimed at the lay public for difficult to understand medical problems. An excellent starting point for the interested parent or family member who may then be motivated to seek more information."
—*Doody's Review Service, 2007*

SEE ALSO *Pregnancy and Birth Sourcebook, 3rd Edition*

Contagious Diseases Sourcebook, 2nd Edition

Basic Consumer Health Information about Diseases Spread from Person to Person through Direct Physical Contact, Airborne Transmissions, Sexual Contact, or Contact with Blood or Other Body Fluids, Including Pneumococcal, Staphylococcal, and Streptococcal Diseases, Colds, Influenza, Lice, Measles, Mumps, Tuberculosis, and Others

Along with Facts about Self-Care and Over-the-Counter Medications, Antibiotics and Drug Resistance, Disease Prevention, Vaccines, and Bioterrorism, a Glossary, and a Directory of Resources for More Information

Edited by Joyce Brennfleck Shannon. 600 pages. 2010. 978-0-7808-1075-4.

SEE ALSO *AIDS Sourcebook, 4th Edition, Hepatitis Sourcebook*

Cosmetic and Reconstructive Surgery Sourcebook, 2nd Edition

Basic Consumer Information about Plastic Surgery and Non-Surgical Appearance-Enhancing Procedures, Including Facts about Botulinum Toxin, Collagen Replacement, Dermabrasion, Chemical Peels, Eyelid Surgery, Nose Reshaping, Lip Augmentation, Liposuction, Breast Enlargement and Reduction, Tummy Tucking, and Other Skin, Hair, Facial, and Body Shaping Procedures

Along with Information about Reconstructive Procedures for Congenital Disorders, Disfiguring Diseases, Burns, and Traumatic Injuries, a Glossary of Related Terms, and a Directory of Additional Resources

Edited by Karen Bellenir. 483 pages. 2007. 978-0-7808-0951-2.

"A comprehensive source for people considering cosmetic surgery... also recommended for medical students who will perform these procedures later in their careers; and public librarians and academic medical librarians who may assist patrons interested in this information."
—*Medical Reference Services Quarterly, Fall '08*

"A practical guide for health care consumers and health care workers... This easy-to-read reference guide would be useful for novice and veteran health care consumers, surgical technology students, nursing students, and perioperative nurses new to plastic and reconstructive surgery. It also may be helpful for medical-surgical nurses as a guide for patient teaching in their practices."
—*AORN Journal, Aug '08*

SEE ALSO *Surgery Sourcebook, 2nd Edition*

Death and Dying Sourcebook, 2nd Edition

Basic Consumer Health Information about End-of-Life Care and Related Perspectives and Ethical Issues, Including End-of-Life Symptoms and Treatments, Pain Management, Quality-of-Life Concerns, the Use of Life Support, Patients' Rights and Privacy Issues, Advance Directives, Physician-Assisted Suicide, Caregiving, Organ and Tissue Donation, Autopsies, Funeral Arrangements, and Grief

Along with Statistical Data, Information about the Leading Causes of Death, a Glossary, and Directories of Support Groups and Other Resources

Edited by Joyce Brennfleck Shannon. 626 pages. 2006. 978-0-7808-0871-3.

Dental Care and Oral Health Sourcebook, 3rd Edition

Basic Consumer Health Information about Dental Care and Oral Health Throughout the Lifespan, Including Facts about Cavities, Bad Breath, Cold and Canker Sores, Dry Mouth, Toothaches, Gum Disease, Malocclusion, Temporomandibular Joint and Muscle Disorders, Oral Cancers, and Dental Emergencies

Along with Information about Mouth Hygiene, Crowns, Bridges, Implants, and Fillings, Surgical, Orthodontic, and Cosmetic Dental Procedures, Pain Management, Health Conditions that Impact Oral Care, a Glossary of Related Terms, and a Directory of Additional Resources

Edited by Amy L. Sutton. 619 pages. 2008. 978-0-7808-1032-7.

"Could serve as turning point in the battle to educate consumers in issues concerning oral health. Tightly written in terms the average person can understand, yet comprehensive in scope and authoritative in tone, it is another excellent sourcebook in the Health Reference Series... Should be in the reference department of all public libraries, and in academic libraries that have a public constituency."
—American Reference Books Annual, 2009

Depression Sourcebook, 2nd Edition

Basic Consumer Health Information about Unipolar Depression, Bipolar Disorder, Dysthymia, Seasonal Affective Disorder, Postpartum Depression, and Other Depressive Disorders, Including Facts about Populations at Special Risk, Coexisting Medical Conditions, Symptoms, Treatment Options, and Suicide Prevention

Along with Statistical Data, a Glossary of Related Terms, and a Directory of Resources for Additional Help and Information

Edited by Sandra J. Judd. 646 pages. 2008. 978-0-7808-1003-7.

"Recommended for public libraries."
—American Reference Books Annual, 2009

SEE ALSO Mental Health Disorders Sourcebook, 4th Edition

Dermatological Disorders Sourcebook, 2nd Edition

Basic Consumer Health Information about Conditions and Disorders Affecting the Skin, Hair, and Nails, Such as Acne, Rosacea, Rashes, Dermatitis, Pigmentation Disorders, Birthmarks, Skin Cancer, Skin Injuries, Psoriasis, Scleroderma, and Hair Loss, Including Facts about Medications and Treatments for Dermatological Disorders and Tips for Maintaining Healthy Skin, Hair, and Nails

Along with Information about How Aging Affects the Skin, a Glossary of Related Terms, and a Directory of Resources for Additional Help and Information

Edited by Amy L. Sutton. 617 pages. 2006. 978-0-7808-0795-2.

"Well organized... presents a plethora of information in a manner that is appropriate in style and readability for the intended audience."
—Physical Therapy, Nov '06

"Helpfully brings together... sources in one convenient place, saving the user hours of research time."
—American Reference Books Annual, 2006

SEE ALSO Burns Sourcebook

Diabetes Sourcebook, 4th Edition

Basic Consumer Health Information about Type 1 and Type 2 Diabetes Mellitus, Gestational Diabetes, Monogenic Forms of Diabetes, and Insulin Resistance, with Guidelines for Lifestyle Modifications and the Medical Management of Diabetes, Including Facts about Insulin, Insulin Delivery Devices, Oral Diabetes Medications, Self-Monitoring of Blood Glucose, Meal Planning, Physical Activity Recommendations, Foot Care, and Treatment Options for People with Kidney Failure

Along with a Section about Diabetes Complications and Co-Occurring Conditions, a Glossary

of Related Terms, and Directories of Resources for Additional Help and Information

Edited by Karen Bellenir. 627 pages. 2008. 978-0-7808-1005-1.

"Completely and comprehensively covering almost everything a student or physician would need to know... well worth the investment."
—*Internet Bookwatch, Dec '08*

SEE ALSO *Endocrine and Metabolic Disorders Sourcebook, 2nd Edition*

■

Diet and Nutrition Sourcebook, 3rd Edition

Basic Consumer Health Information about Dietary Guidelines and the Food Guidance System, Recommended Daily Nutrient Intakes, Serving Proportions, Weight Control, Vitamins and Supplements, Nutrition Issues for Different Life Stages and Lifestyles, and the Needs of People with Specific Medical Concerns, Including Cancer, Celiac Disease, Diabetes, Eating Disorders, Food Allergies, and Cardiovascular Disease

Along with Facts about Federal Nutrition Support Programs, a Glossary of Nutrition and Dietary Terms, and Directories of Additional Resources for More Information about Nutrition

Edited by Joyce Brennfleck Shannon. 605 pages. 2006. 978-0-7808-0800-3.

"A valuable resource tool for any individual."
—*Journal of Dental Hygiene, Apr '07*

"From different recommended eating habits to reduce disease and common ailments to nutrition advice for those with specific conditions, Diet and Nutrition Sourcebook is especially important because so much is changing in this area, and so rapidly."
—*California Bookwatch, Jun '06*

SEE ALSO *Eating Disorders Sourcebook, 2nd Edition, Vegetarian Sourcebook*

■

Digestive Diseases and Disorders Sourcebook

Basic Consumer Health Information about Diseases and Disorders that Impact the Upper and Lower Digestive System, Including Celiac

Disease, Constipation, Crohn's Disease, Cyclic Vomiting Syndrome, Diarrhea, Diverticulosis and Diverticulitis, Gallstones, Heartburn, Hemorrhoids, Hernias, Indigestion (Dyspepsia), Irritable Bowel Syndrome, Lactose Intolerance, Ulcers, and More

Along with Information about Medications and Other Treatments, Tips for Maintaining a Healthy Digestive Tract, a Glossary, and Directory of Digestive Diseases Organizations

Edited by Karen Bellenir. 323 pages. 2000. 978-0-7808-0327-5.

"An excellent addition to all public or patient-research libraries."
—*American Reference Books Annual, 2001*

"Recommended reference source."
—*Booklist, May '00*

SEE ALSO *Gastrointestinal Diseases and Disorders Sourcebook, 2nd Edition*

■

Disabilities Sourcebook

Basic Consumer Health Information about Physical and Psychiatric Disabilities, Including Descriptions of Major Causes of Disability, Assistive and Adaptive Aids, Workplace Issues, and Accessibility Concerns

Along with Information about the Americans with Disabilities Act, a Glossary, and Resources for Additional Help and Information

Edited by Dawn D. Matthews. 602 pages. 2000. 978-0-7808-0389-3.

"A must for libraries with a consumer health section."
—*American Reference Books Annual, 2002*

"A much needed addition to the Omnigraphics Health Reference Series. A current reference work to provide people with disabilities, their families, caregivers or those who work with them, a broad range of information in one volume, has not been available until now... It is recommended for all public and academic library reference collections."
—*E-Streams, May '01*

"An excellent source book in easy-to-read format covering many current topics; highly recommended for all libraries."
—*CHOICE, Jan '01*

■

Disease Management Sourcebook

Basic Consumer Health Information about Coping with Chronic and Serious Illnesses, Navigating the Health Care System, Communicating with Health Care Providers, Assessing Health Care Quality, and Making Informed Health Care Decisions, Including Facts about Second Opinions, Hospitalization, Surgery, and Medications

Along with a Section about Children with Chronic Conditions, Information about Legal, Financial, and Insurance Issues, a Glossary of Related Terms, and Directories of Additional Resources

Edited by Joyce Brennfleck Shannon. 621 pages. 2008. 978-0-7808-1002-0.

"Consumers need to know how to manage their health care the same way they manage anything else in their lives. The text is very readable and is written for the layperson and consumer. The cost is not prohibitive. This book should be in all collections of health care libraries and public libraries."
— *American Reference Books Annual, 2009*

"The information is very current, and the selection of font and layout make the book easy to read. A hardback that will stand up to much usage, this is an excellent resource for consumers... Recommended. General readers."
—*CHOICE, Nov '08*

"Intended for lay readers, this resource clarifies the many confusing and overwhelming details associated with chronic disease care. Meticulous and clearly explained, the book even includes diagrams intended to ease comprehension of over-the-counter medication labels. An essential guide to navigating the health-care rapids."
—*Library Journal, Aug '08*

Domestic Violence Sourcebook, 3rd Edition

Basic Consumer Health Information about Warning Signs, Risk Factors, and Health Consequences of Intimate Partner Violence, Sexual Violence and Rape, Stalking, Human Trafficking, Child Maltreatment, Teen Dating Violence, and Elder Abuse

Along with Facts about Victims and Perpetrators, Strategies for Violence Prevention, and Emergency Interventions, Safety Plans, and Financial and Legal Tips for Victims, a Glossary of Related Terms, and Directories of Resources for Additional Information and Support

Edited by Joyce Brennfleck Shannon. 634 pages. 2009. 978-0-7808-1038-9.

"A recommended pick for any library interested in consumer health and social issues... A 'must' for any serious health collection."
—*California Bookwatch, Jul '09*

SEE ALSO *Child Abuse Sourcebook, 2nd Edition*

Drug Abuse Sourcebook, 3rd Edition

Basic Consumer Health Information about the Abuse of Cocaine, Club Drugs, Hallucinogens, Heroin, Inhalants, Marijuana, and Other Illicit Substances, Prescription Medications, and Over-the-Counter Medicines

Along with Facts about Addiction and Related Health Effects, Drug Abuse Treatment and Recovery, Drug Testing, Prevention Programs, Glossaries of Drug-Related Terms, and Directories of Resources for More Information

Edited by Joyce Brennfleck Shannon. 600 pages. 2010. 978-0-7808-1079-2.

SEE ALSO *Alcoholism Sourcebook, 3rd Edition*

Ear, Nose, and Throat Disorders Sourcebook, 2nd Edition

Basic Consumer Health Information about Disorders of the Ears, Hearing Loss, Vestibular Disorders, Nasal and Sinus Problems, Throat and Vocal Cord Disorders, and Otolaryngologic Cancers, Including Facts about Ear Infections and Injuries, Genetic and Congenital Deafness, Sensorineural Hearing Disorders, Tinnitus, Vertigo, Ménière Disease, Rhinitis, Sinusitis, Snoring, Sore Throats, Hoarseness, and More

Along with Reports on Current Research Initiatives, a Glossary of Related Medical Terms, and a Directory of Sources for Further Help and Information

Edited by Sandra J. Judd. 631 pages. 2007. 978-0-7808-0872-0.

"A resource book for the general public that provides comprehensive coverage of basic up-to-date medical information about the causes, symptoms, diagnosis, and treatment of diseases and disorders that affect the ears, nose, sinuses, throat, and voice... The majority of information is presented in question and answer format, much like questions a patient might ask of a health care provider. An extensive index facilitates the reader's ability to easily access information on any specific topic."
—*Journal of Dental Hygiene*, Oct '07

"A handy compilation of information on common and some not so common ailments of the ears, nose, and throat."
—*Doody's Review Service*, 2007

Eating Disorders Sourcebook, 2nd Edition

Basic Consumer Health Information about Anorexia Nervosa, Bulimia, Binge Eating, Compulsive Exercise, Female Athlete Triad, and Other Eating Disorders, Including Facts about Body Image and Other Cultural and Age-Related Risk Factors, Prevention Efforts, Adverse Health Effects, Treatment Options, and the Recovery Process

Along with Guidelines for Healthy Weight Control, a Glossary, and Directories of Additional Resources

Edited by Joyce Brennfleck Shannon. 557 pages. 2007. 978-0-7808-0948-2.

"Recommended for the reference collection of large public libraries."
—*American Reference Books Annual*, 2008

"A basic health reference any health or general library needs."
—*Internet Bookwatch*, Jun '07

SEE ALSO Diet and Nutrition Sourcebook, 3rd Edition, Mental Health Disorders Sourcebook, 4th Edition

Emergency Medical Services Sourcebook

Basic Consumer Health Information about Preventing, Preparing for, and Managing Emergency Situations, When and Who to Call for Help, What to Expect in the Emergency Room, the Emergency Medical Team, *Patient Issues, and Current Topics in Emergency Medicine*

Along with Statistical Data, a Glossary, and Sources of Additional Help and Information

Edited by Jenni Lynn Colson. 472 pages. 2002. 978-0-7808-0420-3.

"Handy and convenient for home, public, school, and college libraries. Recommended."
—*CHOICE*, Apr '03

"This reference can provide the consumer with answers to most questions about emergency care in the United States, or it will direct them to a resource where the answer can be found."
—*American Reference Books Annual*, 2003

SEE ALSO Injury and Trauma Sourcebook

Endocrine and Metabolic Disorders Sourcebook, 2nd Edition

Basic Consumer Health Information about Hormonal and Metabolic Disorders that Affect the Body's Growth, Development, and Functioning, Including Disorders of the Pancreas, Ovaries and Testes, and Pituitary, Thyroid, Parathyroid, and Adrenal Glands, with Facts about Growth Disorders, Addison Disease, Cushing Syndrome, Conn Syndrome, Diabetic Disorders, Multiple Endocrine Neoplasia, Inborn Errors of Metabolism, and More

Along with Information about Endocrine Functioning, Diagnostic and Screening Tests, a Glossary of Related Terms, and Directories of Additional Resources

Edited by Joyce Brennfleck Shannon. 597 pages. 2007. 978-0-7808-0952-9.

SEE ALSO Diabetes Sourcebook, 4th Edition

Environmental Health Sourcebook, 3rd Edition

Basic Consumer Health Information about the Environment and Its Effects on Human Health, Including Facts about Air, Water, and Soil Contamination, Hazardous Chemicals, Foodborne Hazards and Illnesses, Household Hazards Such as Radon, Mold, and Carbon Monoxide, Consumer Hazards from Toxic Products and Imported Goods, and Disorders

Linked to Environmental Causes, Including Chemical Sensitivity, Cancer, Allergies, and Asthma

Along with Information about the Impact of Environmental Hazards on Specific Populations, a Glossary of Related Terms, and Resources for Additional Help and Information.

Edited by Laura Larsen. 600 pages. 2010. 978-0-7808-1078-5

Ethnic Diseases Sourcebook

Basic Consumer Health Information for Ethnic and Racial Minority Groups in the United States, Including General Health Indicators and Behaviors, Ethnic Diseases, Genetic Testing, the Impact of Chronic Diseases, Women's Health, Mental Health Issues, and Preventive Health Care Services

Along with a Glossary and a Listing of Additional Resources

Edited by Joyce Brennfleck Shannon. 648 pages. 2001. 978-0-7808-0336-7.

"Not many books have been written on this topic to date, and the Ethnic Diseases Sourcebook is a strong addition to the list. It will be an important introductory resource for health consumers, students, health care personnel, and social scientists. It is recommended for public, academic, and large hospital libraries."
— American Reference Books Annual, 2002

"Will prove valuable to any library seeking to maintain a current, comprehensive reference collection of health resources... An excellent source of health information about genetic disorders which affect particular ethnic and racial minorities in the U.S."
—The Bookwatch, Aug '01

Eye Care Sourcebook, 3rd Edition

Basic Consumer Health Information about Eye Care and Eye Disorders, Including Facts about the Diagnosis, Prevention, and Treatment of Refractive Disorders, Cataracts, Glaucoma, Macular Degeneration, and Problems Affecting the Cornea, Retina, and Lacrimal Glands

Along with Advice about Preventing Eye Injuries and Tips for Living with Low Vision or Blindness, a Glossary of Related Terms, and Directories of Resources for More Help and Information

Edited by Amy L. Sutton. 646 pages. 2008. 978-0-7808-1000-6.

"A solid reference tool for eye care and a valuable addition to a collection."
—American Reference Books Annual, 2009

Family Planning Sourcebook

Basic Consumer Health Information about Planning for Pregnancy and Contraception, Including Traditional Methods, Barrier Methods, Hormonal Methods, Permanent Methods, Future Methods, Emergency Contraception, and Birth Control Choices for Women at Each Stage of Life

Along with Statistics, a Glossary, and Sources of Additional Information

Edited by Amy Marcaccio Keyzer. 503 pages. 2001. 978-0-7808-0379-4.

"Recommended for public, health, and undergraduate libraries as part of the circulating collection."
—E-Streams, Mar '02

"Will prove valuable to any library seeking to maintain a current, comprehensive reference collection of health resources... Excellent reference."
—The Bookwatch, Aug '01

SEE ALSO Pregnancy and Birth Sourcebook, 3rd Edition

Fitness and Exercise Sourcebook, 3rd Edition

Basic Consumer Health Information about the Physical and Mental Benefits of Fitness, Including Cardiorespiratory Endurance, Muscular Strength, Muscular Endurance, and Flexibility, with Facts about Sports Nutrition and Exercise-Related Injuries and Tips about Physical Activity and Exercises for People of All Ages and for People with Health Concerns

Along with Advice on Selecting and Using Exercise Equipment, Maintaining Exercise Motivation, a Glossary of Related Terms, and a Directory of Resources for More Help and Information

Edited by Amy L. Sutton. 635 pages. 2007. 978-0-7808-0946-8.

"Updates the consumer information on the physical and mental benefits of physical activity throughout the lifespan offered in earlier editions... Recommended. All readers; all levels."
—*CHOICE, Oct '07*

"An exceptionally well-rounded coverage perfect for any concerned about developing and understanding a fitness program."
—*California Bookwatch, Jun '07*

SEE ALSO *Sports Injuries Sourcebook, 3rd Edition*

Food Safety Sourcebook

Basic Consumer Health Information about the Safe Handling of Meat, Poultry, Seafood, Eggs, Fruit Juices, and Other Food Items, and Facts about Pesticides, Drinking Water, Food Safety Overseas, and the Onset, Duration, and Symptoms of Foodborne Illnesses, Including Types of Pathogenic Bacteria, Parasitic Protozoa, Worms, Viruses, and Natural Toxins

Along with the Role of the Consumer, the Food Handler, and the Government in Food Safety, a Glossary, and Resources for Additional Help and Information

Edited by Dawn D. Matthews. 327 pages. 1999. 978-0-7808-0326-8.

"Recommended reference source."
—*Booklist, May '00*

"This book takes the complex issues of food safety and foodborne pathogens and presents them in an easily understood manner. [It does] an excellent job of covering a large and often confusing topic."
— *American Reference Books Annual, 2000*

Forensic Medicine Sourcebook

Basic Consumer Information for the Layperson about Forensic Medicine, Including Crime Scene Investigation, Evidence Collection and Analysis, Expert Testimony, Computer-Aided Criminal Identification, Digital Imaging in the Courtroom, DNA Profiling, Accident Reconstruction, Autopsies, Ballistics, Drugs and Explosives Detection, Latent Fingerprints,

Product Tampering, and Questioned Document Examination

Along with Statistical Data, a Glossary of Forensics Terminology, and Listings of Sources for Further Help and Information

Edited by Annemarie S. Muth. 574 pages. 1999. 978-0-7808-0232-2.

"Given the expected widespread interest in its content and its easy to read style, this book is recommended for most public and all college and university libraries."
—*E-Streams, Feb '01*

"A wealth of information, useful statistics, references are up-to-date and extremely complete. This wonderful collection of data will help students who are interested in a career in any type of forensic field. It is a great resource for attorneys who need information about types of expert witnesses needed in a particular case. It also offers useful information for fiction and nonfiction writers whose work involves a crime. A fascinating compilation. All levels."
—*CHOICE, Jan '00*

"There are several items that make this book attractive to consumers who are seeking certain forensic data... This is a useful current source for those seeking general forensic medical answers."
—*American Reference Books Annual, 2000*

Gastrointestinal Diseases and Disorders Sourcebook, 2nd Edition

Basic Consumer Health Information about the Upper and Lower Gastrointestinal (GI) Tract, Including the Esophagus, Stomach, Intestines, Rectum, Liver, and Pancreas, with Facts about Gastroesophageal Reflux Disease, Gastritis, Hernias, Ulcers, Celiac Disease, Diverticulitis, Irritable Bowel Syndrome, Hemorrhoids, Gastrointestinal Cancers, and Other Diseases and Disorders Related to the Digestive Process

Along with Information about Commonly Used Diagnostic and Surgical Procedures, Statistics, Reports on Current Research Initiatives and Clinical Trials, a Glossary, and Resources for Additional Help and Information

Edited by Sandra J. Judd. 654 pages. 2006. 978-0-7808-0798-3.

"The text is designed for the general reader seeking information on prevention, disease warning signs, diagnostic and therapeutic questions... It is an excellent resource for the general reader to conveniently locate credible, coordinated and indexed information... The sourcebook will prove very helpful for patients, caregivers and should be available in every physician waiting room."
—*Doody's Review Service, 2006*

SEE ALSO *Diet and Nutrition Sourcebook, 3rd Edition, Digestive Diseases and Disorders Sourcebook*

Genetic Disorders Sourcebook, 4th Edition
Basic Consumer Health Information about Hereditary Diseases and Disorders, Including Facts about the Human Genome, Genetic Inheritance Patterns, Disorders Associated with Specific Genes, Such as Sickle Cell Disease, Hemophilia, and Cystic Fibrosis, Chromosome Disorders, Such as Down Syndrome, Fragile X Syndrome, and Turner Syndrome, and Complex Diseases and Disorders Resulting from the Interaction of Environmental and Genetic Factors, Such as Allergies, Cancer, and Obesity

Along with Facts about Genetic Testing, Suggestions for Parents of Children with Special Needs, Reports on Current Research Initiatives, a Glossary of Genetic Terminology, and Resources for Additional Help and Information

Edited by Sandra J. Judd. 600 pages. 2010. 978-0-7808-1076-1.

Head Trauma Sourcebook
Basic Information for the Layperson about Open-Head and Closed-Head Injuries, Treatment Advances, Recovery, and Rehabilitation

Along with Reports on Current Research Initiatives

Edited by Karen Bellenir. 414 pages. 1997. 978-0-7808-0208-7.

Headache Sourcebook
Basic Consumer Health Information about Migraine, Tension, Cluster, Rebound and Other Types of Headaches, with Facts about the Cause and Prevention of Headaches, the Effects of Stress and the Environment, Headaches during Pregnancy and Menopause, and Childhood Headaches

Along with a Glossary and Other Resources for Additional Help and Information

Edited by Dawn D. Matthews. 342 pages. 2002. 978-0-7808-0337-4.

"Highly recommended for academic and medical reference collections."
—*Library Bookwatch, Sep '02*

SEE ALSO *Pain Sourcebook, 3rd Edition*

Healthy Aging Sourcebook
Basic Consumer Health Information about Maintaining Health through the Aging Process, Including Advice on Nutrition, Exercise, and Sleep, Help in Making Decisions about Midlife Issues and Retirement, and Guidance Concerning Practical and Informed Choices in Health Consumerism

Along with Data Concerning the Theories of Aging, Different Experiences in Aging by Minority Groups, and Facts about Aging Now and Aging in the Future; and Featuring a Glossary, a Guide to Consumer Help, Additional Suggested Reading, and Practical Resource Directory

Edited by Jenifer Swanson. 537 pages. 1999. 978-0-7808-0390-9.

"Recommended reference source."
—*Booklist, Feb '00*

SEE ALSO *Adult Health Sourcebook, Physical and Mental Issues in Aging Sourcebook*

Healthy Children Sourcebook
Basic Consumer Health Information about the Physical and Mental Development of Children between the Ages of 3 and 12, Including Routine Health Care, Preventative Health Services, Safety and First Aid, Healthy Sleep, Dental Care, Nutrition, and Fitness, and Featuring Parenting Tips on Such Topics as Bedwetting, Choosing Day Care, Monitoring TV and Other Media, and Establishing a Foundation for Substance Abuse Prevention

Along with a Glossary of Commonly Used Pediatric Terms and Resources for Additional Help and Information.

Edited by Chad T. Kimball. 624 pages. 2003. 978-0-7808-0247-6.

"Should be required reading for parents and teachers."
—*E-Streams, Jun '04*

"It is hard to imagine that any other single resource exists that would provide such a comprehensive guide of timely information on health promotion and disease prevention for children aged 3 to 12."
—*American Reference Books Annual, 2004*

"This easy-to-read volume is a tremendous resource."
—*AORN Journal, May '05*

SEE ALSO *Childhood Diseases and Disorders Sourcebook, 2nd Edition*

Healthy Heart Sourcebook for Women

Basic Consumer Health Information about Cardiac Issues Specific to Women, Including Facts about Major Risk Factors and Prevention, Treatment and Control Strategies, and Important Dietary Issues

Along with a Special Section Regarding the Pros and Cons of Hormone Replacement Therapy and Its Impact on Heart Health, and Additional Help, Including Recipes, a Glossary, and a Directory of Resources

Edited by Dawn D. Matthews. 321 pages. 2000. 978-0-7808-0329-9.

"A good reference source and recommended for all public, academic, medical, and hospital libraries."
—*Medical Reference Services Quarterly, Summer '01*

"Contains very important information about coronary artery disease that all women should know. The information is current and presented in an easy-to-read format. The book will make a good addition to any library."
—*American Medical Writers Association Journal, Summer '00*

SEE ALSO *Cardiovascular Diseases and Disorders Sourcebook, 4th Edition, Women's Health Concerns Sourcebook, 3rd Edition*

Hepatitis Sourcebook

Basic Consumer Health Information about Hepatitis A, Hepatitis B, Hepatitis C, and Other Forms of Hepatitis, Including Autoimmune Hepatitis, Alcoholic Hepatitis, Nonalcoholic Steatohepatitis, and Toxic Hepatitis, with Facts about Risk Factors, Screening Methods, Diagnostic Tests, and Treatment Options

Along with Information on Liver Health, Tips for People Living with Chronic Hepatitis, Reports on Current Research Initiatives, a Glossary of Terms Related to Hepatitis, and a Directory of Sources for Further Help and Information

Edited by Sandra J. Judd. 570 pages. 2006. 978-0-7808-0749-5.

"The breadth of information found in this one book would not be readily found in another source. Highly recommended."
—*American Reference Books Annual, 2006*

SEE ALSO *Contagious Diseases Sourcebook, 2nd Edition*

Household Safety Sourcebook

Basic Consumer Health Information about Household Safety, Including Information about Poisons, Chemicals, Fire, and Water Hazards in the Home

Along with Advice about the Safe Use of Home Maintenance Equipment, Choosing Toys and Nursery Furniture, Holiday and Recreation Safety, a Glossary, and Resources for Further Help and Information

Edited by Dawn D. Matthews. 587 pages. 2002. 978-0-7808-0338-1.

"As a sourcebook on household safety this book meets its mark. It is encyclopedic in scope and covers a wide range of safety issues that are commonly seen in the home."
—*E-Streams, Jul '02*

Hypertension Sourcebook

Basic Consumer Health Information about the Causes, Diagnosis, and Treatment of High Blood Pressure, with Facts about Consequences, Complications, and Co-Occurring Disorders, Such as Coronary Heart Disease, Diabetes, Stroke, Kidney Disease, and Hypertensive Retinopathy, and Issues in Blood Pressure

Control, Including Dietary Choices, Stress Management, and Medications

Along with Reports on Current Research Initiatives and Clinical Trials, a Glossary, and Resources for Additional Help and Information

Edited by Dawn D. Matthews and Karen Bellenir. 588 pages. 2004. 978-0-7808-0674-0.

"Academic, public, and medical libraries will want to add the Hypertension Sourcebook to their collections."
—E-Streams, Aug '05

"The strength of this source is the wide range of information given about hypertension."
—American Reference Books Annual, 2005

SEE ALSO Stroke Sourcebook, 2nd Edition

Immune System Disorders Sourcebook, 2nd Edition

Basic Consumer Health Information about Disorders of the Immune System, Including Immune System Function and Response, Diagnosis of Immune Disorders, Information about Inherited Immune Disease, Acquired Immune Disease, and Autoimmune Diseases, Including Primary Immune Deficiency, Acquired Immunodeficiency Syndrome (AIDS), Lupus, Multiple Sclerosis, Type 1 Diabetes, Rheumatoid Arthritis, and Graves' Disease

Along with Treatments, Tips for Coping with Immune Disorders, a Glossary, and a Directory of Additional Resources

Edited by Joyce Brennfleck Shannon. 643 pages. 2005. 978-0-7808-0748-8.

"Highly recommended for academic and public libraries."
—American Reference Books Annual, 2006

"The updated second edition is a 'must' for any consumer health library seeking a solid resource covering the treatments, symptoms, and options for immune disorder sufferers... An excellent guide."
—MBR Bookwatch, Jan '06

SEE ALSO AIDS Sourcebook, 4th Edition, Arthritis Sourcebook, 3rd Edition

Infant and Toddler Health Sourcebook

Basic Consumer Health Information about the Physical and Mental Development of Newborns, Infants, and Toddlers, Including Neonatal Concerns, Nutrition Recommendations, Immunization Schedules, Common Pediatric Disorders, Assessments and Milestones, Safety Tips, and Advice for Parents and Other Caregivers

Along with a Glossary of Terms and Resource Listings for Additional Help

Edited by Jenifer Swanson. 570 pages. 2000. 978-0-7808-0246-9.

"As a reference for the general public, this would be useful in any library."
—E-Streams, May '01

"Recommended reference source."
—Booklist, Feb '01

Infectious Diseases Sourcebook

Basic Consumer Health Information about Non-Contagious Bacterial, Viral, Prion, Fungal, and Parasitic Diseases Spread by Food and Water, Insects and Animals, or Environmental Contact, Including Botulism, E. Coli, Encephalitis, Legionnaires' Disease, Lyme Disease, Malaria, Plague, Rabies, Salmonella, Tetanus, and Others, and Facts about Newly Emerging Diseases, Such as Hantavirus, Mad Cow Disease, Monkeypox, and West Nile Virus

Along with Information about Preventing Disease Transmission, the Threat of Bioterrorism, and Current Research Initiatives, with a Glossary and Directory of Resources for More Information

Edited by Karen Bellenir. 610 pages. 2004. 978-0-7808-0675-7.

"This reference continues the excellent tradition of the Health Reference Series in consolidating a wealth of information on a selected topic into a format that is easy to use and accessible to the general public."
—American Reference Books Annual, 2005

"Recommended for public and academic libraries."
—E-Streams, Jan '05

SEE ALSO Environmental Health Sourcebook, 3rd Edition

Injury and Trauma Sourcebook

Basic Consumer Health Information about the Impact of Injury, the Diagnosis and Treatment of Common and Traumatic Injuries, Emergency Care, and Specific Injuries Related to Home, Community, Workplace, Transportation, and Recreation

Along with Guidelines for Injury Prevention, a Glossary, and a Directory of Additional Resources

Edited by Joyce Brennfleck Shannon. 675 pages. 2002. 978-0-7808-0421-0.

"Practitioners should be aware of guides such as this in order to facilitate their use by patients and their families."
—*Doody's Health Sciences Book Review Journal, Sep-Oct '02*

"Recommended reference source."
—*Booklist, Sep '02*

"Highly recommended for academic and medical reference collections."
—*Library Bookwatch, Sep '02*

SEE ALSO *Emergency Medical Services Sourcebook, Sports Injuries Sourcebook, 3rd Edition*

Learning Disabilities Sourcebook, 3rd Edition

Basic Consumer Health Information about Dyslexia, Auditory and Visual Processing Disorders, Communication Disorders, Dyscalculia, Dysgraphia, and Other Conditions That Impede Learning, Including Attention Deficit/ Hyperactivity Disorder, Autism Spectrum Disorders, Hearing and Visual Impairments, Chromosome-Based Disorders, and Brain Injury

Along with Facts about Brain Function, Assessment, Therapy and Remediation, Accommodations, Assistive Technology, Legal Protections, and Tips about Family Life, School Transitions, and Employment Strategies, a Glossary of Related Terms, and Directories of Additional Resources

Edited by Joyce Brennfleck Shannon. 613 pages. 2009. 978-0-7808-1039-6.

"Intended to be a starting point for people who need to know about learning disabilities. Each chapter on a specific disability includes readable, well-organized descriptions... The book is well indexed and a glossary is included. Chapters on organizations and helpful websites will aid the reader who needs more information."
—*American Reference Books Annual, 2009*

"This book provides the necessary information to better understand learning disabilities and work with children who have them... It would be difficult to find another book that so comprehensively explains learning disabilities without becoming incomprehensible to the average parent who needs this information."
—*Doody's Review Service, 2009*

SEE ALSO *Attention Deficit Disorder Sourcebook, Autism and Pervasive Developmental Disorders Sourcebook*

Leukemia Sourcebook

Basic Consumer Health Information about Adult and Childhood Leukemias, Including Acute Lymphocytic Leukemia (ALL), Chronic Lymphocytic Leukemia (CLL), Acute Myelogenous Leukemia (AML), Chronic Myelogenous Leukemia (CML), and Hairy Cell Leukemia, and Treatments Such as Chemotherapy, Radiation Therapy, Peripheral Blood Stem Cell and Marrow Transplantation, and Immunotherapy

Along with Tips for Life During and After Treatment, a Glossary, and Directories of Additional Resources

Edited by Joyce Brennfleck Shannon. 564 pages. 2003. 978-0-7808-0627-6.

"Unlike other medical books for the layperson... the language does not talk down to the reader... This volume is highly recommended for all libraries."
—*American Reference Books Annual, 2004*

"A fine title which ranges from diagnosis to alternative treatments, staging, and tips for life during and after diagnosis."
—*The Bookwatch, Dec '03*

SEE ALSO *Blood & Circulatory Disorders Sourcebook, 3rd Edition, Cancer Sourcebook, 5th Edition*

Liver Disorders Sourcebook

Basic Consumer Health Information about the Liver and How It Works; Liver Diseases, Including Cancer, Cirrhosis, Hepatitis, and

Toxic and Drug Related Diseases; Tips for Maintaining a Healthy Liver; Laboratory Tests, Radiology Tests, and Facts about Liver Transplantation

Along with a Section on Support Groups, a Glossary, and Resource Listings

Edited by Joyce Brennfleck Shannon. 580 pages. 2000. 978-0-7808-0383-1.

"This title is recommended for health sciences and public libraries with consumer health collections."
—*E-Streams, Oct '00*

"Recommended reference source."
—*Booklist, Jun '00*

SEE ALSO *Gastrointestinal Diseases and Disorders Sourcebook, 2nd Edition. Hepatitis Sourcebook*

Lung Disorders Sourcebook

Basic Consumer Health Information about Emphysema, Pneumonia, Tuberculosis, Asthma, Cystic Fibrosis, and Other Lung Disorders, Including Facts about Diagnostic Procedures, Treatment Strategies, Disease Prevention Efforts, and Such Risk Factors as Smoking, Air Pollution, and Exposure to Asbestos, Radon, and Other Agents

Along with a Glossary and Resources for Additional Help and Information

Edited by Dawn D. Matthews. 657 pages. 2002. 978-0-7808-0339-8.

"Highly recommended for academic and medical reference collections."
—*Library Bookwatch, Sep '02*

SEE ALSO *Asthma Sourcebook, 2nd Edition, Respiratory Disorders Sourcebook, 2nd Edition*

Medical Tests Sourcebook, 3rd Edition

Basic Consumer Health Information about X-Rays, Blood Tests, Stool and Urine Tests, Biopsies, Mammography, Endoscopic Procedures, Ultrasound Exams, Computed Tomography, Magnetic Resonance Imaging (MRI), Nuclear Medicine, Genetic Testing, Home-Use Tests, and More

Along with Facts about Preventive Care and Screening Test Guidelines, Screening and

---

Assessment Tests Associated with Such Specific Concerns as Cancer, Heart Disease, Allergies, Diabetes, Thyroid Disfunction, and Infertility, a Glossary of Related Terms, and a Directory of Resources for Additional Help and Information

Edited by Karen Bellenir. 627 pages. 2008. 978-0-7808-1040-2

"This volume has a wide scope that makes it useful... Can be a valuable reference guide."
—*American Reference Books Annual, 2009*

"Would be a valuable contribution to any consumer health or public library."
—*Doody's Book Review Service, 2009*

Men's Health Concerns Sourcebook, 3rd Edition

Basic Consumer Health Information about Wellness in Men and Gender-Related Differences in Health, With Facts about Heart Disease, Cancer, Traumatic Injury, and Other Leading Causes of Death in Men, Reproductive Concerns, Sexual Dysfunction, Disorders of the Prostate, Penis, and Testes, Sex-Linked Genetic Disorders, and Other Medical and Mental Concerns of Men

Along with Statistical Data, a Glossary of Related Terms, and a Directory of Resources for Additional Information

Edited by Sandra J. Judd. 632 pages. 2009. 978-0-7808-1033-4.

"A good addition to any reference shelf in academic, consumer health, or hospital libraries."
—*ARBAOnline, Oct '09*

SEE ALSO *Prostate and Urological Disorders Sourcebook*

Mental Health Disorders Sourcebook, 4th Edition

Basic Consumer Health Information about the Causes and Symptoms of Mental Health Problems, Including Depression, Bipolar Disorder, Anxiety Disorders, Posttraumatic Stress Disorder, Obsessive-Compulsive Disorder, Eating Disorders, Addictions, and Personality and Psychotic Disorders

Along with Information about Medications and Treatments, Mental Health Concerns in

Children, Adolescents, and Adults, Tips on Living with Mental Health Disorders, a Glossary of Related Terms, and a Directory of Resources for Additional Help and Information

Edited by Amy L. Sutton. 680 pages. 2009. 978-0-7808-1041-9.

"Mental health concerns are presented in everyday language and intended for patients and their families as well as the general public... This resource is comprehensive and up to date... The easy-to-understand writing style helps to facilitate assimilation of needed facts and specifics on often challenging topics."
—*ARBAOnline, Oct '09*

"No health collection should be without this resource, which will reach into many a general lending library as well."
—*Internet Bookwatch, Oct '09*

SEE ALSO *Depression Sourcebook, 2nd Edition, Stress-Related Disorders Sourcebook, 2nd Edition*

Mental Retardation Sourcebook

Basic Consumer Health Information about Mental Retardation and Its Causes, Including Down Syndrome, Fetal Alcohol Syndrome, Fragile X Syndrome, Genetic Conditions, Injury, and Environmental Sources

Along with Preventive Strategies, Parenting Issues, Educational Implications, Health Care Needs, Employment and Economic Matters, Legal Issues, a Glossary, and a Resource Listing for Additional Help and Information

Edited by Joyce Brennfleck Shannon. 627 pages. 2000. 978-0-7808-0377-0.

"Public libraries will find the book useful for reference and as a beginning research point for students, parents, and caregivers."
—*American Reference Books Annual, 2001*

"The strength of this work is that it compiles many basic fact sheets and addresses for further information in one volume. It is intended and suitable for the general public."
—*E-Streams, Nov '00*

"An invaluable overview."
—*Reviewer's Bookwatch, Jul '00*

Movement Disorders Sourcebook, 2nd Edition

Basic Consumer Health Information about the Symptoms and Causes of Movement Disorders, Including Parkinson Disease, Amyotrophic Lateral Sclerosis, Cerebral Palsy, Muscular Dystrophy, Multiple Sclerosis, Myasthenia, Myoclonus, Spina Bifida, Dystonia, Essential Tremor, Choreatic Disorders, Huntington Disease, Tourette Syndrome, and Other Disorders That Cause Slowed, Absent, or Excessive Movements

Along with Information about Surgical and Nonsurgical Interventions, Physical Therapies, Strategies for Independent Living, a Glossary of Related Terms, and a Directory of Resources for Additional Help and Information

Edited by Amy L. Sutton. 618 pages. 2009. 978-0-7808-1034-1.

"The second updated edition of Movement Disorders Sourcebook is a winner, providing the latest research and health findings on all kinds of movement disorders in children and adults... a top pick for any health or general lending library's health reference collection."
—*California Bookwatch, Aug '09*

SEE ALSO *Muscular Dystrophy Sourcebook*

Multiple Sclerosis Sourcebook

Basic Consumer Health Information about Multiple Sclerosis (MS) and Its Effects on Mobility, Vision, Bladder Function, Speech, Swallowing, and Cognition, Including Facts about Risk Factors, Causes, Diagnostic Procedures, Pain Management, Drug Treatments, and Physical and Occupational Therapies

Along with Guidelines for Nutrition and Exercise, Tips on Choosing Assistive Equipment, Information about Disability, Work, Financial, and Legal Issues, a Glossary of Related Terms, and a Directory of Additional Resources

Edited by Joyce Brennfleck Shannon. 553 pages. 2007. 978-0-7808-0998-7.

Muscular Dystrophy Sourcebook

Basic Consumer Health Information about Congenital, Childhood-Onset, and Adult-Onset

Forms of Muscular Dystrophy, Such as Duchenne, Becker, Emery-Dreifuss, Distal, Limb-Girdle, Facioscapulohumeral (FSHD), Myotonic, and Ophthalmoplegic Muscular Dystrophies, Including Facts about Diagnostic Tests, Medical and Physical Therapies, Management of Co-Occurring Conditions, and Parenting Guidelines

Along with Practical Tips for Home Care, a Glossary, and Directories of Additional Resources

Edited by Joyce Brennfleck Shannon. 552 pages. 2004. 978-0-7808-0676-4.

"This book is highly recommended for public and academic libraries as well as health care offices that support the information needs of patients and their families."
—*E-Streams, Apr '05*

"Excellent reference."
—*The Bookwatch, Jan '05*

SEE ALSO *Movement Disorders Sourcebook, 2nd Edition*

Obesity Sourcebook

Basic Consumer Health Information about Diseases and Other Problems Associated with Obesity, and Including Facts about Risk Factors, Prevention Issues, and Management Approaches

Along with Statistical and Demographic Data, Information about Special Populations, Research Updates, a Glossary, and Source Listings for Further Help and Information

Edited by Wilma Caldwell and Chad T. Kimball. 360 pages. 2001. 978-0-7808-0333-6.

"The book synthesizes the reliable medical literature on obesity into one easy-to-read and useful resource for the general public."
—*American Reference Books Annual, 2002*

"Well suited for the health reference collection of a public library or an academic health science library that serves the general population."
—*E-Streams, Sep '01*

Osteoporosis Sourcebook

Basic Consumer Health Information about Primary and Secondary Osteoporosis and Juvenile Osteoporosis and Related Conditions, Including Fibrous Dysplasia, Gaucher Disease, Hyperthyroidism, Hypophosphatasia,

Myeloma, Osteopetrosis, Osteogenesis Imperfecta, and Paget's Disease

Along with Information about Risk Factors, Treatments, Traditional and Non-Traditional Pain Management, a Glossary of Related Terms, and a Directory of Resources

Edited by Allan R. Cook. 568 pages. 2001. 978-0-7808-0239-1.

"This resource is recommended as a great reference source for public, health, and academic libraries, and is another triumph for the editors of Omnigraphics."
—*American Reference Books Annual, 2002*

"Will prove valuable to any library seeking to maintain a current, comprehensive reference collection of health resources... From prevention to treatment and associated conditions, this provides an excellent survey."
—*The Bookwatch, Aug '01*

SEE ALSO *Healthy Aging Sourcebook, Women's Health Concerns Sourcebook, 3rd Edition*

Pain Sourcebook, 3rd Edition

Basic Consumer Health Information about Acute and Chronic Pain, Including Nerve Pain, Bone Pain, Muscle Pain, Cancer Pain, and Disorders Characterized by Pain, Such as Arthritis, Temporomandibular Muscle and Joint (TMJ) Disorder, Carpal Tunnel Syndrome, Headaches, Heartburn, Sciatica, and Shingles, and Facts about Diagnostic Tests and Treatment Options for Pain, Including Over-the-Counter and Prescription Drugs, Physical Rehabilitation, Injection and Infusion Therapies, Implantable Technologies, and Complementary Medicine

Along with Tips for Living with Pain, a Glossary of Related Terms, and a Directory of Additional Resources

Edited by Joyce Brennfleck Shannon. 644 pages. 2008. 978-0-7808-1006-8.

"Excellent for ready-reference users and can be used for beginning students in health fields... appropriate for the consumer health collection in both public and academic libraries."
—*American Reference Books Annual, 2009*

SEE ALSO *Arthritis Sourcebook, 3rd Edition; Back and Neck Sourcebook, 2nd Edition;*

Headache Sourcebook; Sports Injuries Sourcebook, 3rd Edition

Pediatric Cancer Sourcebook

Basic Consumer Health Information about Leukemias, Brain Tumors, Sarcomas, Lymphomas, and Other Cancers in Infants, Children, and Adolescents, Including Descriptions of Cancers, Treatments, and Coping Strategies

Along with Suggestions for Parents, Caregivers, and Concerned Relatives, a Glossary of Cancer Terms, and Resource Listings

Edited by Edward J. Prucha. 575 pages. 1999. 978-0-7808-0245-2.

"An excellent source of information. Recommended for public, hospital, and health science libraries with consumer health collections."
—*E-Streams, Jun '00*

"A valuable addition to all libraries specializing in health services and many public libraries."
—*American Reference Books Annual, 2000*

SEE ALSO *Childhood Diseases and Disorders Sourcebook, 2nd Edition, Healthy Children Sourcebook*

Physical and Mental Issues in Aging Sourcebook

Basic Consumer Health Information on Physical and Mental Disorders Associated with the Aging Process, Including Concerns about Cardiovascular Disease, Pulmonary Disease, Oral Health, Digestive Disorders, Musculoskeletal and Skin Disorders, Metabolic Changes, Sexual and Reproductive Issues, and Changes in Vision, Hearing, and Other Senses

Along with Data about Longevity and Causes of Death, Information on Acute and Chronic Pain, Descriptions of Mental Concerns, a Glossary of Terms, and Resource Listings for Additional Help

Edited by Jenifer Swanson. 660 pages. 1999. 978-0-7808-0233-9.

"This is a treasure of health information for the layperson."
—*CHOICE Health Sciences Supplement, May '00*

"Recommended for public libraries."
—*American Reference Books Annual, 2000*

SEE ALSO *Healthy Aging Sourcebook*

Podiatry Sourcebook, 2nd Edition

Basic Consumer Health Information about Disorders, Diseases, and Deformities that Affect the Foot and Ankle, Including Sprains, Corns, Calluses, Bunions, Plantar Warts, Plantar Fasciitis, Neuromas, Clubfoot, Flat Feet, Achilles Tendonitis, and Much More

Along with Information about Selecting a Foot Care Specialist, Foot Fitness, Shoes and Socks, Diagnostic Tests and Corrective Procedures, Financial Assistance for Corrective Devices, a Glossary of Related Terms, and a Directory of Resources for Additional Help and Information

Edited by Ivy L. Alexander. 516 pages. 2007. 978-0-7808-0944-4.

"An excellent resource... Although there have been various types of 'foot books' published in the past, none are as comprehensive as this one. 5 Stars (out of 5)!"
—*Doody's Review Service, 2007*

"Perfect for both health libraries and general-interest lending collections."
—*Internet Bookwatch, Jul '07*

Pregnancy and Birth Sourcebook, 3rd Edition

Basic Consumer Health Information about Pregnancy and Fetal Development, Including Facts about Fertility and Conception, Physical and Emotional Changes during Pregnancy, Prenatal Care and Diagnostic Tests, High-Risk Pregnancies and Complications, Labor, Delivery, and the Postpartum Period

Along with Tips on Maintaining Health and Wellness during Pregnancy and Caring for Newborn Infants, a Glossary of Related Terms, and Directories of Resources for Additional Help and Information

Edited by Amy L. Sutton. 645 pages. 2009. 978-0-7808-1074-7.

SEE ALSO *Breastfeeding Sourcebook, Congenital Disorders Sourcebook, 2nd Edition, Family Planning Sourcebook, Women's Health Concerns Sourcebook, 3rd Edition*

719

Prostate and Urological Disorders Sourcebook

Basic Consumer Health Information about Urogenital and Sexual Disorders in Men, Including Prostate and Other Andrological Cancers, Prostatitis, Benign Prostatic Hyperplasia, Testicular and Penile Trauma, Cryptorchidism, Peyronie Disease, Erectile Dysfunction, and Male Factor Infertility, and Facts about Commonly Used Tests and Procedures, Such as Prostatectomy, Vasectomy, Vasectomy Reversal, Penile Implants, and Semen Analysis

Along with a Glossary of Andrological Terms and a Directory of Resources for Additional Information

Edited by Karen Bellenir. 604 pages. 2006. 978-0-7808-0797-6.

"Certain to be a popular pick among library reference holdings... No prior knowledge is assumed for any of the conditions or terms herein, making it a most accessible general-interest reference."
—*California Bookwatch, Apr '06*

SEE ALSO *Men's Health Concerns Sourcebook, 3rd Edition, Urinary Tract and Kidney Diseases and Disorders Sourcebook, 2nd Edition*

Prostate Cancer Sourcebook

Basic Consumer Health Information about Prostate Cancer, Including Information about the Associated Risk Factors, Detection, Diagnosis, and Treatment of Prostate Cancer

Along with Information on Non-Malignant Prostate Conditions, and Featuring a Section Listing Support and Treatment Centers and a Glossary of Related Terms

Edited by Dawn D. Matthews. 340 pages. 2001. 978-0-7808-0324-4.

"Recommended reference source."
—*Booklist, Jan '02*

"A valuable resource for health care consumers seeking information on the subject... All text is written in a clear, easy-to-understand language that avoids technical jargon. Any library that collects consumer health resources would strengthen their collection with the addition of the Prostate Cancer Sourcebook."
—*American Reference Books Annual, 2002*

SEE ALSO *Cancer Sourcebook, 5th Edition, Men's Health Concerns Sourcebook, 3rd Edition*

Rehabilitation Sourcebook

Basic Consumer Health Information about Rehabilitation for People Recovering from Heart Surgery, Spinal Cord Injury, Stroke, Orthopedic Impairments, Amputation, Pulmonary Impairments, Traumatic Injury, and More, Including Physical Therapy, Occupational Therapy, Speech/Language Therapy, Massage Therapy, Dance Therapy, Art Therapy, and Recreational Therapy

Along with Information on Assistive and Adaptive Devices, a Glossary, and Resources for Additional Help and Information

Edited by Dawn D. Matthews. 519 pages. 2000. 978-0-7808-0236-0.

"This is an excellent resource for public library reference and health collections."
—*American Reference Books Annual, 2001*

"Recommended reference source."
—*Booklist, May '00*

Respiratory Disorders Sourcebook, 2nd Edition

Basic Consumer Health Information about Infectious, Inflammatory, and Chronic Conditions Affecting the Lungs and Respiratory System, Including Pneumonia, Bronchitis, Influenza, Tuberculosis, Sarcoidosis, Asthma, Cystic Fibrosis, Chronic Obstructive Pulmonary Disease, Lung Abscesses, Pulmonary Embolism, Occupational Lung Diseases, and Other Bacterial, Viral, and Fungal Infections

Along with Facts about the Structure and Function of the Lungs and Airways, Methods of Diagnosing Respiratory Disorders, and Treatment and Rehabilitation Options, a Glossary of Related Terms, and a Directory of Resources for Additional Help and Information

Edited by Sandra L. Judd. 638 pages. 2008. 978-0-7808-1007-5.

"An excellent book for patients, their families, or for those who are just curious about respiratory disease. Public libraries and physician offices would find this a valuable resource as well. 4 Stars! (out of 5)"
—*Doody's Review Service, 2009*

"A great addition for public and school libraries because it provides concise health information... readers can start with this reference source and get satisfactory answers before proceeding to other medical reference tools for

more in depth information... A good guide for health education on lung disorders."
—*American Reference Books Annual, 2009*

SEE ALSO *Asthma Sourcebook, 2nd Edition, Lung Disorders Sourcebook*

Sexually Transmitted Diseases Sourcebook, 4th Edition

Basic Consumer Health Information about Chlamydial Infections, Gonorrhea, Hepatitis, Herpes, HIV/AIDS, Human Papillomavirus, Pubic Lice, Scabies, Syphilis, Trichomoniasis, Vaginal Infections, and Other Sexually Transmitted Diseases, Including Facts about Risk Factors, Symptoms, Diagnosis, Treatment, and the Prevention of Sexually Transmitted Infections

Along with Updates on Current Research Initiatives, a Glossary of Related Terms, and Resources for Additional Help and Information

Edited by Laura Larsen. 623 pages. 2009. 978-0-7808-1073-0.

"Extremely beneficial... The question-and-answer format along with the index and table of contents make this well-organized resource extremely easy to reference, read, and comprehend... an invaluable medical reference source for lay readers, and a highly appropriate addition for public library collections, health clinics, and any library with a consumer health collection"
—*ARBAOnline, Oct '09*

SEE ALSO *AIDS Sourcebook, 4th Edition, Contagious Diseases Sourcebook, 2nd Edition, Men's Health Concerns Sourcebook, 3rd Edition, Women's Health Concerns Sourcebook, 3rd Edition*

Sleep Disorders Sourcebook, 3rd Edition

Basic Consumer Health Information about Sleep Disorders, Including Insomnia, Sleep Apnea and Snoring, Jet Lag and Other Circadian Rhythm Disorders, Narcolepsy, and Parasomnias, Such as Sleep Walking and Sleep Talking, and Featuring Facts about Other Health Problems that Affect Sleep, Why Sleep Is Necessary, How Much Sleep Is Needed, the Physical and Mental Effects of Sleep Deprivation, and Pediatric Sleep Issues

Along with Tips for Diagnosing and Treating Sleep Disorders, a Glossary of Related Terms, and a List of Resources for Additional Help and Information

Edited by Sandra J. Judd. 600 pages. 2010. 978-0-7808-1084-6.

Smoking Concerns Sourcebook

Basic Consumer Health Information about Nicotine Addiction and Smoking Cessation, Featuring Facts about the Health Effects of Tobacco Use, Including Lung and Other Cancers, Heart Disease, Stroke, and Respiratory Disorders, Such as Emphysema and Chronic Bronchitis

Along with Information about Smoking Prevention Programs, Suggestions for Achieving and Maintaining a Smoke-Free Lifestyle, Statistics about Tobacco Use, Reports on Current Research Initiatives, a Glossary of Related Terms, and Directories of Resources for Additional Help and Information

Edited by Karen Bellenir. 595 pages. 2004. 978-0-7808-0323-7.

"Provides everything needed for the student or general reader seeking practical details on the effects of tobacco use."
—*The Bookwatch, Mar '05*

"Public libraries and consumer health care libraries will find this work useful."
—*American Reference Books Annual, 2005*

SEE ALSO *Respiratory Disorders Sourcebook, 2nd Edition*

Sports Injuries Sourcebook, 3rd Edition

Basic Consumer Health Information about Sprains and Strains, Fractures, Growth Plate Injuries, Overtraining Injuries, and Injuries to the Head, Face, Shoulders, Elbows, Hands, Spinal Column, Knees, Ankles, and Feet, and with Facts about Heat-Related Illness, Steroids and Sport Supplements, Protective Equipment, Diagnostic Procedures, Treatment Options, and Rehabilitation

Along with a Glossary of Related Terms and a Directory of Resources for Additional Help and Information

Edited by Sandra J. Judd. 623 pages. 2007. 978-0-7808-0949-9.

SEE ALSO *Fitness and Exercise Sourcebook, 3rd Edition, Podiatry Sourcebook, 2nd Edition*

Stress-Related Disorders Sourcebook, 2nd Edition

Basic Consumer Health Information about Stress and Stress-Related Disorders, Including Types of Stress, Sources of Acute and Chronic Stress, the Impact of Stress on the Body's Systems, and Mental and Emotional Health Problems Associated with Stress, Such as Depression, Anxiety Disorders, Substance Abuse, Posttraumatic Stress Disorder, and Suicide

Along with Advice about Getting Help for Stress-Related Disorders, Information about Stress Management Techniques, a Glossary of Stress-Related Terms, and a Directory of Resources for Additional Help and Information

Edited by Amy L. Sutton. 608 pages. 2007. 978-0-7808-0996-3.

"Accessible to the lay reader. Highly recommended for medical and psychiatric collections."
—*Library Journal, Mar '08*

"Well-written for a general readership, the 2nd Edition of Stress-Related Disorders Sourcebook is a useful addition to the health reference literature."
—*American Reference Books Annual, 2008*

SEE ALSO *Mental Health Disorders Sourcebook, 4th Edition*

Stroke Sourcebook, 2nd Edition

Basic Consumer Health Information about Stroke, Including Ischemic, Hemorrhagic, and Mini Strokes, as Well as Risk Factors, Prevention Guidelines, Diagnostic Tests, Medications and Surgical Treatments, and Complications of Stroke

Along with Rehabilitation Techniques and Innovations, Tips on Staying Healthy and Maintaining Independence after Stroke, a Glossary of Related Terms, and a Directory of Resources for Stroke Survivors and Their Families

Edited by Amy L. Sutton. 626 pages. 2008. 978-0-7808-1035-8.

"An encyclopedic handbook on stroke that is written in a language the layperson can understand... This is one of the most helpful, readable books on stroke. This volume is highly recommended and should be in every medical, hospital and public library; in addition, every family practitioner should have a copy in his or her office."
—*American Reference Books Annual, 2009*

SEE ALSO *Brain Disorders Sourcebook, 3rd Edition, Hypertension Sourcebook*

Surgery Sourcebook, 2nd Edition

Basic Consumer Health Information about Common Inpatient and Outpatient Surgeries, Including Critical Care and Trauma, Gastrointestinal, Gynecologic and Obstetric, Cardiac and Vascular, Neurologic, Ophthalmologic, Orthopedic, Reconstructive and Cosmetic, and Other Major and Minor Surgeries

Along with Information about Anesthesia and Pain Relief Options, Risks and Complications, Postoperative Recovery Concerns, and Innovative Surgical Techniques and Tools, a Glossary of Related Terms, and a Directory of Additional Resources

Edited by Amy L. Sutton. 645 pages. 2008. 978-0-7808-1004-4.

"Large public libraries and medical libraries would benefit from this material in their reference collections."
—*American Reference Books Annual, 2009*

SEE ALSO *Cosmetic and Reconstructive Surgery Sourcebook, 2nd Edition*

Thyroid Disorders Sourcebook

Basic Consumer Health Information about Disorders of the Thyroid and Parathyroid Glands, Including Hypothyroidism, Hyperthyroidism, Graves Disease, Hashimoto Thyroiditis, Thyroid Cancer, and Parathyroid Disorders, Featuring Facts about Symptoms, Risk Factors, Tests, and Treatments

Along with Information about the Effects of Thyroid Imbalance on Other Body Systems, Environmental Factors That Affect the Thyroid Gland, a Glossary, and a Directory of Additional Resources

Edited by Joyce Brennfleck Shannon. 573 pages. 2005. 978-0-7808-0745-7.

"Recommended for consumer health collections."
—American Reference Books Annual, 2006

"Highly recommended pick for Basic Consumer health reference holdings at all levels."
—The Bookwatch, Aug '05

SEE ALSO *Endocrine and Metabolic Disorders Sourcebook, 2nd Edition*

Transplantation Sourcebook
Basic Consumer Health Information about Organ and Tissue Transplantation, Including Physical and Financial Preparations, Procedures and Issues Relating to Specific Solid Organ and Tissue Transplants, Rehabilitation, Pediatric Transplant Information, the Future of Transplantation, and Organ and Tissue Donation

Along with a Glossary and Listings of Additional Resources

Edited by Joyce Brennfleck Shannon. 610 pages. 2002. 978-0-7808-0322-0.

"Recommended for libraries with an interest in offering consumer health information."
—E-Streams, Jul '02

"This is a unique and valuable resource for patients facing transplantation and their families."
—Doody's Review Service, Jun '02

Traveler's Health Sourcebook
Basic Consumer Health Information for Travelers, Including Physical and Medical Preparations, Transportation Health and Safety, Essential Information about Food and Water, Sun Exposure, Insect and Snake Bites, Camping and Wilderness Medicine, and Travel with Physical or Medical Disabilities

Along with International Travel Tips, Vaccination Recommendations, Geographical Health Issues, Disease Risks, a Glossary, and a Listing of Additional Resources

Edited by Joyce Brennfleck Shannon. 619 pages. 2000. 978-0-7808-0384-8.

"Recommended reference source."
—Booklist, Feb '01

"This book is recommended for any public library, any travel collection, and especially any collection for the physically disabled."
—American Reference Books Annual, 2001

SEE ALSO *Worldwide Health Sourcebook*

Urinary Tract and Kidney Diseases and Disorders Sourcebook, 2nd Edition
Basic Consumer Health Information about the Urinary System, Including the Bladder, Urethra, Ureters, and Kidneys, with Facts about Urinary Tract Infections, Incontinence, Congenital Disorders, Kidney Stones, Cancers of the Urinary Tract and Kidneys, Kidney Failure, Dialysis, and Kidney Transplantation

Along with Statistical and Demographic Information, Reports on Current Research in Kidney and Urologic Health, a Summary of Commonly Used Diagnostic Tests, a Glossary of Related Terms, and a Directory of Resources for Additional Help and Information

Edited by Ivy L. Alexander. 621 pages. 2005. 978-0-7808-0750-1.

"A good choice for a consumer health information library or for a medical library needing information to refer to their patients."
—American Reference Books Annual, 2006

SEE ALSO *Prostate and Urological Disorders Sourcebook*

Vegetarian Sourcebook
Basic Consumer Health Information about Vegetarian Diets, Lifestyle, and Philosophy, Including Definitions of Vegetarianism and Veganism, Tips about Adopting Vegetarianism, Creating a Vegetarian Pantry, and Meeting Nutritional Needs of Vegetarians, with Facts Regarding Vegetarianism's Effect on Pregnant and Lactating Women, Children, Athletes, and Senior Citizens

Along with a Glossary of Commonly Used Vegetarian Terms and Resources for Additional Help and Information

Edited by Chad T. Kimball. 337 pages. 2002. 978-0-7808-0439-5.

"Organizes into one concise volume the answers to the most common questions concerning vegetarian diets and lifestyles. This title is

recommended for public and secondary school libraries."

—E-Streams, Apr '03

"Invaluable reference for public and school library collections alike."
—Library Bookwatch, Apr '03

"The articles in this volume are easy to read and come from authoritative sources. The book does not necessarily support the vegetarian diet but instead provides the pros and cons of this important decision... Recommended for public libraries and consumer health libraries."
—American Reference Books Annual, 2003

SEE ALSO Diet and Nutrition Sourcebook, 3rd Edition

Women's Health Concerns Sourcebook, 3rd Edition

Basic Consumer Health Information about Issues and Trends in Women's Health and Health Conditions of Special Concern to Women, Including Endometriosis, Uterine Fibroids, Menstrual Irregularities, Menopause, Sexual Dysfunction, Infertility, Cancer in Women, and Other Such Chronic Disorders as Lupus, Fibromyalgia, and Thyroid Disease

Along with Statistical Data, Tips for Maintaining Wellness, a Glossary, and a Directory of Resources for Further Help and Information

Edited by Sandra J. Judd. 679 pages. 2009. 978-0-7808-1036-5.

"This useful resource provides information about a wide range of topics that will help women understand their bodies, prevent or treat disease, and maintain health... A detailed index helps readers locate information. This is a useful addition to public and consumer health library collections"
—ARBAOnline, Jun '09

SEE ALSO Breast Cancer Sourcebook, 3rd Edition, Cancer Sourcebook for Women, 4th Edition, Healthy Heart Sourcebook for Women

Workplace Health and Safety Sourcebook

Basic Consumer Health Information about Workplace Health and Safety, Including the Effect of Workplace Hazards on the Lungs,

Skin, Heart, Ears, Eyes, Brain, Reproductive Organs, Musculoskeletal System, and Other Organs and Body Parts

Along with Information about Occupational Cancer, Personal Protective Equipment, Toxic and Hazardous Chemicals, Child Labor, Stress, and Workplace Violence

Edited by Chad T. Kimball. 610 pages. 2000. 978-0-7808-0231-5.

"As a reference for the general public, this would be useful in any library."
—E-Streams, Jun '01

"Provides helpful information for primary care physicians and other caregivers interested in occupational medicine... General readers; professionals."
—CHOICE, May '01

Worldwide Health Sourcebook

Basic Information about Global Health Issues, Including Malnutrition, Reproductive Health, Disease Dispersion and Prevention, Emerging Diseases, Risky Health Behaviors, and the Leading Causes of Death

Along with Global Health Concerns for Children, Women, and the Elderly, Mental Health Issues, Research and Technology Advancements, and Economic, Environmental, and Political Health Implications, a Glossary, and a Resource Listing for Additional Help and Information

Edited by Joyce Brennfleck Shannon. 597 pages. 2001. 978-0-7808-0330-5.

"Named an Outstanding Academic Title."
—CHOICE, Jan '02

"Yet another handy but also unique compilation in the extensive Health Reference Series, this is a useful work because many of the international publications reprinted or excerpted are not readily available. Highly recommended."
—CHOICE, Nov '01

SEE ALSO Traveler's Health Sourcebook

Teen Health Series
Complete Catalog
List price $69 per volume. School and library price $62 per volume.

Abuse and Violence Information for Teens
Health Tips about the Causes and Consequences of Abusive and Violent Behavior
Including Facts about the Types of Abuse and Violence, the Warning Signs of Abusive and Violent Behavior, Health Concerns of Victims, and Getting Help and Staying Safe

Edited by Sandra Augustyn Lawton. 411 pages. 2008. 978-0-7808-1008-2.

"A useful resource for schools and organizations providing services to teens and may also be a starting point in research projects."
—*Reference and Research Book News, Aug '08*

"Violence is a serious problem for teens... This resource gives teens the information they need to face potential threats and get help—either for themselves or for their friends."
—*American Reference Books Annual, 2009*

Accident and Safety Information for Teens
Health Tips about Medical Emergencies, Traumatic Injuries, and Disaster Preparedness
Including Facts about Motor Vehicle Accidents, Burns, Poisoning, Firearms, Natural Disasters, National Security Threats, and More

Edited by Karen Bellenir. 420 pages. 2008. 978-0-7808-1046-4.

"Aimed at teenage audiences, this guide provides practical information for handling a comprehensive list of emergencies, from sport injuries and auto accidents to alcohol poisoning and natural disasters."
—*Library Journal, Apr 1, '09*

"Useful in the young adult collections of public libraries as well as high school libraries."
—*American Reference Books Annual, 2009*

SEE ALSO Sports Injuries Information for Teens, 2nd Edition

Alcohol Information for Teens, 2nd Edition
Health Tips about Alcohol and Alcoholism
Including Facts about Alcohol's Effects on the Body, Brain, and Behavior, the Consequences of Underage Drinking, Alcohol Abuse Prevention and Treatment, and Coping with Alcoholic Parents

Edited by Lisa Bakewell. 410 pages. 2009. 978-0-7808-1043-3.

"This handbook, written for a teenage audience, provides information on the causes, effects, and preventive measures related to alcohol abuse among teens... The chapters are quick to make a connection to their teenage reading audience. The prose is straightforward and the book lends itself to spot reading. It should be useful both for practical information and for research, and it is suitable for public and school libraries."
—*ARBAOnline, Jun '09*

SEE ALSO Drug Information for Teens, 2nd Edition

Allergy Information for Teens
Health Tips about Allergic Reactions Such as Anaphylaxis, Respiratory Problems, and Rashes
Including Facts about Identifying and Managing Allergies to Food, Pollen, Mold, Animals, Chemicals, Drugs, and Other Substances

Edited by Karen Bellenir. 410 pages. 2006. 978-0-7808-0799-0.

"This is a comprehensive, readable text on the subject of allergic diseases in teenagers. 5 Stars (out of 5)!"
—*Doody's Review Service, Jun '06*

"This authoritative and useful self-help title is a solid addition to YA collections, whether for personal interest or reports."
—*School Library Journal, Jul '06*

Asthma Information for Teens, 2nd Ed.
Health Tips about Managing Asthma and Related Concerns

Including Facts about Asthma Causes, Triggers and Symptoms, Diagnosis, and Treatment

Edited by Kim Wohlenhaus. 400 pages. 2010. 978-0-7808-1086-0.

Body Information for Teens
Health Tips about Maintaining Well-Being for a Lifetime

Including Facts about the Development and Functioning of the Body's Systems, Organs, and Structures and the Health Impact of Lifestyle Choices

Edited by Sandra Augustyn Lawton. 458 pages. 2007. 978-0-7808-0443-2.

Cancer Information for Teens, 2nd Edition
Health Tips about Cancer Awareness, Symptoms, Prevention, Diagnosis, and Treatment

Including Facts about Common Cancers Affecting Teens, Causes, Detection, Coping Strategies, Clinical Trials, Nutrition and Exercise, Cancer in Friends or Family, and More

Edited by Karen Bellenir and Lisa Bakewell. 445 pages. 2010. 978-0-7808-1085-3.

Complementary and Alternative Medicine Information for Teens
Health Tips about Non-Traditional and Non-Western Medical Practices

Including Information about Acupuncture, Chiropractic Medicine, Dietary and Herbal Supplements, Hypnosis, Massage Therapy, Prayer and Spirituality, Reflexology, Yoga, and More

Edited by Sandra Augustyn Lawton. 407 pages. 2007. 978-0-7808-0966-6.

"This volume covers CAM specifically for teenagers but of general use also. It should be a welcome addition to both public and academic libraries."
—*American Reference Books Annual, 2008*

"This volume provides a solid foundation for further investigation of the subject, making it useful for both public and high school libraries."
—*VOYA: Voice of Youth Advocates, Jun '07*

Diabetes Information for Teens
Health Tips about Managing Diabetes and Preventing Related Complications

Including Information about Insulin, Glucose Control, Healthy Eating, Physical Activity, and Learning to Live with Diabetes

Edited by Sandra Augustyn Lawton. 410 pages. 2006. 978-0-7808-0811-9.

"A comprehensive instructional guide for teens... some of the material may also be directed towards parents or teachers. 5 stars (out of 5)!"
—*Doody's Review Service, 2006*

"Students dealing with their own diabetes or that of a friend or family member or those writing reports on the topic will find this a valuable resource."
—*School Library Journal, Aug '06*

"This text is directed to the teen population and would be an excellent library resource for a health class or for the teacher as a reference for class preparation. It can, however, serve a much wider audience. The clinical educator on diabetes may find it valuable to educate the newly diagnosed client regardless of age. It also would be an excellent reference and education tool for a preventive medicine seminar on diabetes."
—*Physical Therapy, Mar '07*

Diet Information for Teens, 2nd Edition
Health Tips about Diet and Nutrition

Including Facts about Dietary Guidelines, Food Groups, Nutrients, Healthy Meals, Snacks, Weight Control, Medical Concerns Related to Diet, and More

Edited by Karen Bellenir. 432 pages. 2006. 978-0-7808-0820-1.

"A very quick and pleasant read in spite of the fact that it is very detailed in the information it gives... A book for anyone concerned about diet and nutrition."
—*American Reference Books Annual, 2007*

SEE ALSO Eating Disorders Information for Teens, 2nd Edition

Drug Information for Teens, 2nd Edition
Health Tips about the Physical and Mental Effects of Substance Abuse
Including Information about Marijuana, Inhalants, Club Drugs, Stimulants, Hallucinogens, Opiates, Prescription and Over-the-Counter Drugs, Herbal Products, Tobacco, Alcohol, and More

Edited by Sandra Augustyn Lawton. 468 pages. 2006. 978-0-7808-0862-1.

"As with earlier installments in Omnigraphics' Teen Health Series, Drug Information for Teens is designed specifically to meet the needs and interests of middle and high school students... Strongly recommended for both academic and public libraries."
—*American Reference Books Annual, 2007*

"Solid thoughtful advice is given about how to handle peer pressure, drug-related health concerns, and treatment strategies."
—*School Library Journal, Dec '06*

SEE ALSO *Alcohol Information for Teens, 2nd Edition, Tobacco Information for Teens, 2nd Edition*

Eating Disorders Information for Teens, 2nd Edition
Health Tips about Anorexia, Bulimia, Binge Eating, And Other Eating Disorders
Including Information about Risk Factors, Diagnosis and Treatment, Prevention, Related Health Concerns, and Other Issues

Edited by Sandra Augustyn Lawton. 377 pages. 2009. 978-0-7808-1044-0.

"This handy reference offers basic information and addresses specific disorders, consequences, prevention, diagnosis and treatment, healthy eating, and more. It is written in a conversational style that is easy to understand... Will provide plenty of facts for reports as well as browsing potential for students with an interest in the topic.
—*School Library Journal, Jun '09*

"Written in a straightforward style that will appeal to its teenage audience. The author does not play down the danger of living with an eating disorder and urges those struggling with this problem to seek professional help.

This work, as well as others in this series, will be a welcome addition to high school and undergraduate libraries."
—*American Reference Books Annual, 2009*

SEE ALSO *Diet Information for Teens, 2nd Edition*

Fitness Information for Teens, 2nd Edition
Health Tips about Exercise, Physical Well-Being, and Health Maintenance
Including Facts about Conditioning, Stretching, Strength Training, Body Shape and Body Image, Sports Nutrition, and Specific Activities for Athletes and Non-Athletes

Edited by Lisa Bakewell. 432 pages. 2009. 978-0-7808-1045-7.

"This no-nonsense guide packs a great deal into its pages... This is a helpful reference for basic diet and exercise information for health reports or personal use."
—*School Library Journal, April 2009*

"An excellent source for general information on why teens should be active, making time to exercise, the equipment people might need, various types of activities to try, how to maintain health and wellness, and how to avoid barriers to becoming healthier... This would still be an excellent addition to a public library ready-reference collection or a high school health library collection."
—*American Reference Books Annual, 2009*

"This easy to read, well-written, up-to-date overview of fitness for teenagers provides excellent wellness and exercise tips, information, and directions... It is a useful tool for them to obtain a base knowledge in fitness topics and different sports."
—*Doody's Review Service, 2009*

SEE ALSO *Diet Information for Teens, 2nd Edition, Sports Injuries Information for Teens, 2nd Edition*

Learning Disabilities Information for Teens
Health Tips about Academic Skills Disorders and Other Disabilities That Affect Learning

Including Information about Common Signs of Learning Disabilities, School Issues, Learning to Live with a Learning Disability, and Other Related Issues

Edited by Sandra Augustyn Lawton. 400 pages. 2006. 978-0-7808-0796-9.

"This book provides a wealth of information for any reader interested in the signs, causes, and consequences of learning disabilities, as well as related legal and educational interventions... Public and academic libraries should want this title for both students and general readers."

—*American Reference Books Annual, 2006*

Mental Health Information for Teens, 3rd Edition
Health Tips about Mental Wellness and Mental Illness
Including Facts about Mental and Emotional Health, Depression and Other Mood Disorders, Anxiety Disorders, Behavior Disorders, Self-Injury, Psychosis, Schizophrenia, and More

Edited by Karen Bellenir. 400 pages. 2010. 978-0-7808-1087-7.

SEE ALSO Stress Information for Teens, Suicide Information for Teens, 2nd Edition

Pregnancy Information for Teens
Health Tips about Teen Pregnancy and Teen Parenting
Including Facts about Prenatal Care, Pregnancy Complications, Labor and Delivery, Postpartum Care, Pregnancy-Related Lifestyle Concerns, and More

Edited by Sandra Augustyn Lawton. 434 pages. 2007. 978-0-7808-0984-0.

Sexual Health Information for Teens, 2nd Edition
Health Tips about Sexual Development, Reproduction, Contraception, and Sexually Transmitted Infections
Including Facts about Puberty, Sexuality, Birth Control, Chlamydia, Gonorrhea, Herpes, Human Papillomavirus, Syphilis, and More

Edited by Sandra Augustyn Lawton. 430 pages. 2008. 978-0-7808-1010-5.

"This offering represents the most up-to-date information available on an array of topics including abstinence-only sexual education and pregnancy-prevention methods... The range of coverage—from puberty and anatomy to sexually transmitted diseases—is thorough and extensive. Each chapter includes a bibliographic citation, and the three back sections containing additional resources, further reading, and the index are all first-rate... This volume will be well used by students in need of the facts, whether for educational or personal reasons."

—*School Library Journal, Nov '08*

"Presents information related to the emotional, physical, and biological development of both males and females that occurs during puberty. It also strives to address some of the issues and questions that may arise... The text is easy to read and understand for young readers, with satisfactory definitions within the text to explain new terms."

—*American Reference Books Annual, 2009*

Skin Health Information for Teens, 2nd Edition
Health Tips about Dermatological Concerns and Skin Cancer Risks
Including Facts about Acne, Warts, Hives, and Other Conditions and Lifestyle Choices, Such as Tanning, Tattooing, and Piercing, That Affect the Skin, Nails, Scalp, and Hair

Edited by Edited by Kim Wohlenhaus. 418 pages. 2009. 978-0-7808-1042-6.

"The material in this work will be easily understood by teenagers and young adults. The publisher has liberally used bulleted lists and sidebars to keep the reader's attention... A useful addition to school and public library collections."

—*ARBAOnline, Oct '09*

Sleep Information for Teens
Health Tips about Adolescent Sleep Requirements, Sleep Disorders, and the Effects of Sleep Deprivation
Including Facts about Why People Need Sleep, Sleep Patterns, Circadian Rhythms, Dreaming, Insomnia, Sleep Apnea, Narcolepsy, and More

Edited by Karen Bellenir. 355 pages. 2008. 978-0-7808-1009-9.

"Clear, concise, and very readable and would be a good source of sleep information for anyone—not just teenagers. This work is highly recommended for medical libraries, public school libraries, and public libraries."
—*American Reference Books Annual, 2009*

SEE ALSO *Body Information for Teens*

Sports Injuries Information for Teens, 2nd Edition
Health Tips about Acute, Traumatic, and Chronic Injuries in Adolescent Athletes
Including Facts about Sprains, Fractures, and Overuse Injuries, Treatment, Rehabilitation, Sport-Specific Safety Guidelines, Fitness Suggestions, and More

Edited by Karen Bellenir. 429 pages. 2008. 978-0-7808-1011-2.

"An engaging selection of informative articles about the prevention and treatment of sports injuries... The value of this book is that the articles have been vetted and are often augmented with inserts of useful facts, definitions of technical terms, and quick tips. Sensitive topics like injuries to genitalia are discussed openly and responsibly. This revised edition contains updated articles and defines sport more broadly than the first edition."
—*School Library Journal, Nov '08*

"This work will be useful in the young adult collections of public libraries as well as high school libraries... A useful resource for student research."
—*American Reference Books Annual, 2009*

SEE ALSO *Accident and Safety Information for Teens*

Stress Information for Teens
Health Tips about the Mental and Physical Consequences of Stress
Including Information about the Different Kinds of Stress, Symptoms of Stress, Frequent Causes of Stress, Stress Management Techniques, and More

Edited by Sandra Augustyn Lawton. 392 pages. 2008. 978-0-7808-1012-9.

"Understanding what stress is, what causes it, how the body and the mind are impacted by it, and what teens can do are the general categories addressed here... The chapters are brief but informative, and the list of community-help organizations is exhaustive. Report writers will find information quickly and easily, as will those who have personal concerns. The print is clear and the format is readable, making this an accessible resource for struggling readers and researchers."
—*School Library Journal, Dec '08*

"The articles selected will specifically appeal to young adults and are designed to answer their most common questions."
— *American Reference Books Annual, 2009*

SEE ALSO *Mental Health Information for Teens, 3rd Edition*

Suicide Information for Teens, 2nd Edition
Health Tips about Suicide Causes and Prevention
Including Facts about Depression, Risk Factors, Getting Help, Survivor Support, and More

Edited by Kim Wohlenhaus. 400 pages. 2010. 978-0-7808-1088-4.

SEE ALSO *Mental Health Information for Teens, 3rd Edition*

Tobacco Information for Teens, 2nd Edition
Health Tips about the Hazards of Using Cigarettes, Smokeless Tobacco, and Other Nicotine Products
Including Facts about Nicotine Addiction, Nicotine Delivery Systems, Secondhand Smoke, Health Consequences of Tobacco Use, Related Cancers, Smoking Cessation, and Tobacco Use Statistics

Edited by Karen Bellenir. 400 pages. 2010. 978-0-7808-1153-9.

SEE ALSO *Drug Information for Teens, 2nd Edition*

Health Reference Series